Therapeutic Reasoning in Occupational Therapy

HOW TO DEVELOP CRITICAL THINKING FOR PRACTICE

Therapeutic Reasoning in Occupational Therapy

HOW TO DEVELOP CRITICAL THINKING FOR PRACTICE

JANE CLIFFORD O'BRIEN, PHD, MS.ED.L, OTR/L, FAOTA

Professor
Occupational Therapy Department
Westbrook College of Health Professions
University of New England
Portland, Maine

MARY ELIZABETH PATNAUDE, DHSC, OTR/L

Associate Clinical Professor, Director of Admissions
Robbins College of Health and Human Sciences
Baylor University
Waco, Texas

TERESSA GARCIA REIDY, MS, OTR/L

Senior Occupational Therapist
Fairmount Rehabilitation Programs
Hunter Nelson Sturge-Weber Syndrome Center
Kennedy Krieger Institute
Baltimore, Maryland

ELSEVIER

ELSEVIER
3251 Riverport Lane
St. Louis, Missouri 63043

THERAPEUTIC REASONING IN OCCUPATIONAL THERAPY   ISBN: 978-0-323-82996-0

Senior Content Strategist: Lauren Willis
Senior Content Development Manager: Lisa Newton
Content Development Specialist: Andrew Schubert
Senior Project Manager: Anne Collett
Design Direction: Brian Salisbury

Printed in India

Last digit is the print number: 9   8   7   6   5   4   3   2   1

Working together
to grow libraries in
developing countries

www.elsevier.com • www.bookaid.org

Nicole Whiston Andrejow, MS, OTR/L
Occupational Therapist
Fairmount Rehabilitation Programs
Kennedy Krieger Institute
Baltimore, Maryland

Alison O'Brien
Theatre Studies
Portland, Maine

Evolve Content Providers

Nicole Whiston Andrejow, MS, OTR/L
Occupational Therapist
Fairmount Rehabilitation Programs
Kennedy Krieger Institute
Baltimore, Maryland

Ted Brown, PhD, MSc, MPA, BScOT(Hons), GCHPE, OT(C), OTR, MRCOT, FOTARA, FAOTA
Professor & Undergraduate Course Coordinator
Department of Occupational Therapy, School of Primary and Allied Health Care
Faculty of Medicine, Nursing and Health Sciences
Monash University–Peninsula Campus
Frankston, Victoria, Australia

Kayla Collins, EdD, OTR/L
Clinical Associate Professor/Director of Curriculum
Baylor University
Waco, Texas

Brittany Conners, OTD, CDWE
Chief Executive Optimist (CEO)
Optimistic Theory, LLC
St. Louis, Missouri

Brendan Cook, OTD (Student)
Washington University School of Medicine
St. Louis, Missouri

Arifa Jahan Ema, MPhil (OT), BSc (OT)
Lecturer in Occupational Therapy
Bangladesh Health Professions Institute (BHPI), CRP
Savar, Dhaka, Bangladesh

Moses Ikiugu, PhD, OTR/L, FAOTA
Professor and Director of Research
Occupational Therapy Department
University of South Dakota
Vermillion, South Dakota

Lynnley W. Moore, MA, CCC-SLP, CBIS
Manager Therapy Services, Senior Speech-Language Pathologist
Fairmount Rehabilitation Programs
Kennedy Krieger Institute
Baltimore, Maryland

Hiromi Nakamura-Thomas, PhD
Saitama Prefectural University
Saitama, Japan

Josh Pastor, MS, OTR/L
Rogue Pediatric Therapies (Private Outpatient OT, PT, SLP clinic)
Ashland, Oregon

Evguenia Popova, PHD, OTR
Assistant Professor
Department of Occupational Therapy
Rush University Medical Center
College of Health Science
Chicago, Illinois

Moshiur Rahman
Lecturer in Occupational Therapy
Department of Occupational Therapy
Bangladesh Health Professions Institute (BHPI)
CRP, Dhaka, Bangladesh

Brenda B. Reagan, MS, OTR'L
Occupational Therapist
Early Advantage
Awendaw, South Carolina
Instructor
Medical University of South Carolina
Charleston, South Carolina

Patricia Tomsic, OTD, OTR/L
Assistant Professor
Lenoir-Rhyne University's School of Occupational Therapy
Hickory, North Carolina

Patricia Turlington, BSc, PT, PCS
Senior Physical Therapist
Fairmount Rehabilitation Programs
Kennedy Krieger Institute
Baltimore, Maryland

Mohammad Mosayed Ullah, PhD, MOT, BSc (Hons) OT
Occupational Therapy Discipline
La Trobe University
Melbourne, Victoria, Australia

Craig Velozo, PhD, OTRL, FAOTA
Division Director, Occupational Therapy
Medical University of South Carolina
College of Health Professions, Department of Rehabilitation Sciences
Charleston, South Carolina

Jarrett Wolske, OTD, OTR/L
Adjunct Clinical Instructor and Occupational Therapist
University of Illinois Chicago
Chicago, Illinois
Academic Support Coach
McHenry County College
Crystal Lake, Illinois

REVIEWERS

Julie Geldner, MSOT Student
Class of 2022
University of New England
Portland, Maine

Jarrett Wolske, OTD, OTR/L
Adjunct Clinical Instructor and Occupational Therapist
Department of Occupational Therapy
University of Illinois Chicago
Academic Support Coach
McHenry County College
Crystal Lake, Illinois
Chicago, Illinois

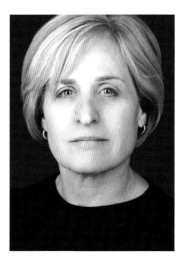

Dr. Jane O'Brien specializes in pediatric occupational therapy where she has worked in hospitals, clinics, early intervention, and home health, and created innovative programs in community settings (e.g., Project ARCH, The FUN program, and Science Night: See, Do, and Learn). She has taught therapeutic reasoning courses for over 20 years, most recently developing the courses that served as the groundwork for this book. She enjoys hiking, kayaking, CrossFit, and spending time with her husband, Mike, and children Scott, Alison, and Molly.

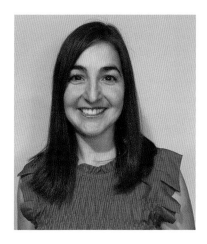

Teressa Garcia Reidy has been an occupational therapist since 2006. Her passion is working with children, especially those with neurological conditions. Her clinical research and publications focus on innovative interventions for children with hemiplegia, constraint induced movement therapy, and clinical outcomes research. She co-developed and was the lead occupational therapist for the first pediatric constraint induced movement therapy program in the Mid-Atlantic region. She has written many chapters, but this is her first experience as an editor. When she is not working, she enjoys spending time with her husband and three young children, cooking with her aunts and sisters, and being outdoors.

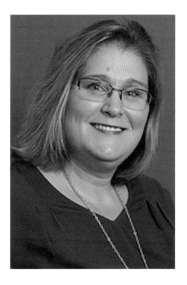

Dr. Mary Beth Patnaude has been an occupational therapist since 1997. She enjoyed working in multiple areas of practice, including pediatrics, acute rehabilitation, psychiatry, and outpatient orthopedics. She has been teaching full time in entry level OT programs since 2013. When not working, she enjoys spending time with her husband, Jeff, and their five sons, Richard, Michael, Aaron, David, and Matthew. She enjoys going to the beach and doing craft projects.

PREFACE

ORGANIZATION

Therapeutic Reasoning in Occupational Therapy: How to Develop Critical Thinking for Practice provides students and OT practitioners with foundational knowledge on critical thinking and clinical reasoning to prepare them to be effective decision-makers in practice. The authors use a practical approach by presenting theory interspersed with case examples, learning activities, and worksheets that can be used in classroom or practice settings to develop therapeutic reasoning. Each chapter provides current materials for class, assessment ideas, and practical information specific to occupational therapy.

Readers develop therapeutic reasoning skills as they work through cases, experiential learning activities, and worksheets. Cases and activities are scaffolded from simple to complex throughout the book to enhance learning. Activities may be adjusted to meet classroom or fieldwork objectives. Each chapter synthesizes current theoretical information and provides examples of how to apply concepts in the classroom or practice setting. The book is designed to be used as a workbook to teach therapeutic reasoning. The authors emphasize key concepts through illustrations, boxes, and tables. The Evolve learning site includes PowerPoints, videoclips, examples for assignments, and additional cases (representing the lifespan and a variety of practice settings) to reinforce reasoning.

The book begins with a review of foundational material (Chapters 1–3) followed by practice considerations (Chapters 4–7), intervention planning (Chapters 8 and 9), and concludes with a discussion of the importance of reflection on therapeutic reasoning (Chapter 10).

Chapter 1 provides an overview of therapeutic reasoning with an emphasis on promoting student success and strategies to create curious learners. Chapter 2 examines occupation as the foundation for reasoning and Chapter 3 describes how to use models of practice and frames of reference to promote therapeutic reasoning.

Next, the authors describe reasoning involved in therapeutic use of self (Chapter 4), evidence-based practice (Chapter 5), and teamwork (Chapter 7). They provide guidelines for selecting assessment tools and making hypotheses based on findings in Chapter 6.

Chapter 8 provides details describing the therapeutic reasoning process used to apply knowledge in practice and Chapter 9 develops these concepts as they inform creative intervention planning. The benefits of reflection in the therapeutic reasoning process along with assessments to measure therapeutic reasoning are provided in Chapter 10.

DISTINCTIVE FEATURES

Each chapter begins with guiding questions to support reading for meaning. The authors include case examples, learning activities, and worksheets to engage readers in the therapeutic reasoning process. The Evolve learning site provides videoclips, additional cases, and resources to promote learning. Distinctive features of the book include the following:

- Dynamic, interactive approach that embeds learning activities within the chapters, which progress from simple to complex to facilitate therapeutic reasoning.
- Clinically relevant learning activities, worksheets, and templates support readers in applying therapeutic reasoning concepts in practice.
- Authentic cases from OT professionals who work with clients across the lifespan highlight a variety of practice settings.
- Short video case contributions from students, practitioners, and educators illustrate diverse perspectives, reinforce content, and provide authentic application opportunities.
- Content reflects the Occupational Therapy Practice Framework (4th edition; AOTA, 2020) and current occupational therapy practice.
- Assessments to measure therapeutic reasoning are described and may be used for self-reflection and to measure reasoning skills in classroom or practice.
- Evolve materials include additional cases, worksheets, templates, video presentations, PowerPoint slides, and reflective activities.

ANCILLARY MATERIALS

Therapeutic Reasoning in Occupational Therapy: How to Develop Critical Thinking for Practice is linked to an Evolve website that provides learning aids and tools for each chapter including the following:

Educator Resources

- PowerPoint slides
- Additional assignments with video presentations

Student and Practitioner Resources

- PDF of in-text worksheets so students can print them
- Video presentations describing therapeutic reasoning from a variety of perspectives. The presentations highlight concepts from each chapter and are associated with assignments to reinforce key concepts.
- Video clips associated with selected learning activities
- Examples of completed learning activities and worksheets
- Reflective activities
- Additional case studies

We dedicate this book to all who foster therapeutic reasoning in future generations of occupational therapists. To the dedicated fieldwork educators, faculty, and colleagues who teach, inspire, and promote new ways to think – we hope that you use this book as a practical resource to promote and enhance therapeutic reasoning. To the clients and families we serve and have served, thank you for sharing your stories and inspiring occupational therapy practitioners to question, analyze, and explore new ways of thinking and doing.

ACKNOWLEDGMENTS

Jane acknowledges the late Dr. Gary Kielhofner and Dr. Jane Case-Smith who influenced her therapeutic reasoning. She thanks Dr. Anita Bundy, Dr. Anne Fisher, Dr. Nancy Carson, Jean Solomon, and all the students, clients, families, and colleagues who mentor, share, and provide learning opportunities to promote her thinking. She appreciates the continued support of her family and friends.

Mary Beth would like to thank her colleagues at Baylor University, Dr. Kayla Collins, and Dr. Kirsten Davin, who contributed cases. She would also like to thank her wonderful husband, Reverend Jeffrey Patnaude, for his support and her sons: Richard, Michael, Aaron, David, and Matthew. You are my world! Finally, she would like to thank her niece Jillian Vincenzo, who allowed us to use a photo of her beautiful son, David Vincenzo, as a cover model.

Teressa would like to thank Dr. Joan Carney and her colleagues at Kennedy Krieger Institute for their immense support and mentorship. She would also like to thank the OT Faculty of Duquesne University, especially Dr. Jaime Munoz and Dr. Jeryl Benson for their support beyond the classroom and for their commitment to creating evidence-based, client-centered, and thoughtful practitioners. She would like to thank her husband, James, and her children, parents, and sisters for their support and encouragement on this project.

The authors would like to thank all the people who contributed cases, assignments, and reviews for this book. It was inspiring working with so many talented professionals. Thank you to Lauren Willis, Anne Collett, Glenys Norquay, Andrew Schubert, Brian Salisbury, and all the people at Elsevier who helped conceive and create this book. It is always enjoyable to work with this team of dedicated professionals.

CONTENTS

Student Success: Therapeutic Reasoning Process

Mary Elizabeth Patnaude

GUIDING QUESTIONS

1. How does curiosity influence the development of therapeutic reasoning?
2. What are the types of therapeutic reasoning?
3. What is the journey from novice to expert practitioner?
4. What are the steps to the therapeutic reasoning process?
5. How is therapeutic reasoning used in the occupational therapy practice?

KEY TERMS

Advanced beginner
Brainstorming
Competent
Conditional reasoning
Ethical dilemma
Ethical distress
Ethical reasoning
Expert
Interactive reasoning
Lived experience

Locus of authority
Narrative reasoning
Novice
Occupational adaptation
Occupational profile
Pragmatic reasoning
Proficient
Scientific reasoning
Socratic questioning
Therapeutic reasoning

INTRODUCTION

The key to being a successful occupational therapist, who empowers clients to reach their goals, is therapeutic reasoning. Therapeutic reasoning is the process of synthesizing information about the client, occupation, and environment to design creative and meaningful occupational therapy intervention. Therapeutic reasoning is a dynamic process that begins with showing a curiosity for learning about another person. Students and practitioners learn to ask many questions often directed by one's model of practice or frame of reference. They use many types of reasoning (i.e., scientific, narrative, pragmatic, interactive, ethical, and conditional) to better understand occupational performance challenges. They reason through each step to generate questions, gather data, identify occupational challenges, create an intervention plan, implement the plan, and assess the outcomes. Using current evidence, experience, and reflection, students and practitioners become more skilled at therapeutic reasoning which benefits clients and their families. The progression from novice to expert practitioner evolves with the development of analytical skills and reflection. Each chapter in this textbook provides content, learning activities, worksheets, and cases to promote therapeutic reasoning. The Evolve site includes cases, videoclips, and guiding questions to reinforce key concepts.

This chapter begins by exploring the role of curiosity in the development of therapeutic reasoning. The author provides an overview of the types, stages, and steps in the process of therapeutic reasoning. A case example is provided to illustrate the therapeutic reasoning process in occupational therapy practice.

In this textbook, occupational therapy (OT) practitioners refer to occupational therapists (OTRs) and occupational therapy assistants (OTAs). OT practitioners enable their clients to engage in meaningful participation through the therapeutic use of everyday occupations (AOTA, 2020b). To fully understand what is meaningful to the client requires that practitioners invest time getting to know the client's interests, values, routines, roles, and environment. This can be done through a formal or informal interview process, known as the occupational profile. The occupational profile outlines "the client's occupational history and experiences, patterns of daily living, interests, values, needs, and relevant contexts" (AOTA, 2020b, p. 80). Box 1.1 provides an example of part of an occupational history for a mother of an infant.

The occupational profile provides the basis for the therapeutic reasoning process. Once the occupational profile is developed, the OT practitioner completes an analysis of occupational performance. After the information is gathered, the therapist collaborates with the client to prioritize goals and assign value and meaning to each of them. The priorities and goals stem from the complex interaction between the client, the environment, and their meaningful occupations. In the example in Box 1.1, it is likely that, in the event of an illness or injury, the client's goals would be focused on returning to caring for her infant. For example, if the client sustained a wrist fracture after falling on ice, the priority for therapy would include adapting her caregiving so she can complete as much as possible within her orthopedic precautions.

Therapeutic reasoning is the process by which the OT practitioner makes clinical decisions based on theory and evaluates the complex ways in which the client, the occupation, and the environment interact to facilitate occupational performance in all settings (AOTA, 2020b; Kielhofner & Forsyth, 2008). See Figure 1.1 for an illustration of this process. Practitioners use therapeutic reasoning to skillfully incorporate these factors into an intervention plan tailored for the client (Benfield & Johnston, 2020). Therapeutic reasoning develops from curiosity that drives students and practitioners to think critically and engage in scholarly inquiry and the discipline that requires they continually return to the literature as a lifelong learner (Benfield & Johnston, 2020; Cain, 2019).

THE ROLE OF CURIOSITY IN THE DEVELOPMENT OF THERAPEUTIC REASONING

Occupational therapy students begin their transformation from student to advanced occupational therapy practitioner by acquiring competence in clinical skills and a knowledge base that sets the stage for future expertise (Benfield & Johnston, 2020). They must develop habits of mind to continually build a knowledge base. As they become more seasoned or expert, they can collect cues about a patient to develop and implement an intervention plan (Benfield & Johnston, 2020). This journey begins with "curiosity, opportunity, breadth and depth, taking risks, and stepping into the future" (Law, 2007, p. 599). Curiosity implies a general sense of wonder and interest in learning about clients, beyond what is required for classroom grades or assignments. Students and practitioners who exhibit curiosity question, hypothesize, reflect, and explore – all important characteristics for developing therapeutic reasoning. This is the basis of client-centered practice and plays a key role in transforming students into advanced practitioners.

Students must be given a multitude of opportunities to study cases about clients from all stages of life, facing diverse challenges such as developmental, chronic mental illness, and

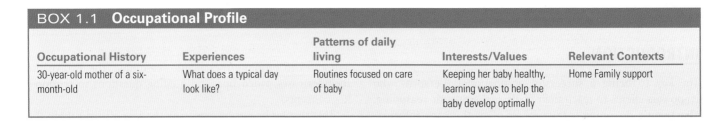

BOX 1.1	Occupational Profile			
Occupational History	**Experiences**	**Patterns of daily living**	**Interests/Values**	**Relevant Contexts**
30-year-old mother of a six-month-old	What does a typical day look like?	Routines focused on care of baby	Keeping her baby healthy, learning ways to help the baby develop optimally	Home Family support

Therapeutic Reasoning Process

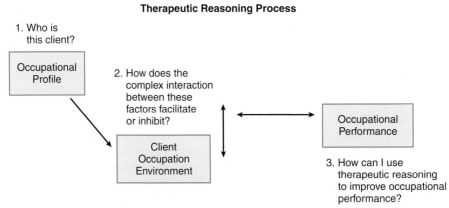

Fig. 1.1 Using Therapeutic Reasoning to Improve Occupational Performance

complex medical conditions. Students need to feel safe to examine in depth aspects of the cases to understand the breadth of the client's experience.

For example, a student on fieldwork presented with the case of a 12-month-old child with low muscle tone due to a genetic condition may first examine what they know about the condition (based on coursework and scientific knowledge). The student also examines the specific occupations in which a child participates that would be affected by the condition, such as the child's inability to play. The student further explores family dynamics, environment, and cultural expectations. Further questions may stimulate curiosity for learning and add to the intervention options for the child and family. Following are some questions that may promote curiosity:

- How are sibling interactions impacted by the child's condition?
- Do older siblings understand the condition and support the child's ability to gain independence?
- What are the parents' goals, dreams, and expectations for the child?
- What community resources are available?
- How does the environment support or hinder the child and family's goals?
- What does the child and family enjoy doing together?
- What does the child like to do? What makes him laugh?
- How can occupational therapy support the child's engagement in family events and traditions?
- How are the parents coping with the child's recent diagnosis? How does this impact their interaction with their child?

Occupational therapy students and practitioners need to develop curiosity to learn as much as they can about the client and family because it underpins the therapeutic reasoning process and is fundamental to understanding the unique perspective of each client (Dyche & Epstein, 2011).

LEARNING ACTIVITY: CURIOSITY

Brainstorming: On the first day of fieldwork, your supervisor asks you to plan a 30-minute activity for a 25-year-old client who was in an accident and lost use of their right side and experienced a head injury. Complete Worksheet 1.2.
- List questions you have regarding this case.
- Organize your questions into categories.
- Develop at least 5 ways to find answers to these questions.
- Without knowing the answers, design the activity.
  - What things are you considering?
  - How will you adapt and change it if the client is not able to engage in it?

Brainstorming allows students and practitioners to safely explore aspects of cases and think through multiple solutions and scenarios. This may facilitate creativity and novelty. Providing a safe space for brainstorming is essential when working to develop curiosity of learning. Socratic questioning is an educational technique to challenge learners to delve more deeply into topics and find their own answers. When using Socratic questioning techniques, educators ask leading questions to stimulate problem-solving and creativity. Instead of searching for the "correct" answer, students search for multiple answers and solutions

(as illustrated in the above learning exercise). This stimulates curiosity and promotes therapeutic reasoning. See Chapter 8 for more information on Socratic questioning and techniques to facilitate therapeutic reasoning.

Curiosity drives individuals to ask tough questions and find creative solutions to solve problems (Cain, 2019). This creative problem-solving is the basis for both the complex reasoning process needed to create and employ effective intervention and the pathway to developing therapeutic reasoning.

While curiosity is fundamental to the development of therapeutic reasoning, it is not always encouraged in the classroom or clinic. The structure of the medical system rewards efficiency which encourages rushing and rapid response that can compromise attention to detail and inhibit thoughtful decision-making (Dyche & Epstein, 2011). Students and practitioners in professional programs need to master a large and specialized body of knowledge (Norman, 2012). This means that educators often utilize a lecture-based approach to convey the sheer volume of information needed for students to acquire the competence to enter the ranks of the profession and are often unable to reward curiosity in favor of rewarding competence (Norman, 2012). The sheer volume of material needed to be covered leads faculty in the health professions to rush through content. This need to rush and work in haste and the passive learning occurring in some didactic programs can dampen curiosity (Dyche & Epstein, 2011).

Educators can allow opportunities for students and practitioners to follow their curiosity by utilizing alternative pathways for learning, such as experiential learning, creative problem-solving assignments, and authentic case scenarios (with varying amounts of information). The learning activities and worksheets provided in this text, along with an array of case studies with videoclips (found in the Evolve Learning Materials) are designed to encourage curiosity. Learners benefit by being introduced to these alternative pathways, and by being assured that they will still reach the desired destination, that of advancing their skills and abilities for practice. Although these alternative learning pathways may be time consuming and feel risky, they allow students to develop lifelong learning skills and therapeutic reasoning for practice (Law, 2007).

Promoting curiosity in the classroom and clinic means that educators allow students and practitioners the opportunity to explore and sometimes fail and this requires they be comfortable with "failure." Failure does not mean the student or practitioner is not competent, but rather they took a risk and now must move in another direction. Failure often leads to feelings of uncertainty. Helping students and practitioners challenge themselves to take risks may require educators to build in assignments that support curiosity but are low stakes. For example, a student or practitioner is more able to design a novel creative intervention on a simulated client when the focus is on the reflection of the session (rather than the grade or outcome). This provides the learner with a safe space to create. Experiencing "failure" as they learn therapeutic reasoning in the classroom or clinic helps students and practitioners learn to face the complexity and uncertainty of therapeutic practice and develop skills to honestly examine their own competence (Dyche & Epstein, 2011). Box 1.2 provides an example of failure that led to learning in a classroom setting.

For students and practitioners to engage in the learning process for therapeutic reasoning, they must move away from feeling comfortable being "fed" information; they must be convinced that asking their own questions is just as important as answering the questions given to them by faculty and professionals (Cain, 2019). In addition, they must be encouraged to find answers to their own questions through scholarly inquiry (Cain, 2019). Finally, students and practitioners need to evaluate the efficacy of the entire process through reflection.

Curiosity builds a depth of understanding that allows the OT practitioner to gain self-awareness and reflection needed to develop therapeutic reasoning (Dyche & Epstein, 2011). For example, students and practitioners benefit from taking the time to evaluate themselves to gauge their ability to delve deeply into concepts and understand how they react to uncertainty. Critical analysis and questioning skills can be learned, and they are essential skills for all OT practitioners (Law, 2007). See Chapter 10 for more on reflection.

TYPES OF THERAPEUTIC REASONING

Therapeutic reasoning requires practitioners to synthesize information from a variety of sources to inform intervention planning. Occupational therapy practitioners examine human performance, which is influenced by many factors and involves both an art (the act of engaging the client in occupational therapy) and science (based on biological, physical, psychoemotional, and social information). There are several types of reasoning: scientific, narrative, pragmatic, ethical, interactive, and conditional. Each type of reasoning provides important guidelines that are helpful in practice.

Scientific Reasoning

Scientific reasoning begins with understanding the client's condition and the possible effects it may have on occupational performance (Boyt-Schell, 2019). It is based on scientific inquiry, which defines and tests hypotheses. Practitioners using this type of reasoning seek to find out the cause, symptoms, and progression of the condition. They base practice decisions on established protocols. Students and new therapists are comfortable with scientific reasoning because it provides answers based on facts that may be learned in traditional didactic coursework. This type of reasoning lends itself to protocols to address occupational performance deficits based on the client's condition. For example, if a client has a complete Spinal Cord Injury (SCI) at the C6 level, it is likely that the client has no sensory or motor function below that level. The practitioner hypothesizes based on the diagnosis that the client is not able to feed themselves without adaptive equipment. While scientific reasoning provides some important information, it does not provide the client's whole story and may limit understanding of how the client experiences the condition.

Narrative Reasoning

Narrative reasoning refers to understanding the client's story from their perspective. When utilizing narrative reasoning, OT practitioners seek to understand the client's experience and perspective of their own situation and use this information to create an intervention plan (Boyt-Schell, 2019). Practitioners learn about the client's lived experience (i.e., how they view their strengths and challenges and engage in daily activities), which informs client-centered intervention plans. For example, when treating a client for a hand injury, an OT practitioner may use narrative reasoning to understand the ways in which the injury affected the client's life story. Furthermore, a client who defines himself as a guitar player who has always performed for family and friends, written songs, and taught guitar lessons for income will want to gain fine motor skills to return to this occupation. The OT practitioner who understands the client's lived experience creates an intervention plan to focus upon finger isolation and strength, bilateral hand skills, timing, sequencing, speed, and dexterity. Knowing information from the client's story allows the OT practitioner to create intervention goals and activities that are meaningful to the client.

Pragmatic Reasoning

Pragmatic reasoning examines the relationship between the therapy itself and the situations surrounding it that may influence decisions (Boyt-Schell, 2019). OT practitioners using pragmatic reasoning consider the payor, referral source, frequency, and duration of services. They also consider the timing of intervention, environment, resources, and costs. They use pragmatic reasoning to skillfully merge the practical factors with the desired intervention outcomes to develop creative solutions that both benefit the client and work with the resources and situations surrounding the intervention.

For example, an OT practitioner working in a school setting uses pragmatic reasoning when determining how the child's therapy sessions fit into the school day. The therapist considers the time of the session, location of intervention (e.g., during classroom instruction, or pull-out model), and the child's strengths, challenges, and goals. The OT practitioner may decide that it is beneficial to complete OT intervention addressing fine motor skills during the writing block in the classroom when it is relatively quiet, and the teacher is helping other children at stations. Conversely the OT practitioner may decide that the child needs a break from the classroom environment during the writing block as this is frustrating for him due to his poor fine motor skills. Alternatively, the OT practitioner may decide to provide therapy in both settings to support both skill development and classroom performance. OT practitioners balance pragmatic reasoning with ethical reasoning to make sure the client's goals are addressed and services are meeting standards of practice.

Ethical Reasoning

Ethical reasoning refers to thinking through what needs to be accomplished in therapy in relation to what should be done (Boyt-Schell, 2019). Occupational therapy practitioners refer to the AOTA Code of Ethics (2020a), which defines ethical principles to promote and maintain high standards of conduct, including beneficence, nonmaleficence, autonomy, justice, veracity, and fidelity. Table 1.1 defines each principle and provides a practice example. Practitioners also rely on knowledge of state and federal laws, and institution or facility policies and procedure (Grajo & Rushanan, 2021).

Common sources of ethical tension in occupational therapy are outlined in Table 1.2. The steps to ethical decision-making are defined in Box 1.3. When facing a challenging situation, practitioners begin by gathering information about the situation, contexts (where and when did this occur), facts, and persons involved. This provides objective data so they can identify the type of ethical problem, which is defined as ethical distress (i.e., practitioner experiences discomfort when prevented from doing what is believed to be right), ethical dilemma (i.e., practitioner must choose between conflicting alternatives), or locus of authority (i.e., practitioner decides who should resolve the ethical issue) (Grajo & Rushanan, 2021; Purtilo, 2005).

Once the practitioner determines the type of ethical problem, they review standards of practice, laws and regulations and define the principles involved according to the Code of Ethics (AOTA, 2020a). They explore possible solutions by considering how the actions may affect each of the involved persons. They decide upon an action, complete the action, and evaluate the process and outcomes.

Interactive Reasoning

The occupational therapy process is highly dependent on effective interpersonal communication and collaboration. Interactive reasoning refers to the ability to therapeutically engage in interactions by giving and receiving cues about how to respond to one another (Boyt-Schell, 2019). OT practitioners carefully consider how their feedback (non-verbal or verbal) and interactions (e.g., body language, body position, use of humor, communication style) promote the therapeutic relationship. They observe how the client responds to them and adjust as needed to maintain a therapeutic relationship so the client achieves their occupational therapy goals.

For example, an OT practitioner using interactive reasoning with a client who experienced a stroke and does not understand language gently approaches the client, makes eye contact, smiles, and says hello and her name, and hands the client a

TABLE 1.1   AOTA (2020a) Code of Ethics Principles

Principle	Description	Practice Example
Beneficence	Concern for well-being and safety of clients; provide services that are good and protect clients from harm	Collaborate with client and family on goals and intervention; provide therapy in accordance with scope of practice
Nonmaleficence	Do not cause harm	Ensure continuity of services; maintain professional boundaries
Autonomy	Respect the right of the individual	Allow clients to make decisions about their needs and services; maintain confidentiality
Justice	Promote fairness and objectivity	Advocate for fair and equitable access to high-quality services; provide high-quality services to all clients
Veracity	Provide comprehensive, accurate, and objective information	Document truthful and accurate representation of services provided; provide honest description of professional qualifications
Fidelity	Be faithful; treat other professionals with respect, fairness, discretion, and integrity	Respect others in the workplace; follow workplace guidelines for conflict resolution

BOX 1.3   Steps to Ethical Decision-Making

1. Gather information
2. Identify the type of ethical problem
3. Use ethical theories or approaches to analyze the problems
4. Explore alternatives
5. Complete the action
6. Evaluate the process and outcome.

washcloth. The therapist provides a simple one-word cue, "wash," to see if the client can respond. The client looks at the therapist and touches the washcloth but does not grasp it. The practitioner looks directly at the client, nods in an encouraging way, and waits to see if the client responds before assisting. He nods slightly as if to indicate he would like to use it. The practitioner gently helps the client wash his hands and smiles at the client. At the end of the encounter, the OT practitioner decides to provide pictures so the client can express his feelings during the session. This example illustrates the use of interactive reasoning by considering one's use of non-verbal and verbal communication. Interactive reasoning involves therapeutic use of self, an essential component of occupational therapy practice. Chapter 4 describes therapeutic use of self and the Intentional Relationship Model (IRM; Taylor, 2020), which examines one's communication styles.

TABLE 1.2 Common Sources of Ethical Tension in Daily Practice (Bushby et al., 2015; Kinsella et al., 2008).	
Source of ethical tension	**Commonly cited clinical examples**
Resource and systemicconstraints – challenges related to providing services in conditions that are not optimal	Inadequate time for intervention with clients or for communication with team, patient, or family members Insufficient levels of staff Overly large caseloads Lack of resources such as appropriate assessment tools or ability to access research to inform practice
Conflicting values between practitioners and clients, between practitioners from different disciplines, and even between students and therapists	Differences of opinion between various team members; these differences frequently involved discharge issues
Witnessing questionable behavior by healthcare practitioners	Disrespectful attitudes, inappropriate language, failure to communicate, breach of confidentiality
Failure to speak up	Common tension experienced as to when to advocate and speak up on behalf of clients or to witness clients "falling through the cracks." Tensions related to speaking up on behalf of clients emerged in the areas of protecting client's rights, facilitating independence, and ensuring safety
Working with vulnerable clients	Tensions experienced when clients are partly competent to make their own choices, and when healthcare practitioners do not involve them in their own health-related decision-making
Client safety	Ethical tensions concerning client safety were identified with respect to discharge planning, knowledge of unsafe behavior, practice errors, clinical education, and involvement in research
Upholding professional standards	Ethical tensions related to upholding professional standards such as implementing client-centered practice, evidence-based practice, competency of occupational therapists

Permission from: Grajo, L., & Rushanan, S. (2021). Ethical decision-making in occupational therapy practice. In J. O'Brien & J. Solomon (Eds.). Occupational Analysis and Group Process (2nd ed., p. 173). Elsevier.

Conditional Reasoning

Conditional reasoning involves examining multiple aspects to evaluate the client's strengths and challenges to create and implement an intervention plan. OT practitioners who use conditional reasoning consider the client's condition as a whole; they synthesize information regarding the person, contexts, and environment. They use knowledge of the client's condition, interaction style, ethics and policies, practical information, and the client's story (including occupational history) to prioritize and establish goals. Practitioners who use conditional reasoning also reason how the client's condition may change. As such, conditional reasoning uses many of the other forms of reasoning. Conditional reasoning is typically used by experienced practitioners who seamlessly adapt to situations that come up in the occupational therapy process.

For example, a therapist working with a client in an acute care setting following an exacerbation of an illness considered sequelae of the condition; progression of illness; client's previous occupational roles, responsibilities, and routines; discharge setting; resources; and the client's goals and interests when creating an intervention plan. She advocated for home health services upon discharge and provided adaptive equipment to allow the client to engage in family activities of meal preparation, walks with spouse, and caring for the dog (all occupations the client valued). The therapist used her knowledge of the hospital loan program to secure equipment at a reasonable rate. The practitioner noted that the client became very quiet and looked away when she discussed the illness and her spouse taking care of her, which prompted the practitioner to suggest a support group with women her age that met nearby (and knowing the client had transportation resources).

LEARNING ACTIVITY: TYPES OF REASONING

Use Worksheet 1.3 and provide examples of how an OT practitioner may use each type of reasoning for the following scenario.

A fieldwork student must create an intervention plan for a 4-year-old boy with a genetic disorder resulting in mild left-sided weakness and dyspraxia, in an outpatient clinic. The child's mother reports he has difficulty completing fasteners, especially initiating a zipper.

The student observes that the child has full range of motion in his left hand but overall weak grip strength and no spontaneous fine grip patterns. He uses his right hand to place the edge of the jacket in his left hand; his left hand slips when gripping the jacket and he is not able to calibrate and sustain his grip long enough to manipulate the other part of the jacket into the base of the zipper. The left hand lacks enough grip to initiate and sustain grasp and the child can not initiate any supination with his left hand while gripping the jacket. He has difficulty moving each hand in different directions. The child has sufficient grip in his right hand.

- Identify questions regarding this scenario that address each type of therapeutic reasoning.

JOURNEY FROM NOVICE TO EXPERT PRACTITIONER

The transformation from novice to expert practitioner requires an understanding of the occupational therapy process. The process is fluid, dynamic, and complex. Occupational therapy practitioners utilize therapeutic reasoning to choose the occupations that will be most effective in achieving the client's goals (AOTA, 2020b). For example, a student may enter occupational therapy school with the understanding of how to strengthen muscles. They know physiologically that challenging the muscle will make it stronger. However, they may not know that hand strength can be improved just as much by kneading thick bread dough as by using theraputty. They may also not know that if a client enjoys making bread, they are more likely to engage in the kneading process for many more minutes than they would completing a series of theraputty exercises. This reasoning process is likely to lead to a more successful outcome for the client.

Over time, therapeutic reasoning develops along a continuum as the practitioner gains experience and reflects on practice. For example, someone with significant years of experience, mentorship, and continuing education in outpatient pediatric practice may be at a proficient or expert level. But, if that same practitioner decides to move into acute care, their therapeutic reasoning abilities may significantly change due to their lack of experience and exposure.

Table 1.3 outlines the stages of progression of therapeutic reasoning from novice to expert practitioner and lists the type of reasoning related to the stage. Novice practitioners generally use scientific reasoning or concepts from coursework to guide their decisions in practice. They focus on learning procedural skills, including assessments, and intervention planning procedures (Carrier et al., 2012; Durning et al., 2011; Dreyfus & Dreyfus, 2004; Fleming, 1991; Kuipers & Grice, 2009; Mitchell & Usworth, 2005). They do not have professional experience so seek out supervision or emulate clinicians who work in the same setting. As practitioners develop their comfort with procedures, see more clients, and reflect upon their work, they become advanced beginners who recognize additional cues and see clients as individuals. The competent practitioner has a broader understanding of the client's problems and is likely to individualize intervention (using narrative reasoning). They see more facts and observe more so they can prioritize goals and intervention. However, they have difficulty with flexibility and creativity. With practice, reflection, and the ability to give and receive feedback, they progress to become proficient practitioners, who view the client's situation as a whole and rely on professional experience to develop

goals. They can modify plans. Expert practitioners recognize and understand the rules of practice and settings to creatively address client issues. The expert practitioner synthesizes information from multiple sources; they identify relevant cues along with knowledge of the client's medical, physical, and psychosocial factors to make practice decisions and design intervention. The expert practitioner understands the personal and environmental factors (contexts) influencing occupational performance and skillfully uses supports in practice, while addressing barriers. Expert practitioners are intuitive and skilled at using conditional reasoning. They consider multiple factors when practicing and attend to details of a client's narrative to create occupation-based interventions (Carrier et al., 2012; Durning et al., 2011; Kuipers & Grice, 2009; Mitchell & Unsworth, 2005). Expert practitioners are able to justify their choices and articulate the evidence to support their decisions.

STEPS TO THE THERAPEUTIC REASONING PROCESS

The purpose of this text is to describe the ways in which students can become proficient in the therapeutic reasoning process. Figure 1.2 illustrates the process. The process includes several steps: using theory to generate questions, gathering information, identifying occupational challenges, creating an intervention plan, implementing the plan and assessing the outcomes. This is a dynamic process which may require revisiting steps throughout. See Chapter 8 regarding applying knowledge to practice. For example, while conducting an intervention new data often arises that may require the OT practitioner to adjust the intervention plan. Learning to continually assess the progress of an intervention and adjust one's plan shows advanced therapeutic reasoning and benefits clients.

OT practitioners use theoretical principles and models of practice to guide the reasoning process. Guided by these theories and models, OT practitioners utilize a logical process to gather information about a client, process the information, integrate it into an understanding of the client's needs, develop an intervention plan, implement the intervention, evaluate the efficacy of the plan, and reflect on the process. This is a cyclical process in which the clinician learns and adjusts as they go along (Leavitt-Jones et al., 2010). Following is an overall description of each step and a case to illustrate its application.

Use Theory to Generate Questions

Step one in the therapeutic reasoning process is for practitioners to generate questions guided by theory. Using theories and models of practice allows students and practitioners to make decisions based on research evidence. Using an occupation-based model of practice such as Model of Human Occupation (MOHO; Taylor, 2017), Person-Environment-Occupation-Performance (PEOP; Baum et al., 2015), Canadian Model of Occupational Performance and Engagement (CMOP-E; CAOT, 1997), or Occupational Adaptation (OA; Schkade & Schultz, 2003) helps OT practitioners understand and explain the complexity of human occupation. See Chapter 3 for more information on occupation-based models of practice

TABLE 1.3 Development of Therapeutic Reasoning Skills		
Stages of Therapeutic Reasoning	**Description**	**Reasoning**
Novice	Adheres to textbook theories, relies on scientific reasoning, follows protocols; focus on procedural skills	Scientific
Advanced Beginner	Beginning to individualize intervention	Pragmatic
Competent	Sees more facts, individualizes intervention, incorporates narrative reasoning	Narrative Ethical
Proficient	Views client as a whole, modifies plans	Interactive
Expert	Intuitive, uses multiple sources to create intervention, articulates evidence, identifies cues	Conditional

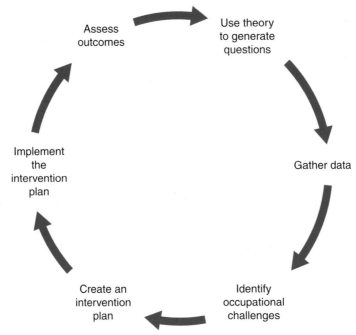

Fig. 1.2 Therapeutic Reasoning Process

and frames of reference. These models were created based on occupational therapy concepts, principles, and assumptions and based on research evidence related to human occupation and change. They help practitioners understand, evaluate and facilitate occupational performance. See Chapter 2 describing the use of occupation in practice.

OT practitioners seek to understand multiple factors influencing a client's occupational performance. The model of practice or frame of reference provides guidance of what types of questions to ask and what type of information the practitioner may want to observe. Table 1.4 provides sample questions based on occupation-based models of practice. For example, a practitioner using Kielhofner's Model of Human Occupation (MOHO; Kielhofner, 2008; Taylor, 2017) will generate questions to gather information on a client's volition, habituation, performance capacity (specifically the lived experience), and environment. A practitioner using the Person-Environment-Occupation-Performance model (Baum et al., 2015) will generate questions regarding the person, environment, occupation and in particular how the client engages in their desired occupations.

Gather Data

OT practitioners gather data from client interviews, observation, and assessment tools. The interview includes information about the client's past performance, experiences, daily activities, interests, needs, and desires. Gathering information about the client's story or narrative is essential to client-centered practice. Throughout the evaluation process, the practitioner observes the client's physical, processing, and social–emotional skills. They may observe the client completing activities, such as making a sandwich, brushing one's teeth, or dressing, and complete a thorough task analysis. OT practitioners use standardized and non-standardized assessments to gather data. See Chapter 6 for more details on evaluation

TABLE 1.4 **Questions Based on Occupation-Based Models of Practice**	
Model of Practice	**Sample Questions**
Model of Human Occupation (MOHO)	
• Volition (values, interests, personal causation)	What things that you do are important to you?
• Habituation (habits, roles, routines)	How do you spend your day?
• Performance capacity (lived experience)	How do you view your abilities?
• Environment (social, physical, institutional, societal)	What is your home, school, work setting like?
Person-Environment-Occupation-Performance Model (PEOP)	
• Person	What is the relationship between psychological factors and well-being and life balance?
• Environment	How does culture influence perceptions of occupational therapy and occupational performance?
• Occupation	How do the environment and stage of life impact performance in meaningful activities?
Canadian Model of Occupational Performance and Engagement (CMOP-E)	
• Person (spirituality, affective, physical, cognitive)	What do you want to accomplish?
• Occupation (self-care, leisure, productivity)	What do you do for leisure activities?
• Environment (physical, institutional, cultural, social)	What are your traditions?

and assessment. The OTR is responsible for the evaluation, but the OTA may engage in data gathering by administering some assessments and completing observations of which they have established clinical competency.

Identify Occupational Challenges

The OT with input from the OTA synthesizes the information to identify the client's strengths and challenges and identify what is interfering with the client's occupational performance. The OT creates this conceptualization using principles (that are based on research evidence) from models of practice and frames of reference to explain factors that support or interfere with occupational performance. OTs and OTAs use current research evidence to decide intervention approaches and strategies. They examine the rationale, method, and techniques based on evidence. See Chapter 5 regarding integrating evidence in practice. Box 1.4 lists some sample hypotheses based on selected models of practice and frames of reference. This stage of the reasoning process challenges the therapist to use therapeutic reasoning to identify factors that need to be addressed in therapy. Therapists may identify multiple reasons for occupational challenges. In this case, the therapist prioritizes where to begin. Together with the client, the practitioner develops goals that address the client's desires and are congruent with the therapist's hypotheses regarding how to promote change.

Create an Intervention Plan

The OT is responsible for developing the intervention plan, but may seek input from the OTA. The intervention plan outlines the strategies, techniques, and activities to address the goals and objectives (that were developed with input from the client). The goals and objectives are measurable occupation-based goals. See Chapter 9 for a discussion of goals and templates for intervention plans. Creating an intervention plan requires knowledge of the models and frames of reference that support the decisions. Specifically, the models and frames of reference define how change occurs in practice, based on research. This information forms the basis for the intervention plan and allows practitioners to adjust techniques, strategies, and their role as needed.

For example, if the therapist hypothesizes that limited strength in both upper extremities is interfering with an older adult's ability to complete his morning routine, the intervention activities are focused upon upper body strengthening. The practitioner relies on research from the biomechanical frame of reference, which states that increasing repetition of movement with additional weight recruits more muscle activity leading to strengthening (Rybski, 2012). If during the intervention the practitioner does not see the intended results, the practitioner may re-evaluate and determine that upper extremity strength may be impaired for another reason, such as poor postural stability leading the practitioner to adjust the intervention plan to address postural stability.

The intervention plan describes the goals (both long and short term), rationale for including these goals, strategies to address the goals, and the role of the OT practitioner. The plan also provides practical information including method of service delivery, length of sessions, time of sessions, type of activities, setting for the information, safety precautions, discharge setting, and any considerations that may influence the plan. The plan may include information related to re-evaluation or outcomes measurements. See Chapter 9 for detailed information about the intervention plan.

Implement the Intervention Plan

Engaging the client in the activities to address the goals as outlined in the intervention plan includes engaging clients in meaningful occupations and activities, interventions to support occupations, education and training, advocacy, group interventions, and virtual interventions (AOTA, 2020b). The process includes establishing a therapeutic relationship with the client, so that the client benefits from the intervention activities and reaches the established goals. See Chapter 4 for more information on the therapeutic relationship. OT intervention requires both knowledge of the art (e.g., therapeutic use of self) and science (e.g., physical, process, and social). The intervention session allows the OT practitioner to use creativity in choosing activities that address each client's goal. Practitioners may choose to promote occupational performance by creating opportunities, establishing or restoring skills or abilities, maintaining performance through supports, or modifying or preventing disability (AOTA, 2020b). OT practitioners must adapt and modify activities to promote the "just-right" challenge so that clients benefit from the intervention. Reading cues and responding to them require the practitioner to pay attention to the client, surroundings, and address the client's needs and goals. The practitioner carefully monitors the client's response during the intervention and modifies activities and the intervention plan as needed.

BOX 1.4	**Sample Hypotheses**	
Model of Practice/Frame of Reference	**Principle**	**Hypothesis**
Model of Human Occupation	Change in any aspect of volition, habituation, performance capacity, and/or the environment can result in a change in one's thoughts, feelings, and actions (Kielhofner, 2008; O'Brien & Kielhofner, 2017).	Client's poor self-efficacy (belief in one's abilities) interferes with their ability to engage in novel activities resulting in poor performance.
Biomechanical	To increase muscle strength, the muscle must be overloaded to the point of fatigue, which requires more motor units and causes hypertrophy and hyperplasia of glycolic type II fast-twitch muscle fibers (Rybski, 2012).	Weak dominant (right) arm and hand strength since immobilization from injury limit the client's ability to complete desired daily activities.

Assess Outcomes

The OT practitioner reviews the client's progress throughout the process and measures the outcomes of intervention using assessment tools and comparing occupational performance after therapy compared to initial evaluation findings. The practitioner measures the client's progress on goals. OT practitioners may want to examine client, caregiver, or group satisfaction with OT services to determine the success of outcomes. The practitioner may gain important information by measuring the influence of the OT intervention on caregiver, groups, or populations. For example, it may be important to know if the intervention improved the caregiver's quality of life, improved wellness in the community, or changed attitudes towards persons with disability. Reflecting upon the outcomes and debriefing with team members may provide additional data for the next intervention. Chapter 10 describes reflection techniques.

CASE ILLUSTRATION OF THE THERAPEUTIC REASONING PROCESS

The following case by Brendan Cook illustrates the therapeutic reasoning process. The full evaluation and intervention plan are included in Box 1.5. For a short reflection from the student therapist, see Evolve site Videoclip 1.1 (Brendan). Brendan works with a team of professionals and considers their observations and assessments in his plan. See Chapter 7 describing techniques to promote therapeutic reasoning in teams.

Use Theory to Generate Questions

Brendan organized his evaluation using occupation-based models of practice, the Person-Environment-Occupation-Performance (PEOP) and the Model of Human Occupation (MOHO). PEOP allowed him to get a complete picture of the client's (David) occupational needs within the context of the environment (setting, societal attitudes, occupational justice) and MOHO allowed him to identify what David most wants to accomplish, his habits and routines, his lived experience, and the influence of the environment on his daily life. He generated the following questions:

Person

- What is David's occupational history?
- What does David want to accomplish? What are his concerns?
- What are his motor, process, and social interaction abilities?
- How does cognitive, and psychological functioning influence his occupational performance?

BOX 1.5   Occupational Therapy Case Study by Brendan Cook, OTD Student

Client's Name (changed to protect personal identity): David Bland

Date of report: 10/15/2020

DOB: 01/09/1972

Chronological age: 49 Years

Setting: Community Independence Occupational Therapy Outpatient Clinic

Primary Diagnosis: Psychosis

Reason for referral to OT: David was referred to occupational therapy by his case manager 6 months ago when he was residing in a homeless shelter. He has now secured placement in his own independent apartment and has been living there for 2 weeks. You are the occupational therapist assigned to complete a routine re-evaluation today in his apartment today.

Client history

Comorbidities: Hypertension, Diabetes II, Depression, Anxiety, and Fatigue

Medical: David's primary medical concerns are hypertension and diabetes. He has diabetic neuropathy with associated pain, primarily in the lower extremities; because of this, he walks with a cane, but sometimes forgets to use it.

Family: David currently lives by himself in a senior apartment that is paid through a homeless shelter service. David reports that he has no family members living in town, and the closest family member lives in Arkansas (5 hours away). David reports that he has some church members and associates that can assist him if he asks. However, David states "I am mostly by myself, and would much rather like to keep it that way."

Educational: David graduated from St. Louis High School. David always wanted to go to college, and/or get a GED but always felt that there was not enough time.

Environment: David currently lives in a senior, one-bedroom, apartment in St. Louis. His apartment is on the first level, and there are no steps. David has a standard tub shower and a grab bar within the shower.

Background information from other professionals

Case Manager Report: "Prior to obtaining his new apartment, David had been homeless for about 2 years. At the homeless shelter, we provide temporary housing at the shelter, full cooked meals, and various resources for our clients. While at the homeless shelter, David attended some of the group classes, such as mindfulness and job training. David always displayed a positive attitude and kindness towards staff members and other clients. After conversing with David, we granted him permanent housing at a local senior apartment. David still attends the medical clinic to manage his healthcare needs. It is noted in our documents that he has a disability case still open, but we do not know how long it would take to get the approval. After meeting with David two weeks ago, I still believe that there is room for improvement on his everyday skills: household management, leisure activity, cooking, and or daily routines that might improve his health and safety, and much more."

Primary Care Doctor Report: "David's primary medical concerns are his hypertension and diabetes. We are fearful that he has not been taking his medication as prescribed. David also has diabetic neuropathy with associated pain, primarily in the lower extremities and he walks with a cane sometimes because of this. We see David a few times per year to check vital signs and to monitor any disease progression."

Psychiatrist Report: "In 2016 David was diagnosed with psychosis, anxiety, and depression. David mentioned that prior to 2016 he did experience symptoms and episodes of psychosis. However, David has not experienced an acute episode of psychosis since May of 2019. He has been functioning well with the addition of his current medications. David is currently prescribed with a mood stabilizer and an antidepressant. I last saw David 3 weeks ago. He did not report difficulties with sleep, but mentioned that he seems fatigued when conducting his activities of daily living and has an overall decreased motivation. David also displays some cognition deficits such as attention, executive functioning, and memory. I believe that because David went undiagnosed for a long period, the results are these cognitive deficits within daily function. I am curious to hear how well he is doing with his ADLs and IADLs, as he has now moved into a new apartment."

BOX 1.5 Occupational Therapy Case Study by Brendan Cook, OTD Student—cont'd

Volition

Client's Concerns/Goals: David reports that he gets lonely and feels depressed living in his apartment by himself. He reports "Some days I just don't feel like it. I do not feel like cooking, taking a shower, or cleaning. I just want to sit and do nothing." David also reports, "Some days I just feel very weak. My legs hurt; I am just so tired."

Client/Family Interests: David enjoys going to church, watching TV, riding the bus around town, and eating food at restaurants. David also enjoys listening to music and playing card games with his church members.

Habituation

Typical day: David states that every day he wakes up around 9:00AM, takes a shower, brushes teeth, and lays right back down in bed to look out the window until his favorite TV show comes on at 11am. If he gets hungry, he says that he will make a peanut butter and jelly sandwich; or go to the homeless shelter to get food and see his friends. He states that he sometimes goes walking around 3:00PM or will ride the bus around town.

Work and leisure activities: Before being diagnosed in 2019, David worked as a janitor in a local high school. Currently David does not have a job and cannot work due to him being in the process of obtaining his disability check. With regards to leisure activities, David stated that he enjoys listening to music and playing card games with his church members.

Description of assessments

Activity Card Sort-Advancing Inclusive Participation (ACS-AIP): Occupational performance assessment that looks at a range of activities of daily living (ADL), IADL, leisure, and social activities and is designed to be used with individuals experiencing homelessness. The inclusion of non-sanctioned occupations, such as those deemed socially unacceptable, unhealthy, or illegal, in the assessment process promotes occupational justice and facilitates holistic care within the homeless population.

Performance Assessment of Self-Care Skills (PASS): Performance-based tool designed to objectively measure and document functional mobility, basic activities of daily living, instrumental activities of daily living with a cognitive emphasis, and instrumental activities of daily living with a physical emphasis in the home or clinic setting. Items can be individually administered, and all items yield an adequacy, safety, and independence score. Only the medication management activities were administered for this evaluation.

Assessment Findings and Behavioral Observations

Assessment	Results	Findings	Behavioral Observations
ACS-AIP	Top 5 goals 1. Traveling 2. Playing sports 3. Looking for jobs 4. Dancing 5. Pursuing a partner	**Activities of Daily Living (ADLs)** David reports that he is able to maintain and participate in many of his ADLs. However, David does report that most of his hygiene products and food are provided through the homeless shelter. **Instrumental Activities of Daily Living (IADLs)** David reported that he participated in many of the areas listed within the IADL category. However, he did mention that when he is lonely, or fatigued, he doesn't like to do anything (e.g. household management) **Rest and Sleep** David mentioned that with the new apartment, and new bed, he still is having trouble sleeping. This is an interesting comment because oftentimes people who experience homelessness have a hard time adjusting to new environments. **Leisure/Social Participation** David stated that he sometimes engages with social friends and activities but is now having a hard time doing that. He gets lonely being in his apartment and rarely communicates to any friends.	During the assessment, David displayed some attention deficits, and required many verbal cues to stay on topic. David also displayed some memory deficits by asking the therapist "what am I supposed to do again?" During the assessment, David fell asleep, displaying signs of fatigue and attention deficits.
PASS (Medication Management)		David reported the next time the medication was supposed to be taken and opened the pill bottle. Throughout the assessment, David required verbal cues to stay on task, displaying some attention deficits.	Ultimately, David has the fine motor ability to open and close his pill bottle. However, his executive functioning deficits cause him to often forget steps in initiating tasks or completing tasks. This may result in him failing to take his medications appropriately.

Continued

BOX 1.5 Occupational Therapy Case Study by Brendan Cook, OTD Student—cont'd

Intervention Plan

Long Term Goal A: David will independently participate in 1 new leisure occupation of his choosing, for a minimum of 30 minutes per week by discharge.

Long Term Goal B: David will be able to independently manage his daily medications for 1 week using a pill planner system by discharge.

Frame of Reference: Cognitive Orientation to daily Occupational Performance (CO-OP)

Short-Term Goals (2)	FOR Principle Used to Address Goals	Intervention Approach/Methods
(A) David will identify the environmental demands for 3 leisure activities within the community, with minimal indirect verbal cues by session two.	Occupational adaptation occurs when the client understands the environmental requirements to engage in the desired occupation. Understanding the environmental requirements is necessary to determine the feasibility for engaging in the leisure occupation.	Although David reports having church friends, he still feels lonely and depressed being by himself in his apartment. This information can be used to explore occupations for David to do that he finds meaningful. The therapist will provide indirect verbal cues, such as "what do you like to do for fun" and use information gathered from the ACS-AIP to support leisure exploration.
(B) With minimal indirect verbal cues, David will document taking the correct medication daily × 3 days.	*Goal* – Create a goal *Plan* – Collaborate with the client on how to achieve the goal. *Do* – Carry out the task of taking and documenting the correct medication with the usage of planned strategy. *Check* – Evaluate on how the process went with the client.	With the goal being documenting and taking the correct medicine, the client can develop a plan to complete the task. During the plan portion, the therapist can provide indirect verbal cues to assist them in solidifying a plan such as "What could you use to help you carry out this task?" After solidifying the plan, and carrying out the task, the therapist will reevaluate with the client on how everything went.

Environmental Factors

- What are some community resources that may support David?
- Where does he live now? Is it accessible?
- Does he have access to services at the homeless shelter?
- What are his social supports?

Occupation Factors

- What are his desired occupations?
- What are David's routines and patterns of occupations?

Performance Factors

- What are David's strengths and challenges?
- How is his mental health (psychosis) interfering with his ability to engage in occupations?
- What medical issues may interfere with his occupational performance?

Gather Data

Brendan completed a client interview to build a rapport and obtain information regarding David's history. He administered the Activity Card Sort – Advancing Inclusive Participation (ACS-AIP; Tyminski et al., 2020) to examine the range of occupations (i.e., instrumental activities of daily living, activities of daily living, social participation, leisure and rest and sleep) and the Performance Assessment of Self-Care Skills (PASS; Rogers et al., 2016) to measure adequacy, safety, and independence with medication management. Brendan gathered information through observation and interaction as well. He noted David fell asleep at one point, displayed difficulty paying attention, and showed memory deficits. David forgot steps and had trouble initiating activities (such as medication management task).

Identify Occupational Challenges

Brendan synthesized all the data and considered David's strengths (e.g., history of being involved in social activities at church; works well in groups per case manager; well-liked by peers) and challenges (e.g., memory, planning, routines, feeling lonely, lack of motivation) within the environment (e.g., homeless for 2 years, recently moved into an independent apartment). Brendan hypothesized that David's current occupations do not support social participation resulting in isolation and feelings of loneliness which interfere with feelings of self-efficacy (belief in oneself) and may also result in apathy or cognitive processing difficulties. Brendan noted that David's difficulties with cognition, specifically initiation and planning, may interfere with his medication management routine.

Create an Intervention Plan

Brendan created two long-term goals to address social participation within the local community and medication management. Brendan considered the local environment when creating the goal and intervention session. David was to identify, select, and engage in one 30-minute new leisure occupation of his choosing per week. This goal encourages David to explore the community, take public transportation, and interact with people at different events. With the therapist's support and guidance, David may find new leisure activities he enjoys that provide him with social contacts. Engaging in light physical activities may serve to motivate David to engage in community activities, while providing opportunities for him to feel successful, building his self-efficacy. This serves to promote occupational adaptation as a person becomes more competent and successful within their environment. Therapy sessions addressing this goal included promoting initiation, planning, and cognitive skills while engaging in leisure exploration activities, such as playing Jenga. Brendan also asked the client reflective questions to promote problem solving and self-evaluation.

Brendan addressed the second goal, "David will independently manage his daily medication for 1 week using a pill planner system, by discharge," using the Cognitive Orientation to daily Occupational Performance (CO-OP) (Polatajko et al., 2001) model. CO-OP is a client-centered approach that empowers clients to engage in cognitive strategies to address their goals. Clients are taught to meet their goals by going through the Goal, Plan, Do, Check process. See Box 1.6 for examples for David.

Implement the Plan

Brendan implemented the intervention plan by establishing a rapport with the client and being mindful of his therapeutic use of self. He carefully chose language that did not include jargon and encouraged David through non-verbal and verbal cues. Brendan sought to empower David by encouraging him to engage in the process. They worked together collaboratively on activities. The activities selected (such as Jenga) were appropriate for David and the setting. They discussed activities in the community that could be completed in 30 minutes and that did not require much money, such as exploring an art museum on the "free day" and park events. David began to use the cognitive strategies from the Goal, Plan, Do, Check process to address his goal for social participation.

Assess Outcomes

David required minimal verbal cues to complete his medication management routine. He participated in a weekly 30-minute leisure activity in the community and expressed satisfaction with engaging in church activities once again. He showed Brendan that he could complete the Goal, Plan, Do, Check process with leisure activities, suggesting he may be able to use this strategy for future goals. David reported feeling more motivated to engage in community activities.

BOX 1.6   Goal-Plan-Do-Check

CO-OP Step	Description	David's example
Goal	Create a meaningful and measurable goal	David will independently complete the pill planner of his choosing to correctly identify his medication for the week.
Plan	Collaborate and decide how to achieve the goal	Discuss how to use the pill planner, cognitive strategies to adhere to the routine, and discuss how to achieve the goal.
Do	Carry out the task	Correctly place medication in pill planner, take correct medication daily and document.
Check	Evaluate the process	Evaluate how many days the system worked and how the process could be revised for better outcomes.

▌ SUMMARY

Students and practitioners who are curious to know about human occupation and methods and techniques ask questions and seek answers that facilitate therapeutic reasoning. Therapeutic reasoning is the process of synthesizing information about the client, occupation, and environment to design creative and meaningful occupational therapy intervention. OT practitioners use many types of therapeutic reasoning (i.e., scientific, narrative, pragmatic, interactive, ethical, and conditional) to better understand clients' occupational performance challenges. As students and practitioners gain experience, reflect upon decisions, and learn more through discussion, reading, and education, they progress from novice, advanced beginner, competent, proficient to expert practitioner. Expert practitioners read many cues, practice based on intuition, and are able to articulate their rationale for decisions. They

modify and adapt intervention to better address the client's goals. The steps of therapeutic reasoning include use theory to generate questions, gather data, identify occupational challenges, create an intervention plan, implement the plan, and assess the outcomes. Therapeutic reasoning is a dynamic process that evolves based on current research and evidence. OT practitioners who stay open to learning, show curiosity about concepts, reflect upon intervention choices, analyze their interactions with clients, gain knowledge on current research evidence, and have a desire to make a difference with clients of all ages will develop therapeutic reasoning skills. The chapters in this textbook provide case examples and learning activities to facilitate therapeutic reasoning. The Evolve learning site has video clips and case examples to provide additional learning opportunities.

REFERENCES

American Occupational Therapy Association. (2020a). Occupational therapy code of ethics. *American Journal of Occupational Therapy, 74*(Suppl. 3). 7413410005.

American Occupational Therapy Association. (2020b). *Occupational therapy practice framework: Domain and process* (4th ed.). North Bethesda, MD: AOTA.

Baum, C. M., Christiansen, C. H., & Bass, D. (2015). The person-environment-occupation-performance (PEOP) model. In C. Christiansen, C. M. Baum, & J. D. Bass (Eds.), *Occupational therapy: performance, participation, and well-being* (4th ed., pp. 49–55). Thorofare, NJ: SLACK Inc.

Benfield, A. M., & Johnston, M. V. (2020). Initial development of a measure of evidence-informed professional thinking. *Australian Occupational Therapy Journal, 67*, 309–319.

Boyt-Schell, B. A. (2019). Professional reasoning in practice. In B. A. B. Schell & G. Gillen (Eds.), *Willard and Spackman's occupational therapy* (13th ed., pp. 482–497). Philadelphia: Wolters Kluwer.

Bushby, K., Chan, J., Druif, H., Ho, K., & Kinsella, E. A. (2015). Ethical tensions in occupational therapy practice: A scoping review. *British Journal of Occupational Therapy, 8*(4), 212–221.

Cain, J. (2019). We should pay more attention to student curiosity. *Currents in Pharmacy Teaching and Learning, 11*, 651–654.

Canadian Association of Occupational Therapists. (1997). *Enabling occupation: an occupational therapy perspective.* Ottawa, ON: CAOT Publications ACE.

Carrier, A., Levasseur, M., Bedard, D., & Desrosiers, J. (2012). Clinical reasoning process underlying choice of teaching strategies: A framework to improve occupational therapists' transfer skill interventions. *Australian Occupational Therapy Journal, 59*, 355–366.

Dreyfus, H., & Dreyfus, S. (2004). The ethical implications of the five-stage-skill acquisition model. *Bulletin of Science, Technology & Society, 24*(3), 251–264.

Durning, S., Artino, A. R., Pangaro, L., van der Vleuten, S. P. M., & Schuwirth, L. (2011). Context and clinical reasoning: Understanding the perspective of the expert's voice. *Medical Education, 45*, 927–938.

Dyche, L., & Epstein, R. M. (2011). Curiosity and medical education. *Medical Education, 45*, 663–668.

Fleming, M. H. (1991). The therapist with the three-track mind. *American Journal of Occupational Therapy, 45*, 1007–1014.

Grajo, L., & Rushanan, S. (2021). Ethical decision-making in occupational therapy practice. In J. O'Brien & J. Solomon (Eds.). *Occupational Analysis and Group Process* (2nd ed., pp. 173). St. Louis, MO: Elsevier.

Kielhofner, G., & Forsyth, K. (2008). Therapeutic reasoning: Planning, implementing, and evaluating outcomes of therapy. In G. Kielhofner (Ed.), *Model of human occupation: Theory and application* (4th ed.). Philadelphia, PA: Lippincott, William & Wilkins.

Kielhofner, G. (2008). *Model of human occupation: Theory and application* (4th ed.). Philadelphia, PA: Lippincott, Williams & Wilkins.

Kinsella, E. A., Park, A., Appiagyei, J., Chang, E., & Chow, D. (2008). Through the eyes of students: Ethical tensions in occupational therapy practice. *Canadian Journal of Occupational Therapy, 75*(3), 176–183.

Kuipers, K., & Grice, J. (2009). The structure of novice and expert occupational therapists' clinical reasoning before and after exposure to a domain-specific protocol. *Australian Occupational Therapy Journal, 56*, 418–427.

Law, M. C. (2007). A firm persuasion in our work. Occupational therapy: A journey driven by curiosity. *American Journal of Occupational Therapy, 61*, 599–602.

Leavitt-Jones, T., Hoffman, K., Dempsey, J., Jeong, S. Y. S., Noble, D., Norton, C. A., Roche, J., & Hickey, N. (2010). The 'five rights' of clinical reasoning: An educational model to enhance nursing students ability to identify and manage clinically 'at risk' patients. *Nurse Education Today, 30*(6), 515–520.

Mitchell, R., & Unsworth, C. A. (2005). Clinical reasoning during community health home visits: Expert and novice differences. *British Journal of Occupational Therapy, 68*(5), 215–223.

Norman, G. (2012). On competence, curiosity and creativity. *Advances in Health Science Education, 17*, 611–613.

O'Brien, J., & Kielhofner, G. (2017). The dynamics of human occupation. In R. Taylor (Ed.), *Kielhofner's model of human occupation* (5th ed., pp. 24–37). Philadelphia, PA: Wolters Kluwer.

Polatajko, H., Mandich, A. D., Miller, L. T., et al. (2001). Cognitive orientation to daily occupational performance (CO-OP): Part II – the evidence. *Physical & Occupational Therapy in Pediatrics, 30*, 83–106.

Purtilo, R. (2005). *Ethical dimensions in the health professions* (4th ed.). North Bethesda, MD: American Occupational Therapy Association (AOTA).

Rogers, J. C., Holm, M. B., & Chisolm, D. (2016). *Performance Assessment of Self-Care Skills (PASS) Version 4.1.* Pittsburgh, PA: University of Pittsburgh. Assessment manual can be found at: https://bit.ly/2Y5Gwg4.

Rybski, M. (2012). Biomechanical intervention approach. In: *Kinesiology for occupational therapy* (pp. 309–354). Thorofare, NJ: SLACK Inc.

Schkade, J. K., & Schultz, S. (2003). Occupational adaptation. In P. Kramer, J. Hinojosa, & C. B. Royeen (Eds.), *Perspectives in human occupation, participation in life* (pp. 181–221). Philadelphia, PA: Lippincott, Williams & Wilkins.

Taylor, R. (2017). *Kielhofner's model of human occupation.* (5th ed.). WolterKluwer Health/Philadelphia, PA: Lippincott Williams & Wilkins.

Taylor, R. (2020). *The intentional relationship model* (2nd ed.). Philadelphia, PA: FA Davis.

Tyminski, Q. P., Drummond, R. R., Heisey, C. F., Evans, S. K., Hendrix, A., Jaegers, L. A., & Baum, C. M. (2020). Initial development of the Activity Card Sort-Advancing Inclusive Participation from a homeless population perspective. *Occupational Therapy International, 2020*, 9083082.

WORKSHEET 1.1: OCCUPATIONAL PROFILE (AOTA, 2020b)

Brainstorm how different clients may describe their experiences, patterns, interests and values, and contexts.
- Describe how the categories may altered by an illness or an injury.
- What else would you like to learn about the client?

Parts of the Occupational Profile				
Occupational History	Experiences	Patterns of Daily Living	Interests/Values	Relevant Contexts
30-year-old mother of a six-month-old	Wakes early, feeds baby, eats breakfast, plays with baby, takes care of household tasks, calls friend, takes walk, feeds baby, etc.	Routines focused on care of baby	Keeping her baby healthy, learning ways to help the baby develop optimally	Home Family support
60-year-old man working at a restaurant as a chef				
12-year-old child in the 7th grade				
95-year-old woman living in independent retirement village				

WORKSHEET 1.2: CURIOSITY

Brainstorming

On the first day of fieldwork, your supervisor asks you to plan a 30-minute activity for a 25-year-old client who was in an accident and lost use of their right side and experienced a head injury.

Curiosity
List questions you have regarding this case.
Organize your questions into categories and determine how you would find the answers.
Develop at least 5 ways to find answers.
Without knowing the answers, design the activity.   • What things are you considering?   • How will you adapt and change it if the client is not able to engage in it?

WORKSHEET 1.3: TYPES OF REASONING

Provide examples of how an OT practitioner may use each type of reasoning for the case scenario.

- Identify questions regarding this scenario that address each type of therapeutic reasoning.

Types of Reasoning		
Type of Reasoning	Examples from case	Questions
Scientific		
Narrative		
Pragmatic		
Ethical		
Interactive		
Conditional		

2

Occupation as the Foundation for Therapeutic Reasoning

Mary Elizabeth Patnaude and Jane O'Brien

GUIDING QUESTIONS

1. How does occupation serve as the foundation for therapeutic reasoning?
2. How do OT practitioners use occupation as both a modality and an outcome?
3. How do factors (e.g., personal, environmental, occupation) influence therapeutic reasoning?
4. What cognitive processing skills and attributes support therapeutic reasoning?
5. How are various types of reasoning (i.e., scientific, pragmatic, narrative, interactive, ethical, and conditional) used in the occupational therapy process (i.e., evaluation, intervention, and outcomes)?

KEY TERMS

Context-dependent decisions
Dynamic systems theory
Emotional intelligence
External factors
Internal factors
Intuition
Occupational adaptation

Occupational analysis
Occupational engagement
Occupational identity
Reflective thinking
Self-awareness
Tacit knowledge
Therapeutic use of self

INTRODUCTION

Occupational therapy (OT) is a complex profession whose practitioners provide assessment and intervention for clients from a multitude of cultures in a variety of practice settings, from the intensive care unit to the community (Unsworth & Baker, 2016). To navigate the complexity of practice, OT practitioners employ therapeutic reasoning as they engage in the entire occupational therapy process of evaluation, intervention, and assessment of outcomes. They develop an intervention plan for a client based on factors discovered in the interview and evaluation process, implement the intervention, reflect on its effectiveness, and evaluate the outcomes (Benfield & Johnston, 2020). The therapeutic reasoning process provides a link between theory and practice (Kristensen & Petersen, 2016; Unsworth & Baker, 2016).

A foundational belief of the profession is that humans are occupational beings whose health and well-being depends upon the ability to engage in meaningful occupations and that occupational participation sustains health, while occupational deprivation inhibits health (Kristensen & Petersen, 2016; Mee et al., 2004). Participation in meaningful occupations provides the basis for clients to be content and live a balanced life (AOTA, 2020; Mee et al., 2004). Therefore,

occupation is both a method to address a client's challenges (i.e., modality) and the desired result of the intervention process (i.e., outcome).

OT practitioners engage in different types of reasoning (i.e., conditional, ethical, interactive, narrative, pragmatic, and scientific) to understand a client's occupational challenges. This requires they use a variety of cognitive processes to analyze, anticipate, decide, hypothesize, judge, perceive, prioritize, problem-solve, and read cues. OT practitioners rely on emotional intelligence, intuition, reflection, self-awareness, and therapeutic use of self during the occupational therapy process.

The authors describe occupation, its complexity, and its relationship to health and well-being. They review factors influencing occupational performance and emphasize the role of occupation both as a therapeutic modality (i.e., means) and outcome (i.e., ends) of the therapy process. The relationship between occupation, cognitive processing skills and attributes provides insight into the therapeutic reasoning process. The authors examine the types of therapeutic reasoning used to facilitate occupational engagement. Case examples and learning activities illustrate how occupation influences therapeutic reasoning in practice.

OCCUPATION AS A FOUNDATION

Engaging in one's desired occupations influences health and well-being (Creek & Hughes, 2008; Mee et al., 2004; Stav et al., 2012). Occupational engagement refers to the "client's doing, thinking, and feeling under certain environmental conditions in the midst of or as a planned consequence of therapy" (Kielhofner, 2008, p. 184). Occupational engagement promotes physical, cognitive, social, and emotional activity and is considered part of one's identity. Researchers report strong evidence linking physical activity to health (Creek & Hughes, 2008; Rajarajeswaran & Vishnupriya, 2009; Stav et al., 2012). Physical activity provided when engaging in occupation improves mental health and well-being as observed in improvements in mood, physical self-perception, self-esteem, and socialization (Creek & Hughes, 2008). For example, taking a walk every day may decrease one's chance of developing certain types of cancer but walking with a close friend may lead to more relational satisfaction (Rajarajeswaran & Vishnupriya, 2009). OT practitioners create intervention plans to promote occupational engagement.

Engagement in meaningful occupations contributes to the health and well-being of people across the lifespan (Kristensen & Petersen, 2016; Mee et al., 2004; Rajarajeswaran & Vishnupriya, 2009; Stav et al., 2012; Weinstock-Zlotnick & Mehta, 2018). Mee and colleagues (2004) found that clients with mental illness valued occupational participation to acquire new skills, cope with challenges, and experience the satisfaction of achievement. For example, when completing a woodworking task, clients stated that they improved their coordination and gained specific skills related to the object they created, which led to feelings of accomplishment. Clients felt encouraged to continue working on the project, which led to greater skill acquisition and satisfaction (Mee et al., 2004). Community-dwelling older adults reported better health and quality of life when engaging in work, leisure, and social activities in the community (Stav et al., 2012). Engaging clients experiencing musculoskeletal disorders in occupations has several benefits. The ways in which the upper extremities are used during everyday tasks (i.e., occupations) involves more diverse movements than rote exercise (Weinstock-Zlotnick & Mehta, 2018). The engaging nature of participating in desired occupations may empower the client to ignore pain and anxiety caused by moving an injured limb that may prevent or ameliorate learned disuse (Weinstock-Zlotnick & Mehta, 2018).

Finally, clients are motivated by occupations that contribute to achieving their goals, and in which they find satisfaction in mastery (Mee et al., 2004; Stav et al., 2012). For example, if a client wants to improve hand function to bake cookies to give away, they may be more likely to participate in therapy utilizing cookie dough rather than theraputty for exercise.

The primary occupation of children is play, which promotes motor, social, and cognitive skill development. Facilitating play allows children with disabilities to take part in a much desired occupation with peers. OT practitioners use knowledge of the factors influencing play and therapeutic reasoning to determine how to creatively engage children and their families. They consider the environment, tasks, and the child's strengths and challenges. Children are highly motivated by novel and interesting play activities, which can be adjusted to promote success. OT practitioners working with children also address occupations of feeding, dressing, bathing, toileting, academics, care of pets, and social participation.

Engaging in therapeutic reasoning that reflects the importance of occupation, which is a core value of the profession, leads OT practitioners to effectively choose the most beneficial interventions for their clients (Kristensen & Petersen, 2016). The focus on occupation encourages and supports clients in leading balanced, contented lives (Mee et al., 2004; Stav et al., 2012).

COMPLEXITY OF OCCUPATION

Several theories, such as chaos theory, dynamic systems theory and complexity theory, address the complex, non-linear processes associated with occupation (Aldrich, 2008; Bird & Strachan, 2020; Ramshaw, 2020). A central tenet of systems theory is that systems tend toward equilibrium by moving towards attractors, which organize the system, and moving away from repellers, which destabilize the system (Aldrich, 2008). Occupational therapists view equilibrium as the client's ability to make the necessary changes to engage in desired occupations over time, which is referred to as occupational adaptation. If a person's abilities (i.e., internal factors) are not sufficient to return the person to a state or sense of occupational adaptation, the person will depend upon their interactions with the environment (i.e., external factors) to return to a sense of occupational adaptation (Aldrich, 2008).

The dynamic interaction that occurs between the person's cognitive and neural systems and the environment during occupation helps to bring about changes that results in occupational adaptation. For example, a person can pick up a coffee cup because they have previously learned unconscious information that helps discern the weight of the object. The brain has a system of feedback that remembers when the person last picked up a similar object, and it prepares the hand to grasp the cup. Neural pathways integrate motor and sensory information rapidly to make postural adjustments to lift the cup without throwing it over one's head or losing balance as one picks it up. During the task of picking up one's coffee, the person processes the environment, size of cup, previous motor experiences, sensory stimuli (such as visual, auditory, smells, tactile, vestibular) to create the desired response. Figure. 2.1 illustrates the complexity of occupation using the example of enjoying a cup of coffee.

Since occupations are dynamic and provide the impetus for individuals to pursue a fulfilling life, they are inherently meaningful and motivating (Lazzarini, 2004). The dynamic nature of occupation provides a strong force for neural change due to the motivation provided by the human being's drive for occupational balance and self-organization (Aldrich, 2008; Lazzarini, 2004). Participation in simple, meaningful occupations, such as getting up every day and getting dressed is so powerful, that it can slow the cognitive decline seen in conditions such as Alzheimer's disease (Lazzarini, 2004; Stav et al., 2012). The power of participation in everyday activities is demonstrated by the fact that occupational engagement can produce practice-dependent cortical change and improved cognitive performance (Gillen, 2013; Sorman et al., 2019). Engagement in activities that stimulate the

mind and the body improves fluid intelligence (i.e., the ability to reason quickly and to think abstractly) and executive functioning (i.e., working memory, flexible thinking, and self-control) (Sorman et al., 2019).

OCCUPATIONAL ANALYSIS

OT practitioners use therapeutic reasoning to analyze, problem-solve, and decide on intervention goals as they complete an occupational analysis. An occupational analysis details the skills, performance patterns, sequence, activity demands, contexts, and client factors required to complete a desired occupation. The *Occupational Therapy Practice Framework* (4th ed) (AOTA, 2020) provides a comprehensive listing and definitions of terms that may help practitioners organize the analysis. Occupational analyses may also be structured based on a selected model of practice or frame of reference (O'Brien & Solomon, 2022) (Worksheet 2.3). For example, an occupational analysis may be comprehensive or examine cognitive, physical, social–emotional, or contextual factors influencing occupation. See Worksheets 2.3, 2.4, and 2.5 for sample Occupational Analyses. The OT practitioner decides what type of occupational analysis to complete.

Table 2.1 provides examples of the results of an occupational analysis of scrapbooking at home by identifying how the findings of the analysis inform occupation and OT intervention for a 50-year-old woman with carpometacarpal osteoarthritis.

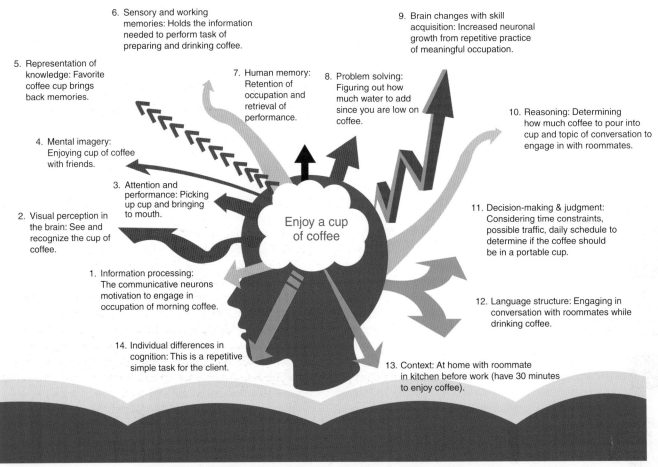

6. Sensory and working memories: Holds the information needed to perform task of preparing and drinking coffee.

9. Brain changes with skill acquisition: Increased neuronal growth from repetitive practice of meaningful occupation.

5. Representation of knowledge: Favorite coffee cup brings back memories.

7. Human memory: Retention of occupation and retrieval of performance.

8. Problem solving: Figuring out how much water to add since you are low on coffee.

10. Reasoning: Determining how much coffee to pour into cup and topic of conversation to engage in with roommates.

4. Mental imagery: Enjoying cup of coffee with friends.

3. Attention and performance: Picking up cup and bringing to mouth.

Enjoy a cup of coffee

11. Decision-making & judgment: Considering time constraints, possible traffic, daily schedule to determine if the coffee should be in a portable cup.

2. Visual perception in the brain: See and recognize the cup of coffee.

1. Information processing: The communicative neurons motivation to engage in occupation of morning coffee.

12. Language structure: Engaging in conversation with roommates while drinking coffee.

14. Individual differences in cognition: This is a repetitive simple task for the client.

13. Context: At home with roommate in kitchen before work (have 30 minutes to enjoy coffee).

Fig. 2.1 Complexity of Occupation: Process of Engaging in Occupation

TABLE 2.1 Results of Occupational Analysis: Scrapbooking

Type of reasoning	Relationship to occupation	OT Intervention
Scientific	Examine how joint changes in the hand facilitate or inhibit tasks required to complete occupation.	Provide larger tools to prevent joint strain. Provide joint protection education to allow the client to complete the task without feeling like she is causing damage to her joints.
Narrative	Explore stories about items chosen to include in scrapbook and how the client became interested in scrapbooking. Identify how the client feels about the ways in which scrapbooking may affect her joints.	Ask the client to tell the story of the page completed to better understand the client. Allow the client to explain how scrapbooking affects her sense of self.
Pragmatic	The client attends therapy at a clinic, where she may not have many tools and scrapbooking items.	The therapist secures tools and items for scrapbooking, including adapted tools which may allow the client to continue scrapbooking, with less pain or damage to joints.
Conditional	The therapist examines the physical, social, and cognitive requirements of scrapbooking within the context of the clinic and home environment. The therapist analyzes the activity demands and determines if the activity should be completed in a group or individual session. The therapist considers financial, transportation needs when referring the client to a women's group in the community.	Use adaptive tools, joint protection training, and orthotics to manage edema and joint deformation to improve the client's ability to engage in scrapbooking with a group of women in the community.
Ethical	The therapist considers the therapeutic benefits of engaging in the activity in a group (beneficence). The therapist allows the client to have choice in the activity and if she is in a group or individual session (autonomy). During the session, the therapist is mindful to provide fair and equitable services (Justice).	The therapist is mindful of the client's right to privacy during therapy sessions. The therapist does not reveal information about the client's diagnoses or plan of care. The therapist allows the client choices.
Interactive	The therapist observes and responds to the client's personality, communication style, body language, and responses to directions. The therapist observes (and intervenes as needed) interactions between group members and signs of frustration, bullying, power struggles, or aggression, as well as positive interactions.	The therapist may position members of groups close together to support each other. During individual sessions, the therapist is mindful of how they are communicating with the client and how they are being perceived.

LEARNING ACTIVITY: ANALYZING OCCUPATIONS

Complete Worksheet 2.3 to complete a comprehensive occupational analysis of an occupation of your choice (complete as if you are completing the activity).
- How would this analysis inform an intervention activity for a 6-year-old girl who is unable to use her right upper extremity (R UE) and experiences mild cognitive impairment?

LEARNING ACTIVITY: OCCUPATIONAL ANALYSIS BASED ON SELECTED FRAMES OF REFERENCE

Complete Worksheet 2.4 to analyze the aspects of an occupation as related to a selected frame of reference of your choice.
- How does a frame of reference inform the occupational analysis?

LEARNING ACTIVITY: CONTEXTUAL ANALYSIS

Complete Worksheet 2.5 to analyze the contextual aspects of an occupation of your choice (complete as if you are completing the activity in a familiar setting).
- Describe how changing the context(s) of the activity, changes the performance demands.

OCCUPATION AS A THERAPEUTIC MODALITY AND AS THE OUTCOME OF THERAPY

The use of occupation-based intervention promotes motor recovery and improves cognitive function (Gillen, 2013; Sorman et al., 2019). Occupation remodels the brain through repetitive practice of everyday tasks which promote neuronal growth (Gillen, 2013). In addition, people value occupations in which they choose to engage and consequently they will participate in the occupation for longer periods of time (Persson et al., 2001). Clients value performing the desired occupation and benefit therapeutically by engaging in the occupation (Persson et al., 2001, Stav et al., 2012).

Engaging in desired occupations is the goal or desired outcome of occupational therapy. For example, to improve a child's ability to play with peers at school, OT practitioners engage the child in role play activities to develop skills with the goal of playing with peers. The practitioner facilitates a play session with one peer and promotes positive play behaviors. Engaging in play activities graded to challenge the child requires therapeutic reasoning. This is an example of an occupation (play with peers) outcome of therapy.

OT practitioners may also engage clients in occupations to address performance challenges. For example, the practitioners may engage a child in play activities to improve upper extremity functioning for self-care and academics. They may engage children in games (such as "red light, green light") to address attention to verbal directions. Playing the game is an occupation. In this example, the game (i.e., occupation) is the modality to improve the child's ability to pay attention to directions.

OT practitioners create intervention which flexibly uses occupation as both the modality and outcome. Engaging a client in the occupation provides insight into adaptations, progress, and self-awareness, while working on the skills and performance aspects that need to be addressed. The therapist may decide to measure the client's progress in completing the occupation or developing performance skills. The practitioner may intersperse sessions targeting the performance components needed to successfully complete the occupation. Fisher (1998) urges practitioners to move quickly to occupation-based interventions so that clients can use multiple cues for performance. The following case illustrates the process of using occupation as a modality and as an outcome in practice.

Case Application: Occupation as a Modality and an Outcome

Vincent is a 69-year-old gentleman whose favorite occupation is cooking Sunday dinner for his children and grandchildren. He experienced a mild right cerebrovascular accident (R CVA) which led to weakness in the left upper extremity, decreased balance, and impaired problem-solving. His goal is to cook Sunday dinner at home for his family.

Therapeutic reasoning involves making context-dependent decisions to design individually tailored interventions that benefit the client (Kristensen & Petersen, 2016). Each individual constructs their occupational identity based on what is most meaningful to them (Unruh, 2004). For example, the OT practitioner collaborates with Vincent and they establish the following goals.

Home Long-Term Goal: With minimal assistance from his grandson, Vincent will cook a 5-item meal at home for 10 people

This long-term goal will be completed after discharge. The OT practitioner used pragmatic reasoning (considering the therapy kitchen, length of stay, and Vincent's current abilities) to create a hospital therapy outcome (See hospital long-term goal below).

Hospital Long-Term Goal: With minimal assistance from the OT practitioner, Vincent will cook a 3-item meal within 1 hour in the OT kitchen for 4 people

Both long-term goals address occupation (i.e., meal preparation) as the outcome of therapy. The hospital long-term goal relates to the home long-term goal, but the OT practitioner used pragmatic reasoning to adjust the goal, including space, time, and the social aspects. The practitioner added a time constraint to the hospital goal to challenge Vincent's cognitive processing skills when creating a realistic menu. The home long-term goal considers the physical (e.g., Vincent's familiar kitchen at home) and social (e.g., grandson likes to assist his grandfather in the kitchen) contexts.

The OT practitioner identified performance skills, client factors, and activity demands that may interfere with Vincent's ability to cook a large meal for his family or complete a 3-course meal in the OT kitchen for 4 people. They used cooking tasks and adjusted activities so Vincent challenged his abilities without failing or becoming frustrated. The following short-term goals will be addressed through a variety of cooking tasks. This is an example of using occupation (i.e., meal preparation) as the modality or means of intervention. Meal preparation is the activity in which Vincent will develop performance skills as indicated in the following short-term goals.

Short-Term Goal 1: Improve left upper extremity strength to hold 3 pounds during meal preparation. The OT practitioner decides to have Vincent start by making soup. This is a simple task, and he can sit down for most of it. Since he currently has weakness in his left upper extremity, the OT practitioner will assist him as needed and vary the weights of materials so he may be successful. Vincent will work on upper extremity strength throughout this activity as he lifts cans of broth, carries chicken from refrigerator to stove, retrieves 1-pound bags of rice from cupboard, and lifts pots, pans, and dishes.

Short-Term Goal 2: Improve dynamic standing balance to maintain upright position for 30 minutes during meal preparation in the OT kitchen. The OT practitioner anticipates that Vincent will have difficulty moving in a crowded kitchen at home due to issues with dynamic balance since his CVA. The activities associated with this goal provide a safe environment to address balance. Vincent will engage in a cooking activity where he must pick up multiple items placed throughout the space. The OT practitioner grades the activities to challenge his abilities while allowing him to be successful. For example, the practitioner schedules the session so Vincent is the only person in the kitchen. He must gather objects to make a salad (one at a time) and return them to the table. This challenges his dynamic balance while he visually scans the kitchen for items. He must reach, bend, twist, carry, and release objects. The OT practitioner will adjust the requirements as needed by adding or removing obstacles, changing the degree of movement required, and altering the number and type of items he must retrieve.

Short-Term Goal 3: Demonstrate improved problem-solving by listing food and items necessary for a simple 2-item lunch for 2 people. Vincent will need to plan menus and list food items for a large group when preparing for the Sunday meal at home (his long-term home goal). The OT practitioner observed that Vincent had difficulty problem-solving, and this is often present when a person has experienced a CVA. The practitioner will design activities to facilitate problem-solving by having Vincent list items needed for various recipes. The OT practitioner anticipates that Vincent may have visual difficulties, so they create large printed and laminated recipe cards for Vincent to circle all the food items. This allows the practitioner to observe his problem-solving and scanning skills. There are many tasks and skills that can be centered around this activity. For example, the practitioner may re-arrange the steps to the recipe and ask Vincent to reorder the steps to address sequencing skills.

The complexity of occupation influences therapeutic reasoning. OT practitioners examine the big picture and the small details of occupational engagement. In the above example, the therapist focuses on the macro (meal preparation activities) and the micro (performance skills needed to complete each activity). The experienced practitioner moves back and forth between macro and micro views to create intervention activities. Figure 2.2 shows this process. For example, the therapist addresses meal preparation in one session. In a subsequent session, the therapist may focus on one component of this task, such as upper extremity motor control or standing balance. The activities involved in meal preparation inform the reasoning process and allow the practitioner to also examine the performance skills, patterns, client factors, and activity demands needed to complete the activities while also considering the environment in which the occupations occur. The therapeutic reasoning process requires that the OT practitioner continually problem-solve how to address the occupation while analyzing the details that attribute to the client's engagement in those occupations. The practitioner makes decisions on when to adapt and change tasks so clients can improve their abilities to engage in things for which they find meaning. The following sections explain the therapeutic reasoning processes, terminology and types of reasoning, cognitive processing skills, and attributes to apply knowledge of occupation in practice.

THERAPEUTIC REASONING TERMINOLOGY

The term *clinical reasoning*, used in medical education generally refers to the process of thinking critically about the diagnosis and patient management (Bissessur et al., 2009) or the integration of one's own (biomedical and clinical) knowledge with initial patient information to form a case representation of the problem (Gruppen, 2017). The term *professional reasoning* describes the process of thinking through situations and creating intervention plans (Benfield & Johnston, 2020). *Critical thinking* emphasizes the thought process used during the reasoning process (Rochmawati & Wiechula, 2010). *Therapeutic reasoning* refers to the process by which therapists

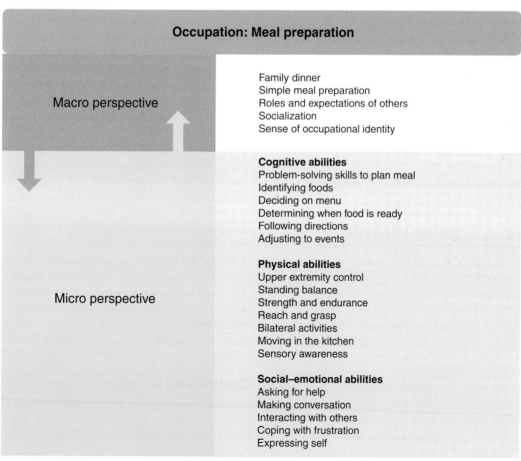

Occupation: Meal preparation

Macro perspective

Family dinner
Simple meal preparation
Roles and expectations of others
Socialization
Sense of occupational identity

Cognitive abilities
Problem-solving skills to plan meal
Identifying foods
Deciding on menu
Determining when food is ready
Following directions
Adjusting to events

Physical abilities
Upper extremity control
Standing balance
Strength and endurance
Reach and grasp
Bilateral activities
Moving in the kitchen
Sensory awareness

Micro perspective

Social–emotional abilities
Asking for help
Making conversation
Interacting with others
Coping with frustration
Expressing self

Fig. 2.2 Occupation in Practice

"collect cues, gather data, process the information, come to an understanding of a patient problem or situation, plan and implement interventions, evaluate outcomes, and reflect on and learn from the process" (Levett-Jones et al., 2010, p. 516). The authors of this textbook use this broad definition of *therapeutic reasoning* which includes the steps and types of reasoning, cognitive processes, skills, attributes, and strategies OT practitioners employ to understand a client's occupational challenges, plan and implement intervention, and measure outcomes.

Types of Reasoning

OT practitioners use a variety of types of reasoning (e.g., scientific, narrative, conditional, ethical, interactive, pragmatic) as they engage in the steps of therapeutic reasoning, which have been identified as: generate questions, gather data, identify occupational challenges, create an intervention plan, implement the plan, and assess outcomes (Kielhofner, 2008). Chapter 1 provides a description of the steps and types of reasoning. For example, OT practitioners draw upon scientific reasoning to determine the model of practice or frame of reference to generate questions and gather information about the client. They use narrative reasoning to understand the client's lived experience to identify occupational challenges. OT practitioners use conditional reasoning to synthesize information from scientific and narrative reasoning for prioritizing information and creating meaningful intervention that matches the client's personal and environmental contexts. As OT practitioners implement intervention plans, they apply interactive reasoning to choose body language, words, communication style, and support strategies that match the client's personality and style. An OT practitioner participates in ethical reasoning to plan and implement high quality services within the domain of occupational therapy, treat all clients fairly, and remain truthful in documentation. They employ scientific reasoning to measure outcomes of intervention. They rely on pragmatic reasoning to consider training, space, materials, time, and feasibility of intervention plans within the setting. During each step of the therapeutic reasoning process, OT practitioners use many types of reasoning.

THERAPEUTIC REASONING PROCESS

Therapeutic reasoning is a complex multifaceted process that involves synthesizing information gained from multiple sources and creating a conceptualization of the client's occupational performance challenges to create and implement an occupational therapy plan and reflect upon the outcomes. See Figure 2.3 for a diagram of the therapeutic reasoning process.

As OT practitioners engage in the steps of therapeutic reasoning, they examine the client's personal factors (e.g., experience, background, motives, beliefs, interests, and personality style) along with environmental factors (e.g., setting, policies, attitudes, rules, research evidence, and cultural factors). They use a variety of types of reasoning and cognitive

processing skills to synthesize information from an occupational analysis (which identifies factors influencing the client's performance). They base decisions on their knowledge, experiences, and cognitive processing attributes (such as emotional intelligence) and in consideration of the client's goals, condition, and occupational history. They judge, read cues, perceive, and prioritize information throughout the therapy process. Creating the intervention plan involves synthesizing all the information to hypothesize factors that may be interfering with the client's occupational engagement and developing a conceptualization of how intervention may promote occupational engagement. OT practitioners use therapeutic reasoning throughout the entire process as they critically analyze their decisions, reflect upon outcomes, and adjust strategies and therapy to provide best practice to support clients in reaching their goals.

Contexts

Therapeutic reasoning involves judgment, insight, and experience (Durning et al., 2011) within the specific situation or context. In occupational therapy, context is a broad construct that includes personal factors (e.g., age, sexual orientation, gender identity, person's background, life experiences, culture, lifestyle) and environmental factors (i.e., physical environment, social or physical supports, attitudes, resources, services) that influence one's occupational participation (AOTA, 2020).

Durning and colleagues (2011) found that physicians made practice decisions based on personal factors (i.e., credibility of source, emotions, appointment goals); environmental factors (i.e., resources including time, consultation with colleagues, or testing materials); and influence of the encounter setting (balancing goals of patient and practitioner, interaction; consequences of contextual factors for patient care). These themes resonate with OT practitioners as they consider personal and environmental factors as an important part of the reasoning process.

Carrier et al. (2012) also described personal and environmental factors that influence the therapeutic reasoning process. They identified personal factors of the therapist (internal factors) including knowledge and experiences (i.e., professional and personal), personal habits, preparation, and availability (i.e., emotional, cognitive physical) (Carrier et al., 2012). They also identified factors external to the therapist as including the client's characteristics (e.g., emotional, cognitive, physical), environment (e.g., social, physical, and practice contexts), task (e.g., content, objective) and the interactions between the factors. OT practitioners use knowledge, experiences, and practice setting information to identify patterns, sort information, and make decisions during each step of the therapeutic reasoning process.

Occupational Analysis

OT practitioners gather information on a client's performance patterns (acquired habits, routines, roles, and rituals), performance skills (observable goal-directed actions), and client factors (specific capabilities, characteristics, or beliefs) (AOTA,

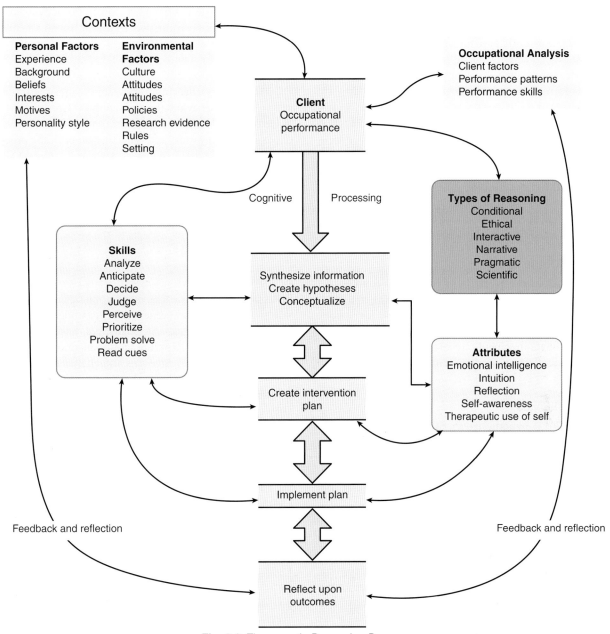

Fig. 2.3 Therapeutic Reasoning Process

2020). Performance skills include motor, process, and social interaction. Client factors include values, beliefs, and spirituality, body functions and body structures. OT practitioners evaluate and analyze the factors influencing a client's occupational engagement.

Novice therapists rely on scientific or procedural reasoning and rely on textbook findings and protocols (Durning et al., 2011). However, clients (even with the same diagnoses) have varying occupational performance needs. Expert clinicians have experience and a well-developed knowledge base to flexibly adapt and intuitively change direction to allow the occupational therapy process to progress. They use conditional,

interactive, and narrative reasoning to understand the client's experience and needs while skillfully integrating scientific reasoning (Carrier et al., 2012; Durning et al., 2011).

Cognitive Processing Skills and Attributes

Therapeutic reasoning is a *cognitive process* that requires that the OT practitioner use cognitive skills (e.g., analyze, anticipate, decide, judge, perceive, prioritize, problem-solve, and read cues) and cognitive attributes (e.g., emotional intelligence, intuition, reflection, self-awareness, therapeutic use of self) to synthesize information, create hypotheses, and conceptualize those factors interfering with a client's occupational performance.

For example, as they complete the initial evaluation and collect data, OT practitioners rely on cognitive skills to analyze the information, anticipate future performance, decide on where to investigate further, judge how the client performs, perceive aspects of occupations that may be problematic, prioritize areas of strengths and challenges, problem-solve how to intervene, and read the client's cues. They consistently examine their decisions as new evidence arises and as the situation or client's performance changes. For example, the OT practitioner may decide to add a goal of community mobility after learning the client has no transportation once leaving the hospital. Together the client and therapist problem-solve ways to address this goal. On a separate occasion, the practitioner uses skills in perception as they sense the client is becoming distant or uninterested in addressing therapy goals.

Cognitive Attributes

OT practitioners possess a variety of cognitive attributes that contribute to therapeutic reasoning, including emotional intelligence, intuition, reflection, self-awareness, and therapeutic use of self. OT practitioners can develop and enhance these attributes to facilitate therapeutic relationships through education, experience, reflection, feedback from others and self, and mentorship.

Emotional Intelligence

Chaffey et al. (2012) hypothesize that the emotions and intuition that influence therapeutic reasoning are part of emotional intelligence. Emotional intelligence is awareness and understanding of one's own emotions (Howe, 2008) and includes the propensity to allow emotions to drive cognition and action (Palmer & Stough, 2001 in Chaffey et al., 2012). Thinking on one's feet or acting "in the moment" involves gathering evidence from the activity, interaction, and occupational analysis to adjust or change course (Dougherty et al., 2016). This takes time to develop and requires a higher level of therapeutic reasoning. Work in class with simulated actors and clients, opportunities to observe experienced therapists, and low stakes opportunities for "practice" help students and practitioners gain confidence in their abilities and develop therapeutic reasoning skills (such as problem-solving, decision-making, judgment, reading cues) (Bowyer et al., 2018).

Intuition

The flexibility to think on one's feet, make quick decisions, and evaluate outcomes requires tacit knowledge and intuition (Fleming, 1994; Schell & Schell, 2008; Unsworth, 2001; Chaffey et al., 2012). Tacit knowledge can be defined as skills, ideas and experiences that people have but may not necessarily be easily expressed (Chugh, 2015). For example, tacit knowledge is shared between fieldwork educators and students through extensive personal contact, regular interaction, and trust (Chugh, 2015). It includes one's intuition, which is knowledge that is immediate and accessed without a conscious awareness of reasoning (Chaffey et al., 2010). For example, an experienced therapist gently cues a client to encourage a movement or slows down the movement before the client fatigues or stops the session to

change direction as the therapist reasons the activity is too frustrating and counterproductive. Intuition has an affective component (Chaffey et al., 2010).

Reflection

OT practitioners reflect upon and examine their own therapeutic reasoning and behaviors throughout the OT process (Mattingly & Fleming, 1994). Reflective thinking involves thinking while doing, being self-aware, and reflecting on both the process and outcomes (Schon, 1983; Mattingly, 1991). Oftentimes OT practitioners reflect in practice, requiring that they think and respond quickly. They monitor and evaluate their client's involvement in each session, adjust and modify directions or cues as needed, change activities to promote engagement and attend to both the physical and interactive aspects of the session. See Chapter 10 for more on reflection.

Self-awareness

Reflection on one's practice, during practice and after, requires self-awareness. Self-awareness refers to understanding oneself, interpersonal strengths, and challenges, and identifying one's role in relationships. Expert practitioners understand their personal and professional strengths and challenges (Taylor, 2020). They evaluate their role in the therapeutic relationship and identify strategies and techniques to support clients in practice. They can hear and assess feedback from others. Self-awareness allows OT practitioners to evaluate all aspects of the occupational therapy process to identify how therapeutic use of self may have influenced the process and outcomes. See Chapter 10 for more on self-assessment.

Therapeutic Use of Self

Therapeutic use of self requires practitioners to be self-aware and reflect on their thoughts and actions in practice to determine how to relate and interact with the client. Therapeutic use of self refers to using one's own personality, communication style, and experiences to engage clients in the therapeutic process. The Intentional Relationship Model (Taylor, 2020) identifies six communication modes, advocating, collaborating, encouraging, empathizing, problem-solving, and instructing, as essential for use of self. Therapeutic use of self involves providing and reading verbal and nonverbal cues, actively attending to the client, and adjusting one's interaction styles as needed to promote the therapeutic relationship. See Chapter 4 for more information on therapeutic use of self.

LEARNING ACTIVITY: COGNITIVE PROCESSING SKILLS AND ATTRIBUTES

Complete Worksheet 2.7. Define each cognitive processing skill and attribute listed and provide a personal example of how it is used in practice (or in your life).
- What is the advantage of providing a personal example?
- How does defining terms help you understand the cognitive process used in therapeutic reasoning?

Application of Therapeutic Reasoning Process

The following case provides an example of the ways in which chronic pain can impede occupational performance and life satisfaction in an adolescent and illustrates the therapeutic reasoning process. For a full case report, see the Evolve site.

Marlee is a 16-year-old girl who is receiving occupational therapy in an outpatient hospital setting. She presents with diagnoses of chronic pain and postural orthostatic tachycardia syndrome (POTS). Chronic pain, such as the chronic headaches experienced by Marlee, seriously affect engagement in activities of daily living (ADL) and can negatively affect emotions (Nieuwenhuizen et al., 2014). Marlee reports that she spends most of her day resting and texting friends. Before her injury, she engaged in the occupations of cheerleading, socializing, and volunteering at a pet shelter. Although she had previous diagnoses of anxiety and eating disorder, she was independent in all ADLs and IADLs, such as simple meal preparation.

The OT practitioner administered the Canadian Occupational Therapy Performance Measure (COPM) (Polatajko et al., 2002) to identify Marlee's self-reported challenges in occupational engagement. The COPM is useful for engaging verbal clients in identifying their perceived difficulties. The COPM allows Marlee, who presents with chronic pain, to focus on improvement of performance and participation, rather than bodily processes. Clients identify areas of concerns and rate their performance and satisfaction on a scale of 1 (low) to 10 (high). The specific occupations and category of concerns for Marlee are outlined in Table 2.2, with ratings listed in Table 2.3.

Conceptualization

The OT practitioner analyzed the findings from the interview, where Marlee described herself as an active and social teen until recently. The practitioner perceived Marlee was angry that she could not attend school, even though Marlee said it did not matter to her. The practitioner used information gained from the narrative, and scientific knowledge of adolescents' roles, and the diagnostic information to create hypotheses regarding Marlee's current occupational

TABLE 2.3   Canadian Occupational Performance Measure: Marlee's Occupational Performance Ratings

Occupational Performance	Performance Scores	Satisfaction Scores
Showering in under 60 minutes with no breaks	1	7
Going to the mall to try on clothes	1	1
Keeping room clean	1	4
Cleaning bathroom and doing chores	1	4
Going to school for a full day	1	1
Babysitting/finding camp counselor job	5	5
Total/Problems	10/6	22/6
Score	1.6	3.6

performance. The practitioner hypothesized that Marlee's chronic pain, anxiety and POTS limited her engagement in preferred occupations. Furthermore, the OT practitioner hypothesized that Marlee's environmental factors (i.e., community resources, school friends, leisure activities, family support) along with her personal factors (i.e., teen, history of being social, interests in being active, success in academics) support occupational engagement.

The OT practitioner completed an analysis of client factors (e.g., physical, social, and cognitive), performance skills and patterns and hypothesized that the changes in her physical capabilities due to the POTS interfere with both her social engagement (as she can not attend school and socialize with friends) and Marlee's physical activities (since she is unable to participate in physical activities currently) and that this disruption results in a loss of occupational identity. Since Marlee is not able to attend school, something that she is successful at, she is losing confidence in her abilities and is showing decreased self-efficacy (i.e., belief in her skills and abilities), which may also be contributing to her anxiety.

The OT practitioner prioritized goals for Marlee to complete her personal care, increase her ability to attend school, and socialize with friends. The OT practitioner collaborated with Marlee and together they developed strategies to increase her activity levels, provide her frequent breaks, and allow her to gain strategies to support academic success. The OT practitioner worked closely with Marlee and was aware of therapeutic modes. For example, she empathized by listening to Marlee discuss missing out on events (such as cheerleading, sports activities, and school). She encouraged Marlee when they tried to take a longer walk one day. And she advocated with the school occupational therapist that Marlee return to school one morning a week with supports at school.

Table 2.4 outlines the therapeutic reasoning process utilized by the OT practitioner in Marlee's intervention plan.

Marlee's case illustrates the role that daily occupations play in the health and well-being of a teen with physical and psychosocial challenges. Marlee is not engaging in self-care, social participation with friends, and academics due to POTS and post-concussion. Marlee has decreased physical endurance. The following long-term goals were created:

1. Marlee will complete her morning dressing routine in 30 minutes with no more than 1 rest break.
2. Marlee will plan and participate in 1–2 leisure activities each weekend.

TABLE 2.2   Canadian Occupational Performance Measure: Marlee's Findings

Occupation	Category	Client Concerns
Self-care	Personal Care	Showers Dressing upper and lower body
	Functional Mobility	Dizzy spells and falls
	Community Mobility	Endurance for going to the mall Cheerleading competitions
Productivity	Paid/Unpaid Work	Volunteering at pet shelter Babysitting
Household Management		Cleaning room Cleaning bathroom Making a meal/snack Emptying dishwasher
Play/School		Going to school all day
Leisure	Quiet Recreation	(No problems reported)
	Active Recreation	Going to football and basketball games Hanging out with friends at school Cheerleading practice
	Socialization	Going over to a friend's house

Continued

CASE STUDY—cont'd

TABLE 2.4   Therapeutic Reasoning Process: Marlee

Type of reasoning	Relationship to occupation	OT Intervention
Scientific	POTS resulted in frequent episodes of light headedness, falling, and low back pain. She fell down the stairs. Recent fall and POTS limits her ability to engage in occupations of cheerleading, socializing, and volunteering at a pet shelter, and attend school. She is not attending to her ADL consistently.	Complete ADL training in a variety of settings and grade the activities. 1. To decrease task demands, she can complete the ADL of painting nails while sitting. 2. To increase task demands, she can complete the ADL of bathing and dressing at the locker room at her swimming session.
Narrative Reasoning	Understand fears and hopes about recovery. She is fearful of falling (and embarrassing herself again) and she has low back pain interfering with her ability to engage in physical activity.	1. Incrementally adding more activity to her day. 2. Understand that her love of animals may increase her motivation to participate in functional mobility if done while walking a dog.
Pragmatic Reasoning	Client is being treated in outpatient rehabilitation setting. She receives OT 3 times weekly for 1 hour. She lives close to the mall and enjoys going to school. How could other disciplines, such as PT and social work, augment the OT intervention and improve goal achievement?	1. Referral to psychologist to assist with severe anxiety. 2. Referral to a nutritionist due to decreased engagement in meal preparation and feeding and eating. 3. Recommendation of referral for a formal educational evaluation to better understand the effects of her concussion on her educational performance and anxiety around completing schoolwork.
Conditional Reasoning	The therapist examines the physical, social, and cognitive requirements of chosen occupations within the context of the home as contrasted by the outside environment. Occupations outside the home provoked greater anxiety than those inside the home.	1. Complete an OT session after her aquatic PT session, to reinforce strategies discussed in PT, and provide opportunity to complete occupations outside the home in a supportive way. 2. Utilize a visually pleasing schedule to give the client a graphic picture of how her occupational deprivation impacts her quality of life and encourage her to add more occupation to her life.
Interactive Reasoning	Marlee was initially quiet but easily warmed up to the therapist and showed a sense of humor. She is verbal and attentive to others. Marlee is very critical of herself and has high expectations. She is easily frustrated.	Use empathizing and collaborating modes to engage Marlee in sessions. She may need advocating mode to receive services at school.
Ethical Reasoning	Provide high-quality services to Marlee by setting goals with her, following through with plan, and reflecting upon progress. Maintain confidentiality by not discussing case with her friends (who visit often).	Consult with team members who have expertise in eating disorders and anxiety if needed.

3. Marlee will participate in 2–3 household chores per week with distant supervision.
4. Marlee will demonstrate independence in moderate level healthy meal preparation including clean up 1×/week.
5. Marlee will participate in community outing to shop for and try on clothing 1–2 times with therapist supervision.
6. Marlee will return to school × 1 day a week.

Throughout the intervention period, the OT practitioner reflected on the session activities and Marlee's participation. The practitioner adjusted activities and incorporated Marlee's feedback into sessions. The OT practitioner frequently used encouraging mode which Marlee did not appreciate as she interpreted this as disingenuous. The OT practitioner worked to avoid using encouraging words, but rather smiled and asked Marlee what she thought of the activity or performance. This collaborating mode worked better with Marlee and promoted her belief in her skills and abilities.

At discharge, Marlee reported that she was now spending most of her time in work and recreation activities, taking shorter rest breaks, and playing with the other teens in the neighborhood. Her schoolwork improved as well, as she was getting caught up on her assignments and had started using the asynchronous learning tools provided by her school. She was starting to visualize continued improvement by planning to attend school in person two full days a week, when previously she was attending school virtually. She expressed the desire to gradually increase her in-person school days to 5 days a week.

LEARNING ACTIVITY: APPLICATION OF COGNITIVE PROCESSING

Complete Worksheet 2.8 to identify examples of cognitive processing (i.e., types of reasoning, cognitive processing skills, cognitive processing attributes) that were used in Marlee's case.
• What type of reasoning might you use and why?

• What cognitive processing skills might you incorporate into the occupational therapy intervention?
• What skills and attributes would you expand upon to provide intervention?

SUMMARY

The ability to engage in meaningful occupation is linked to health and wellness. OT practitioners work with clients of all ages and abilities to promote occupational adaptation so that clients can engage in occupations that are meaningful to them and provide them a sense of identity. Each person engages in their own patterns and types of occupations. OT practitioners utilize meaningful occupations both as the method of intervention (modality) and as the desired outcome of therapy. When engaging in therapeutic reasoning, OT practitioners examine personal and environmental factors along with client factors, performance skills and patterns. They use cognitive processing skills (e.g., analyze, anticipate, decide, judge, perceive, prioritize, problem-solve, read cues) and attributes (e.g., emotional intelligence, intuition, reflection, self-awareness, therapeutic use of self) during each step of the process. Practitioners use a variety of types of reasoning throughout the OT process.

REFERENCES

Aldrich, R. (2008). From complexity theory to transactionalism: Moving occupational science forward in theorizing the complexity of behavior. *Journal of Occupational Science, 15*(3), 147–156.

American Occupational Therapy Association. (2020). *Occupational therapy practice framework: Domain and process* (4th ed.). North Bethesda, MD: AOTA.

Benfield, A. M., & Johnston, M. V. (2020). Initial development of a measure of evidence-informed professional thinking. *Australian Occupational Therapy Journal, 67*, 309–319.

Bird, M., & Strachan, P. H. (2020). Complexity science education for clinical nurse researchers. *Journal of Professional Nursing, 36*(2), 50–55.

Bissessur, S. W., Geijteman, E. C. T., Al-Dulaimy, M., Teunlssen, P. W., Richir, M., Arnold, A. E. R., & de Vries, T. P. G. M. (2009). Therapeutic reasoning: from hiatus to hypothetical model. *Journal of Evaluation in Clinical Practice, 15*(6), 985–989.

Bowyer, P., Munoz, L., Morriss, M., Moore, C. C., & Tiongco, C. G. (2018). Long term impact of model of human occupation training on therapeutic reasoning. *Journal of Allied Health, 48*(3), 188–193.

Carrier, A., Levasseur, M., Bedard, D., & Desrosiers, J. (2012). Clinical reasoning process underlying choice of teaching strategies: A framework to improve occupational therapists' transfer skill interventions. *Australian Occupational Therapy Journal, 59*, 355–366.

Chaffey, L., Unsworth, C. A., & Fossey, E. (2010). A grounded theory of intuition among occupational therapist in mental health practice. *British Journal of Occupational Therapy, 73*, 300–308.

Chaffey, L., Unsworth, C. A., & Fossey, E. (2012). Relationship between intuition and emotional intelligence in occupational therapists in mental health practice. *American Journal of Occupational Therapy, 66*, 88–96.

Creek, J., & Hughes, A. (2008). Occupation and health: A review of selected literature. *British Journal of Occupational Therapy, 71*(11), 456–468.

Chugh, R. (2015). Do Australian universities encourage tacit knowledge transfer? *Proceedings of the 7th International Joint Conference on Knowledge Discovery, 3*, 128–135. doi:10.5220/0005585901280135.

Dougherty, D. A., Toth-Cohen, S. E., & Tomlin, G. S. (2016). Beyond research literature: Occupational therapists' perspectives on and uses of "evidence" in everyday practice. *Canadian Journal of Occupational Therapy, 83*(5), 288–296.

Durning, S., Artino, A. R., Pangaro, L., van der Vleuten, S. P. M., & Schuwirth, L. (2011). Context and clinical reasoning: Understanding the perspective of the expert's voice. *Medical Education, 45*, 927–938.

Fleming, M. H. (1994). The search for tacit knowledge. In C. Mattingly & M. H. Fleming (Eds.), *Clinical reasoning: Forms of inquiry in a therapeutic practice* (pp. 21–45). Philadelphia, PA: FA Davis.

Fisher, A. G. (1998). Uniting practice and theory in an occupational framework. *American Journal of Occupational Therapy, 52*(7), 509–521.

Gillen, G. (2013). 2013 Eleanor Clarke Slagle lecture: A fork in the road: An occupational hazard? *American Journal of Occupational Therapy, 6*(67), 643–652.

Gruppen, L. (2017). Clinical reasoning: Defining it, teaching it, assessing it, studying it [editorial]. *Western Journal of Emergency Medicine, 18*(1), 4–7.

Howe, D. (2008). *The emotionally intelligent social worker.* London: Palgrave Press.

Kielhofner, G. (2008). *A Model of Human Occupation: Theory and Application* (4th ed.). Philadelphia, PA: Lippincott, Williams & Wilkins.

Kristensen, H. K., & Petersen, K. S. (2016). Occupational science: An important contributor to occupational therapists' clinical reasoning. *Scandinavian Journal of Occupational Therapy, 23*(3), 240–243.

Lazzarini, I. (2004). Neuro-occupation: the nonlinear dynamics of intention, meaning, and perception. *British Journal of Occupational Therapy, 67*(8), 342–352.

Levett-Jones, T., Hoffman, K., Dempsey, J., Jeong, S. Y. -S., Nobel, D., Norton, C. A., et al. (2010). The 'five rights of clinical reasoning: An educational model to enhance nursing students' ability to identify and manage clinically 'at risk' patients. *Nurse Education Today, 30*, 515–520.

Mattingly, C. (1991). The narrative nature of clinical reasoning. *American Journal of Occupational Therapy, 45*(11), 998–1005.

Mattingly, C., & Fleming, M. H. (Eds.). (1994). *Clinical reasoning: Forms of inquiry in a therapeutic practice.* Philadelphia, PA: FA Davis.

Mee, J., Sumsion, T., & Craik, C. (2004). Mental health clients confirm the value of occupation in building competence and self-identity. *British Journal of Occupational Therapy, 67*(5), 225–233.

Nieuwenhuizen, M. G., deGroot, S., Janssen, T. W., van der Maas, L. C., & Beckerman, H. (2014). Canadian occupational performance measure performance scale: Validity and responsiveness in chronic pain. *Journal of Rehabilitation Research and Development, 51*(5), 727–746.

O'Brien, J., & Solomon, J. (2022). Clinical application: Exercises and worksheets. In J. O'Brien & J. Solomon (Eds.), *Occupational analysis and group process* (2nd ed., pp. 307–312; 341–343). Elsevier.

Palmer, B., & Stough, C. (2001). *SUEIT: Swinburne University Emotional Intelligence Test: Interim technical manual.* Melbourne, Victoria, Australia: Swinburne University Organizational Psychology Research Unit.

Persson, D., Erlandsen, L. K., Eklund, M., & Iwareson, S. (2001). Value dimensions, meaning, and complexity in human occupation-A tentative structure for analysis. *Scandinavian Journal of Occupational Therapy, 8*, 7–18.

Polatajko, H. J., Townsend, E. A., & Craik, J. (2002). Canadian Model of Occupational Performance and Engagement. In E. A. Townsend & H. J. Polatajko (Eds.). *Enabling occupation II: Advicing an occupational therapy vision for health, well-being, and justice through occupation.* CAOT ACE.

Ramshaw, B. (2020). Ag systems and complexity science to real patient care. *Journal of Evaluation in Clinical Practice, 26*(5), 1559–1563.

Rochmawati, E., & Wiechula, R. (2010). Education strategies to foster health professional students' clinical reasoning skills. *Nursing and Health Sciences, 12*, 244–250.

Rajarajeswaran, P., & Vishnupriya, R. (2009). Exercise in cancer. *Indian journal of medical and paediatric oncology: official journal of Indian Society of Medical & Paediatric Oncology, 30*(2), 61–70.

Schell, J. W., & Schell, B. A. B. (2008). Teaching for expert practice. In B. A. B. Schell & J. W. Schell (Eds.), *Clinical and professional reasoning in occupational therapy* (pp. 258–288). Philadelphia, PA: Lippincott Williams & Wilkins.

Schon, D. A. (1983). *The reflective practitioner: How professionals think in action.* New York: Basic Books, Inc.

Sorman, D. E., Hansson, P., Pritshke, I., & Ljungberg, J. K. (2019). Complexity of primary lifetime occupation and cognitive processing. *Frontiers in Psychology, 10*, 1–12.

Stav, W. B., Hallenen, T., Lane, J., & Arbesman, M. (2012). Systematic review of occupational engagement and health outcomes among community dwelling older adults. *The American Journal of Occupational Therapy, 66*(3), 301–310.

Taylor, R. (2020). *The intentional relationship model* (2nd ed.). Philadelphia, PA: FA Davis.

Unruh, A. M. (2004). Reflections on: 'so…what do you do?' Occupation and the construction of identity. *Canadian Journal of Occupational Therapy, 71*, 290–295.

Unsworth, C. A. (2001). The clinical reasoning of novice and expert occupational therapist. *Scandinavian Journal of Occupational Therapy, 6*, 198–207.

Unsworth, C., & Baker, A. (2016). A systematic review of professional reasoning literature in occupational therapy. *British Journal of Occupational Therapy, 79*(1), 5–16.

Weinstock-Zlotnick, G., & Mehta, S. (2018). A systematic review of the benefits of occupation-based intervention for patients with upper extremity musculoskeletal disorders. *Journal of Hand Therapy, 32*, 141–152.

Worksheets

WORKSHEET 2.1: UNDERSTANDING OCCUPATIONAL CHOICES

List occupations that you do to feel healthy. Then list occupations that you do which may impede your health.
1) How can you increase the health-promoting occupations and decrease the health-inhibiting occupations?
2) How do you feel when your ability to engage in meaningful healthy occupations is prevented?

Understanding Occupational Choices
Name:
List occupations that you do to feel healthy.
• Describe how often you engage in those occupations.
• Describe how you feel when engaging in these occupations.
• Identify the benefits and challenges of these occupations.
List some occupations you engage in that may impede your health.
• Describe how often you engage in these occupations.
• Describe how you feel when engaging in these occupations.
• Identify the benefits and challenges of these occupations.
Describe how you might increase the health promoting occupations and decrease the health inhibiting occupations.
Describe how you feel when you are not able to engage in meaningful healthy occupations.

WORKSHEET 2.2: VALUE OF OCCUPATION

Summarize the findings from a research article that examines the benefits of participation in one's desired activities (i.e., occupations).

Value of Occupation
Name:
Reference:
Overview:
Findings:
Describe the benefits of participating in this occupation.
Describe clients who may benefit from engaging in this occupation.
Discuss how an OT practitioner could incorporate this occupation into practice.
Describe the importance of this occupation to you.
Describe clients who may find this occupation important.

WORKSHEET 2.3: ANALYZING OCCUPATIONS

Complete a comprehensive occupational analysis of an occupation of your choice (complete as if you are completing the activity).
- How would this analysis inform an intervention activity for a 6-year-old girl who is unable to use her right upper extremity (R UE) and experiences mild cognitive impairment?

Comprehensive Activity Analysis (O'Brien & Solomon, 2022)		
	Explanation	**Description of how item is used for specific activity**
Occupation/Activity or Task	Describe the selected occupation, activity, or task.	
Client's Goal	Client's priorities, interests, and desires to be addressed in therapy.	
Rationale for Selection	Describe who the client is (person, group, or population) and how the occupation, activity, or task addresses the client's goal.	
Relevance and Importance	Describe the meaning (consider culture, symbolic, subjective)	
Successful Outcome	How will you know it was successful?	
Sequence of Steps	List sequence of steps to complete. Describe any timing requirements.	
Preparation	Describe how the client and/or therapist need to prepare.	
Equipment	Identify large objects that remain in setting and are needed for activity, such as table and chairs.	
Technology	List low or high technology needs.	
Materials/Supplies and their Properties	Identify materials and supplies needed and properties (i.e., texture, consistency, size, purpose, shape, color, sensory).	
Space	Describe setting in which activity occurs (e.g., outdoors, large space for physical activity).	
Social	Describe the social and altitudinal requirements.	
Costs	Fees or additional costs.	
Precautions	Include safety, medication effects, supervision needs, dietary requirements, motor, or emotional triggers.	
Performance Skills (observable goal-directed actions that allow client to perform)		
• **Motor**	Describe actions related to moving and interacting with objects (e.g., grips objects; reaches for items)	
• **Process**	Describe actions related to making decisions to select and interact and use objects, carry out steps and problem-solve to engage in and complete activity (e.g., selects correct object for task; seeks help when needed).	
• **Social interaction**	Describes actions related to communicating and interacting with others (e.g., makes eye contact; acknowledges others).	

Comprehensive Activity Analysis (O'Brien & Solomon, 2022)—cont'd		
	Explanation	**Description of how item is used for specific activity**
Client Factors (Describe key factors that influence performance).		
Body Function: values, beliefs, spirituality	One's perceptions, motivations, and related meaning that influence occupational performance.	
Body Function: Mental Functions		
• **Specific mental functions**	Includes higher-level cognitive, attention, memory, perception, thought, sequencing, emotional and self-awareness.	
• **Global mental functions**	Includes awareness, orientation, psychosocial, temperament and personality, energy, and sleep.	
• **Sensory functions**	Includes visual, hearing, vestibular, taste, smell, touch, proprioception, pain, interoception, temperature and pressure.	
Body Function: Neuromusculoskeletal and Movement-Related Functions (Describe movement required for performance).		
• **Functions of joints and bones**	Describe ROM, integrity of joints for performance.	
• **Muscle functions**	Includes muscle power, and endurance for performance.	
• **Movement functions**	Describe voluntary movement and gait requirements for performance.	
Body Function: cardiovascular, hematological, immunological, respiratory system functions	Describe how systems may influence performance (e.g., is the intensity level appropriate for client with cardiovascular impairment?).	
Body Function: voice and speech functions	Describe requirements of voice and speech functions.	
Body Function: skin and related structures	Describe skin and related structures in relationship to occupation, activity, or task.	
Body Structures	Anatomical parts of the body that support body function. Describe what is required when completing occupation, activity or task.	
Transfer of Learning	How will this activity transfer to daily living.	

Reference: American Occupational Therapy Association. (2020). Occupational therapy practice framework: Domain and process (4th ed.). *American Journal of Occupational Therapy, 71*(Suppl.2), S1–S96.
From: O'Brien, J., & Solomon, J. (2022). Clinical application: Exercises and worksheets. In J. OBrien and J. Solomon (Eds.). *Occupational analysis and group process* (2nd ed.; pp. 341–343). Elsevier.

WORKSHEET 2.4: OCCUPATIONAL ANALYSIS BASED ON SELECTED FRAME OF REFERENCE

Analyze the aspects of an occupation as related to a selected frame of reference of your choice. Discuss how the frame of reference informed the occupational analysis.

Occupational Analysis based on selected Frame of Reference (O'Brien & Solomon, 2022)		
	Explanation	**Description of how item is used for specific occupation using the selected Frame of Reference**
Frame of Reference	Provide a brief description of frame of reference.	
Occupation/Activity or Task	Describe the selected occupation, activity, or task.	
Client's Goal	Client's priorities, interests, and desires to be addressed in therapy.	
Rationale for Selection	Describe who the client is (person, group, or population) and how the occupation, activity, or task address the client's goal.	
Relevance and Importance	Describe the meaning (consider culture, symbolic, subjective)	
Sequence of Steps	List sequence of steps to complete. Describe any timing requirements.	
Preparation	Describe how the client and/or therapist need to prepare.	
Equipment	Identify large objects that remain in setting and are needed for activity, such as table and chairs.	
Technology	List low or high technology needs.	
Materials/Supplies and their Properties	Identify materials and supplies needed and properties (i.e., texture, consistency, size, purpose, shape, color, sensory).	
Space	Describe setting in which activity occurs (e.g., outdoors, large space for physical activity).	
Social	Describe the social and altitudinal requirements.	
Costs	Fees or additional costs.	
Precautions	Include safety, medication effects, supervision needs, dietary requirements, motor, or emotional triggers.	
Performance Skills (observable goal-directed actions that allow client to perform)		
• **Motor**	Describe actions related to moving and interacting with objects (e.g., grips objects; reaches for items)	
• **Process**	Describe actions related to making decisions to select and interact and use objects, carry out steps and problem-solve to engage in and complete activity (e.g., selects correct object for task; seeks help when needed).	
• **Social interaction**	Describes actions related to communicating and interacting with others (e.g., makes eye contact; acknowledges others).	

Occupational Analysis based on selected Frame of Reference (O'Brien & Solomon, 2022)—cont'd		
	Explanation	Description of how item is used for specific occupation using the selected Frame of Reference
Client Factors (Describe key factors that influence performance).		
Body Function: values, beliefs, spirituality	One's perceptions, motivations, and related meaning that influence occupational performance.	
Body Function: Mental Functions		
• Specific mental functions	Includes higher-level cognitive, attention, memory, perception, thought, sequencing, emotional and self-awareness.	
• Global mental functions	Includes awareness, orientation, psychosocial, temperament and personality, energy, and sleep.	
• Sensory functions	Includes visual, hearing, vestibular, taste, smell, touch, proprioception, pain, interoception, temperature and pressure.	
Body Function: Neuromusculoskeletal and Movement-Related Functions (Describe movement required for performance).		
• Functions of joints and bones	Describe ROM, integrity of joints for performance.	
• Muscle functions	Includes muscle power, and endurance for performance.	
• Movement functions	Describe voluntary movement and gait requirements for performance.	
Body Function: cardiovascular, hematological, immunological, respiratory system functions	Describe how systems may influence performance (e.g., is the intensity level appropriate for client with cardiovascular impairment?).	
Body Function: voice and speech functions	Describe requirements of voice and speech functions.	
Body Function: skin and related structures	Describe skin and related structures in relationship to occupation, activity, or task.	
Body Structures	Anatomical parts of the body that support body function. Describe what is required when completing occupation, activity or task.	

Reference: American Therapy Association. (2020). Occupational therapy practice framework: Domain and process (4th ed.). *American Journal of Occupational Therapy, 71*(Suppl.2), S1–S96.
From: O'Brien, J., & Solomon, J. (2022). Clinical application: Exercises and worksheets. In J. OBrien and J. Solomon (Eds.). *Occupational analysis and group process* (2nd ed.; pp. 215–217). Elsevier.

WORKSHEET 2.5: CONTEXTUAL ANALYSIS

Analyze the contextual aspects of an occupation of your choice (complete as if you are completing the activity in a familiar setting).
- Describe how changing the context(s) of the activity, changes the performance demands.
  Refer to the *Occupational Therapy Practice Framework* (4th ed.) (AOTA, 2020) for further definition of environmental and personal factors.

Contextual Analysis (O'Brien & Solomon, 2022)	
Activity Description:	
Goal:	
Meaning Describe the meaning and importance of activity	
Sequence of Steps List sequence of steps to complete.	
Materials/Supplies and their Properties Identify materials and their properties (i.e., texture; consistency; size; purpose; shape; color; and sensory properties)	
Space Describe setting in which activity occurs (e.g., outdoors, large space for physical activity).	
Social Describe social and attitudinal requirements.	
Performance Skills	
Motor Skills Describe actions related to moving and manipulating objects.	
Process Skills Describe actions related to selecting, interacting, and using objects (e.g., problem solving).	
Social Interaction Skills Describes actions related to communicating and interacting with others (e.g., makes eye contact; acknowledges others).	
Contexts: Environmental Factors (Describe how the environment influences performance in this activity)	
Physical (e.g., setting, surroundings)	
Technology	
Social (e.g., supports, attitudes)	
Institution (e.g., services, systems, policies)	

Contextual Analysis (O'Brien & Solomon, 2022) — cont'd	
Contexts: Personal Factors (Describe how client's experiences influence performance)	
Background Consider age, experiences, education, gender identity and history.	
Culture Describe family culture, identification.	
Social Describe past and current lifestyle choices and interactions.	
Habits and Routines Describe past and present habits and routines.	
Professional Identity Describe how client views professional roles and expectations.	
Strengths and Challenges Describe psychological strengths and challenges.	
Other Describe other health conditions and fitness as they influence performance.	
Summarize contextual supports and hindrances.	
How could you change the contextual aspects of the activity?	

Reference: American Occupational Therapy Association. (2020). Occupational therapy practice framework: Domain and process (4th ed.). *American Journal of Occupational Therapy, 71*(Suppl.2), S1–S96.
From: O'Brien, J., & Solomon, J. (2022). Clinical application: Exercises and worksheets. In J. OBrien and J. Solomon (Eds.). *Occupational analysis and group process* (2nd ed.; pp. 311–312). Elsevier

WORKSHEET 2.6: GOALS ADDRESSING OCCUPATION AS A MODALITY AND OUTCOME

Create goals that address occupation as the modality to improve occupational performance and goals that identify occupation as the desired outcome.
- Provide examples of activities for each goal.
- Identify how the activities could be modified or adapted to meet the individual client's needs.

Goals addressing occupation as a modality and outcome		
	Occupation as Modality	**Occupation as Outcome**
Goal		
Sample activities		
Modification to activities		

WORKSHEET 2.7: COGNITIVE PROCESSING SKILLS AND ATTRIBUTES

Define each cognitive processing skill and attribute listed and provide a personal example of how it is used in practice (or in your life).
- What is the advantage of providing a personal example?
- How does defining terms help you understand the cognitive process used in therapeutic reasoning?

Cognitive Processing Skills and Attributes		
Cognitive skill or attribute	Definition	Personal Example
Analyze		
Anticipate		
Decide		
Judge		
Perceive		
Prioritize		
Problem-solve		
Read cues		
Synthesize information		
Create hypotheses		
Conceptualize		
Emotional intelligence		
Intuition		
Reflection		
Self-awareness		
Therapeutic use of self		

WORKSHEET 2.8: APPLICATION OF COGNITIVE PROCESSING

Identify examples of the cognitive processing (i.e., types of reasoning, cognitive processing skills, cognitive processing attributes) that were used in Marlee's case.

- What type of reasoning might you use and why?
- What cognitive processing skills might you incorporate into the occupational therapy intervention?
- What skills and attributes would you expand upon to provide intervention?

Application of Cognitive Processing	
Cognitive term	**Example from Case Description**
Analyze	
Anticipate	
Decide	
Judge	
Perceive	
Prioritize	
Problem-solve	
Read cues	
Synthesize information	
Create hypotheses	
Conceptualize	
Emotional intelligence	
Intuition	
Reflection	
Self-awareness	
Therapeutic use of self	

Application of Cognitive Processing—cont'd	
Types of Therapeutic Reasoning	
Scientific	
Narrative	
Conditional	
Ethical	
Interactive	
Pragmatic	
What other cognitive processes might you incorporate into the occupational therapy intervention?	
What skills and attributes would you expand upon to provide intervention?	

Models of Practice and Frames of Reference: Essential Concepts for Therapeutic Reasoning

Jane O'Brien

GUIDING QUESTIONS

1. How do OT practitioners use occupation-based models of practice and frames of reference to inform therapeutic reasoning?
2. What is meant by eclecticism?
3. How are organizing and complementary models of practice used to inform therapeutic reasoning?
4. How do OT practitioners use knowledge of conceptual practice models to guide assessment and intervention planning?

KEY TERMS

Biomechanical frame of reference
Complementary models
Conceptual practice models
Eclecticism
Frames of reference
Lived experience
Model of Human Occupation

Occupational adaptation
Occupation-based models of practice
Occupational competence
Occupational identity
Organizing models
Principles

INTRODUCTION

"How does using a model of practice or frame of reference help my practice? How can they help me more effectively reason for my clients and families?"

Students and OT practitioners seek answers to intervention questions. Models of practice and frames of reference are based upon theory and research evidence and explain concepts that inform practice decisions. For example, models of practice explain human occupation and how to structure and organize one's thinking to understand the client and family. Frames of references provide evidence to explain the role of the practitioner, intervention strategies, and expectations for change. Models of practice and frames of reference guide occupational therapy practice by providing information based on theory and research to use when making practice decisions.

Occupational therapy practitioners see a range of people experiencing physical, emotional, and cognitive difficulties interfering with their ability to participate in daily activities. The goal of occupational therapy is to enable people to return to those things that they find meaningful within the context of their environment. This is a complex task which requires synthesizing information from many sources to assess, establish goals and objectives, create and implement effective intervention plans, and evaluate the progress and outcomes of therapy.

Kielhofner (2004) used the term conceptual practice models to describe diverse concepts organized into unique

occupational therapy theory that provide rationale and guide practice. Using this broad definition, for example, rehabilitation, medical model, Model of Human Occupation, Canadian Model of Occupational Performance and Engagement, biomechanical, and sensory integration are all considered conceptual models of practice.

To further describe practice models, some authors (Gillen, 2014; O'Brien, 2018) differentiate between general conceptual practice models (such as Model of Human Occupation, Canadian Model of Occupational Performance and Engagement, Person-Environment-Occupation-Participation, Rehabilitation) that are used to structure one's perspectives of the client and frames of references or approaches, that are used to explain principles, theory, and strategies for intervention.

The authors of this textbook use the terms models of practice to describe general conceptual practice models. They further define the models created to explain human occupation by using the term occupation-based models of practice.

Occupation-based models of practice provide structure to organize one's thinking regarding the myriad of factors influencing a client's ability to engage in desired activities and in so doing, inform therapeutic reasoning. Occupation-based models of practice focus on explaining concepts related to occupations and remain true to occupational therapy philosophy (Wong & Fisher, 2015). Frames of reference provide research evidence to explain function and dysfunction, assessment, the role of the therapist, strategies and techniques for intervention, and underlying components (Wong & Fisher, 2015). Frames of reference provide information to facilitate therapeutic reasoning to create an action plan. Figure 3.1 shows a schematic of the relationship between occupation-based models of practice and frames of reference. Often practitioners use multiple models or frames of reference together, referred to as *multimodal* or eclectic reasoning (Ikiugu et al., 2009; Turpin & Iwama, 2011).

After defining and describing occupation-based models of practice and frames of reference, the author outlines how they guide therapeutic reasoning. The author describes the importance of using principles derived from the models and frames of reference to explain concepts in practice, identify intervention strategies, describe the role of the OT practitioner, define change, and inform evaluation and intervention processes. A variety of case examples and learning activities are provided throughout the chapter to reinforce concepts.

OCCUPATION-BASED MODELS OF PRACTICE

Models of practice provide an organized structure to explain complex concepts and theories. Some models, such as the medical model, rehabilitative model, or cognitive behavioral model, may inform occupational therapy practice, but they do not focus on occupation and may leave OT practitioners wondering how occupational therapy distinctly contributes to the team. For example, the medical model suggests a problem-solving approach that includes identifying the problem by examining signs, symptoms, and body systems and creating a plan to address areas of concern. While the medical model promotes a plan of care that involves following protocols, it may not adequately define the role of an OT practitioner.

Occupation-based models of practice integrate research and information from occupational therapy philosophy, values, and process to describe the complexity of occupational performance (Wong & Fisher, 2015). Since OT professionals value occupation as both the central outcome of intervention and the means to reach the desired outcome, occupation-based models of practice provide a depth and breadth of information to clearly define the role of occupational therapy and strengthen the assessment and intervention process. Table 3.1 provides a brief description of the concepts and guiding principles of occupation-based models of practice. Readers are advised to seek out more detailed information about each model by reviewing the original sources.

As OT students and practitioners engage in therapeutic reasoning, they use knowledge of the profession, theory, and research to make sense of human occupation. An occupation-based model of practice defines concepts and organizes complex information from multiple sources to explain occupational performance. Occupation-based models of practice emphasize understanding the interactions between the person, occupation,

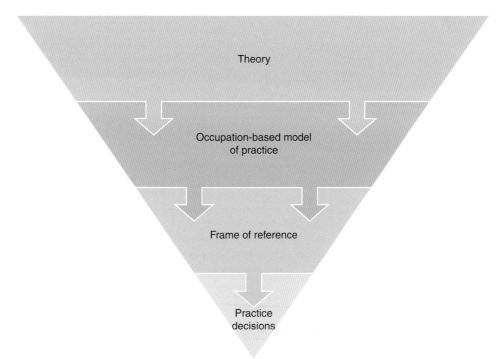

Fig. 3.1 Relationship between Models of Practice and Frames of Reference

TABLE 3.1   Occupation-Based Models of Practice

Model	Authors	Components	Guiding principles
Model of Human Occupation (MOHO) (Kielhofner, 2008; Taylor, 2017)	Dr. Gary Kielhofner	Volition Habituation Performance Capacity Environment	• Occupational actions, thoughts and emotions always arise out of the dynamic interaction of volition, habituation, performance capacity, and environmental context. • Change in any aspect of volition, habituation, performance capacity, and/or the environment can result in a change in the thoughts, feelings, and doing. • Volition, habituation and performance capacity are maintained and changed through what one does and what one thinks and feels about doing. • A pattern of volition, habituation and performance capacity will be maintained so long as the underlying thoughts, feelings, and actions are consistently repeated in a supporting environment. • Change requires that novel thoughts, feelings, and actions emerge and be sufficiently repeated in a supportive environment to coalesce into a new organized pattern (Kielhofner, 2008; O'Brien & Kielhofner, 2017).
Person-Environment-Occupation-Performance (PEOP) (Bass et al., 2017; Baum et al., 2015; Christiansen et al., 2015)	Dr. Caroline Baum Dr. Charles Christiansen	Person Environment Occupation Performance	• "Each life situation may be examined in terms of person, environment, occupation and performance factors that support (or limit) participation and contribute to the narratives of individuals, organizations, and groups" (Bass et al., 2017, p. 167). • PEOP emphasizes the active "doing" of occupational performance. • Collaboration is essential to the intervention process. • Person, occupation, and environment interact with each other. • Client-centered practice (the client's choices, interests, and contexts) drive decision-making, goal setting, and intervention planning.
Canadian Model of Occupational Performance and Engagement (CMOP-E) (CAOT, 1997; Polatajko et al., 2007)	Dr. Helene Polatajko Dr. Elizabeth Townsend Dr. Janet Craik Canadian Association of Occupational Therapists	Person (spirituality is core) Environment Occupation	• Client-centered practice is a collaborative practice between the client and therapist that facilitates enabling occupations (CAOT, 1997, p. 180) • Limitations within the person or an unsupportive environment decrease occupational performance. • Limited occupational opportunities lead to decreased occupational engagement. • Spirituality is the core. • Occupational engagement and experience are important for life satisfaction. • Cognitive, affective, and physical factors interact within an environment for occupational performance. Change in one component results in change in another. • Occupational therapists enable occupation by identifying gaps between desired and actual occupational participation and intervening.
Occupational Adaptation (OA) (Grajo, 2017; Schkade & Schultz, 2003)	Dr. Janette Schkade Dr. Sally Schultz	Press for mastery (occupational challenges, responses, role demands, roles) Contexts (physical, social, cultural, temporal, personal, virtual) Occupational adaptation Occupational participation	• The person is an occupational being who has a desire to master his or her environment (by participating in occupations). • The occupational environment demands mastery from the person. These demands enable or restrict participation in occupations. • The person's level of mastery and the environment's level of demand for mastery create occupational roles and role demands or expectations, occupational challenges, and responses from the person (referred to as *press for mastery*). • To navigate the press for mastery, the person goes through the process of occupational adaptation. • The occupational therapist enables the client to participate in occupations, facilitates the environment, and uses occupations to empower the occupational adaptation process (Grajo, 2017).
Kawa Model (Iwami, 2006)	Dr. Michael Iwami	Client's narrative using metaphor of river to identify: • Life flow and priorities • Environment and contexts (social and physical) • Obstacles and challenges • Influencing factors in one's life • Opportunities to enhance flow (occupations)	• Client's viewpoint is the ultimate perspective. • Using a metaphor (life is a river) to describe one's life journey allows clients to think more deeply about their life circumstances and reflect. • All elements in nature are profoundly connected, and people seek ways to live in harmony with nature and circumstances. Therefore, the metaphor of a river helps them discover things about themselves to help them engage in life. • Environment is part of the person (not a separate entity). • Disability is a collective experience. It affects the environment and the people surrounding the person with disability. • The strategy of rehabilitation is not to confront the perceived problems directly and rationally, but to bend, adapt, and flex one's circumstances to the surrounding environment. • How OT practitioners work with their clients is largely dependent on the client's values.

O'Brien, J. & Kuhaneck, H. (2020). Using occupational therapy models and frames of reference. In J. O'Brien & H. Kuhaneck (Eds.). *Case-Smith's Occupational Therapy for Children and Adolescents* (8th ed., p. 23). Elsevier.
O'Brien, J., Stoffel, A., Fisher, G., & Iwami, M. (2020). Occupation-centered practice models. In N. Carson (Ed.). *Psychosocial Occupational Therapy* (p. 47–75). Elsevier.

and environment and the dynamic nature of human performance (Wong & Fisher, 2015). Each model differs in the focus of intervention and desired outcomes. Occupation-based models provide descriptions of:

- theory and research evidence to support concepts,
- factors influencing occupational engagement, adaptation, or participation,
- principles explaining the interactions among factors,
- assessments to measure components,
- guidelines for implementing intervention, and
- expected outcomes of therapy.

OT practitioners are urged to use occupation-based models of practice to guide their reasoning. A description of applying the Model of Human Occupation in practice follows and may serve as a template to the process.

LEARNING ACTIVITY: EXAMINING THE LITERATURE

Use Worksheet 3.2 to summarize findings from a current research article that describes the use of an occupation-based model of practice in an occupational therapy setting.

- Describe the purpose of the research.
- Summarize the methodology.
- What factors or components of the model did the authors address?
- Describe the principles (if any) outlined in the study.
- What were the findings of the research?
- What did you learn about the occupation-based model of practice from this study?

APPLICATION OF THE MODEL OF HUMAN OCCUPATION IN PRACTICE

Kielhofner's Model of Human Occupation (Taylor, 2017) identifies person factors as volition (one's values, interests, and personal causation); habituation (routines, habits, and roles); and performance capacity (skills, abilities, and lived experience). The model emphasizes the importance of the environment (personal, physical, social, political) in supporting or hindering one's occupational performance. Humans engage in routines and roles that are reinforced by doing; one's belief in one's roles and expectations is central to occupational performance. The MOHO differs from other models in that it provides concepts and operational definitions of volition and habituation; considers the person's subjective view of their experience, that is the lived experience as part of performance capacity; and expands one's view of the environment (Kielhofner, 2008; Taylor, 2017).

According to Model of Human Occupation theory, the interaction between the systems (volition, habituation, performance capacity, and environment) lead to one's occupational identity (sense of self). One's occupational identity is reinforced over time as one is successful in performing those desired occupations (occupational competence). Having an established occupational identity and achieving occupational competence allows a person to change and adapt flexibly to challenges (occupational adaptation). Kielhofner suggests that since the systems are interactive and dynamic, changing one system affects the others and therefore OT practitioners may prioritize intervention to address any component.

Box 3.1 presents a case report illustrating the use of the Model of Human Occupation to structure the occupational therapy evaluation and intervention plan.

LEARNING ACTIVITY: COMPARING OCCUPATION-BASED MODELS OF PRACTICE

The process of comparing models encourages students and practitioners to carefully analyze the concepts from each model and promotes therapeutic reasoning. Use Worksheet 3.3 to compare three models using the case example (Grace).

Case example: Grace is a 90-year-old woman living on her own in a small ranch home in rural Maine, where she has lived for the past 60 years. Grace lost her husband 15 years ago and they did not have any children. Both of her sisters and all her nieces and nephews have passed away. Her family (grand nieces, grand nephews, and their children) live nearby in the small town. Grace enjoys daily visits from family and catching up on the "news". She cooks for herself and maintains her home. Grace recently sustained a stroke which resulted in right upper extremity hemiplegia interfering with her ability to dress, feed, and complete daily routines. When she had her stroke, she hit the garage door (while driving). She reports "Something happened, and the car lunged forward. I guess I can't drive anymore." She is concerned that she cannot use her right arm adequately, drive to get groceries, and pick up cleaning supplies.

- How are the models similar and different from each other?
- Which model do you prefer? why?
- How do the models organize or structure your therapeutic reasoning?

BOX 3.1   Case Report: Applying the Model of Human Occupation

Client's Name: Ken Smith

Date of report: 9/16/2016

Date of referral: 9/14/2016

DOB: 3/15/1959

Primary intervention diagnosis/concern: muscular sclerosis (MS) – progressive relapsing

Secondary diagnosis/concern: depression with suicidal ideation

Precautions/contraindications: falls, dysphagia, peripheral nerve damage

Reason for referral to OT: Activities of Daily Living (ADL) training

Occupational profile: Mr. Smith is a 58-year-old man with a history of MS (diagnosed at age 22). Mr. Smith lives with his wife (his primary caregiver) in a one-story home. He is an unemployed carpenter (for the last 2 years) secondary to MS. Mr. Smith presents with a staggered gait, dragging his feet with each step; slurred speech; and slow movements with little eye contact. He speaks softly and states he does not really care about the future. His wife states he has become less involved with home activities within the year and does not seem to have any interests. She is concerned that he is giving up. His last exacerbation was 3 months ago.

Continued

BOX 3.1   Case Report: Applying the Model of Human Occupation—cont'd

Concerns: Mr. Smith's wife is concerned that he does not want to be involved in life activities.

Assessment (descriptions and findings): *Interest Checklist* (modified) (Kielhofner & Neville, 1983) gathers information on a client's strength of interest and engagement in 68 activities in the past, currently, and in the future. The focus is on leisure interests that influence activity choices.

INTEREST CHECKLIST

Level of interest	Findings: Interests	Interpretation
Past 10 years	Strong: walking, golf, dancing, swimming, reading, writing, family, concerts, barbeques	Mr. Smith had a variety of active interests with family and friends.
Past year	Strong: walking, reading, writing, family	Mr. Smith is not engaging in as many social activities outside of the family. Overall, he reports engaging in less activities.
Currently	Walking, reading, writing, family, television	Mr. Smith currently engages in less physically active interests. He is still walking and hopes to continue this.
Future	Walking, swimming, family, concerts, movies	Mr. Smith noted many activities that he would like to pursue in the future, some of them were past interests.

Occupational Self-assessment (OSA) (Baron et al., 2006) is a self-report measure to assess how well a client feels they perform (occupational competence) and how important the activity is to them (values). The therapist examines patterns of scores. Large gaps in not being able to perform those things that one values may indicate areas in need of intervention. The OSA key forms provide client measures for both scales (occupational competence and values) which may be used to document and measure outcomes.

OCCUPATIONAL SELF-ASSESSMENT

	Total score	Measure (error)	Interpretation of scores/findings
Competence	45	38 ± 2	Mr. Smith reports low belief in his skills. He scored many items low in terms of his belief that he could accomplish the activity.
Values	52	48 ± 3	Ms. Smith reported that a variety of activities were important to him.

Client priorities as reported high value and low competency on OSA:
- Handling my responsibilities
- Physically doing what I need to do
- Managing my basic needs (food, medicine)

Clinical observations provided information on ADL and physical functioning. Mr. Smith engaged in several tasks to assess his physical abilities.

Performance	Observation/ Findings	Interpretation
Washing face and hands	Swayed while at sink; had to hold onto countertop; used gross grasp to grab hand cloth and had difficulty manipulating cloth to wash face.	Postural control and bilateral (B) lower extremities (LE) weakness [especially right (R) LE] noted; R upper extremity (UE) in-hand manipulation difficulty interfering with ability to complete ADLs.
Walking over to sink and getting glass from cabinet	Walked with wide gait and right foot drop noted; held onto counter when reached above head; not able to extend to toes to reach above; held glass in palmar grasp; able to bring to mouth but not smooth.	B LE weakness and coordination deficits; B UE coordination difficulty; force modulation issues (put glass down forcefully) and spilled water when bringing to mouth are interfering with ADL performance.
Putting on his coat	Grasped coat with both hands; difficulty zipping coat and buttoning; took over 5 minutes to put on coat.	Fine motor coordination impaired as he struggled with buttoning and zipping. Fine motor coordination interferes with ADL performance.

The following information was obtained during a 30-minute interview with the client. Mr. Smith engaged in conversation and answered questions when asked.

Occupations

Mr. Smith has difficulty completing his morning routine and no longer works. He does not take walks anymore and typically spends the day watching television. His wife performs household duties.

Volition

Mr. Smith worked as a carpenter for 25 years before he stopped this year when his MS became severe. He built the cabinets and furniture in his house and spoke proudly of his work. He enjoyed walks in the woods, sitting by the lake, and spending time with family at camp. He reports that he no longer wants to do any of those things, and he feels useless. Findings from the *Interest Checklist* indicate that Mr. Smith stopped engaging in activities that he found meaningful. He expressed no desire to re-engage in these interests.

Habituation (habits and roles)

Mr. Smith spends days at home with his wife. She assists him with dressing and bathing. They eat breakfast together and then he watches television, while she does errands or goes to work (she works 9 am to 3 pm weekdays). Mr. Smith uses a commode for toileting needs when he is alone. He walks with a walker. He states he spends most of his day watching television and waiting for his wife to come home from work. He plays on the computer periodically. Once his wife comes home, they have lunch and talk. After dinner, they watch television, and he goes to bed around 9 pm. His wife helps him undress and get ready for bed.

BOX 3.1 **Case Report: Applying the Model of Human Occupation—cont'd**

Sometimes family visits and he used to enjoy this. Mr. Smith does not drive or use public transportation. Mr. Smith moves slowly and has difficulty grasping objects. He walks with an unsteady gait and uses a walker.

Performance capacity
- *Subjective experience:* Mr. Smith stated "*I can no longer do anything right, and it is frustrating. I don't want to do anything.*" He admitted that he was good at woodworking and proud of the furniture and cabinets he built at home. He feels like a "loser husband" and is not sure why his wife stays with him. He stated he had no friends, just family.
- *Performance skills:* Mr. Smith can walk short distances with his rolling walker. He speaks with a slurred pattern. He requires assistance with dressing/undressing as he has difficulty with fine motor coordination (buttoning, zipping). Mr. Smith follows simple verbal directions and can sequence 4 steps. He uses an iPad.
- *Performance patterns:* Mr. Smith spends most of the day in passive activities such as watching television and using his iPad. He relies on his wife to help him with ADL, meals, and home management. Lately, his wife notes that Mr. Smith does not want to socialize or engage in activities outside of the home.
- *Client factors:* Mr. Smith has poor fine motor coordination, limited muscle endurance (fatigues after walking 5 feet) and has a wide-based gait with R LE foot drop. He slurs his speech and has difficulty completing daily tasks such as washing his face and hands. Mr. Smith uses adaptive equipment at home (such as Reacher, remote control, and adapted toilet seat). Mr. Smith answered questions, made eye contact, and show a sense of humor (towards the end of the session). He expressed a desire to change things, "It's just not working for me. I would like to see if I could do more again."

Environment
Mr. Smith lives with his wife in a 1 story apartment in the city, close to a park. The environment is close to stores and a YMCA. Family lives nearby. Mr. Smith has limited income.

Interpretation
According to the *Occupational Self-Assessment*, Mr. Smith no longer engages in those activities (woodworking, social participation, hiking, cooking) that he enjoys. He reported these items were of high importance, yet he was not able to do them well. This discrepancy between wanting to do things that you are unable to do may result in feelings of incompetence and lead to low feelings of self-worth (as is often found in depression). He reports strong past interests in which he is no longer engaging. His physical abilities have declined within the past year (per his report and medical record), interfering with his ability to engage in daily activities and he has lost his identity as a worker (this year). The progressive nature of MS (with periods of remission) and his current physical status (as determined through clinical observations) require that Mr. Smith adapt and accommodate activities so that he can continue to participate in those things he finds meaningful.

Strengths
- Environment supports his physical and emotional needs (per report).
- Resources exist within the community to provide transportation to local events.
- Mr. Smith identified future goals.
- Mr. Smith easily engaged in conversation, and occasionally showed a sense of humor.

Weaknesses
- He is experiencing physical decline in strength and endurance.
- Decline in physical abilities interferes with ADL performance.

- Loss of worker role and occupational identity associated with work.
- Client is not engaging in social activities.
- Progressive nature of MS may require adaptation, compensation, and assistive technology.

Long-term goal
1. Mr. Smith will independently complete his morning routine within 1 hour × 7 days a week using adaptive equipment.

Short-term Goals (2)	FOR Principle Used to Address Goals	Intervention Approach/Methods
With set up, Mr. Smith will feed himself independently breakfast × 7 days, using adapted equipment.	Model of Human Occupation. *Change in any aspect of volition, habituation, performance capacity, and/or the environment can result in change in the thoughts, feelings, and doing that make up one's occupation.* (Taylor, 2017, p. 26).	Target change in habits. Developing a routine of feeding himself breakfast using adapted equipment promotes physical performance while establishing a new habit to allow Ken to re-engage in daily activities.
Mr. Smith will engage in 15 minutes of brushing hair, washing face and hands, and brushing teeth × 3 days, using adapted equipment.	Same as above.	Target performance capacity (endurance for standing activity) by increasing the amount of time he can engage in activity (in standing position). Increase the time of activity to build his endurance (work to the point of fatigue but not past it).
Mr. Smith will independently wash his face and hands, each morning (× 7 days) while seated at the sink, using adapted equipment.	Same as above.	Target change in habits to build self-competency and performance. Through doing the activity, Mr. Smith will fulfill his role in home and rely less on his wife for basic needs. This will help him to re-establish his role as husband.

Precautions during the session
Clients with MS should work to the point of fatigue but not past it. Monitor depressive thoughts and report to the team.

Analysis of Therapeutic Reasoning using MOHO Theory
Mr. Smith is not completing his basic needs due to decreased performance capacity (e.g., poor endurance, physical declines due to MS). This may be causing low motivation (volition) for engagement in daily activities, leading to feelings of low self-efficacy, decreased quality of life, and depression. Engaging him in basic ADL activities with support (e.g., assistive equipment, compensatory techniques) will help him create a sense of efficacy and identity so that he can engage in those things he found meaningful (e.g., social activities with wife) leading to positive feelings of occupational competency and increased life satisfaction.

Continued

BOX 3.1   Case Report: Applying the Model of Human Occupation—cont'd

The long-term goal focuses on habituation (i.e., habits, routines, and roles) while addressing performance capacity (i.e., decline in physical skills) and adapting how he completes activities and providing adapted equipment. Mr. Smith expressed the desire to take care of his basic needs. He also expressed frustration with his role as husband. The long-term goal allows Mr. Smith to re-engage in his role as husband by taking care of his basic care needs and completing his morning ADL routine, without relying on his wife. Changing this pattern may help him gain feelings of self-competence leading to improved self-identity and quality of life.

Early success can be motivating in therapy so the OT practitioner grades activities accordingly, while developing a trusting therapeutic relationship. As the OT practitioner learns about the client's values, personality, style, and interactions, they may challenge Mr. Smith to engage in previous occupations or even find new occupational interests. The OT practitioner evaluates the success of the intervention process by measuring the client's changes based on the Occupational Self-Assessment and progress towards goals. Using the Model of Human Occupation helps the OT practitioner make sound therapeutic decisions using a client-centered, occupation-based approach, based on current research evidence.

FRAMES OF REFERENCE

Frames of reference provide information based on research to guide evaluation and intervention planning. Frames of reference address a specific area or client factor (such as strength, movement, or cognition). OT practitioners use knowledge of frames of reference to inform therapeutic reasoning. Frames of reference include descriptions of:

1. Population
2. Nature of function and dysfunction
3. Role of the therapist
4. Assessment tools
5. Principles
6. Strategies and techniques

Table 3.2 provides a description of some frames of reference and their guiding principles. Many frames of reference used in occupational therapy are not developed by occupational therapists. Rather, occupational therapists apply frames of reference using knowledge of occupational therapy's domain and practice (AOTA, 2020). For example, the developmental approach is used by numerous disciplines and was created from psychology research. Each profession that uses this frame of reference views development in terms of their discipline and determines how the frame of reference can provide support to address the professional domain in practice. Using an occupation-based model of practice helps the OT practitioner determine how to apply the frame of reference in one's professional domain.

OT practitioners use information from the frame of reference to identify factors interfering with occupational performance and select intervention strategies to elicit change. For example, practitioners using the developmental approach measure the client's ability to engage in the desired occupation (such as dressing, feeding, bathing, play) based on their developmental level. Intervention using a developmental approach follows the "neuro-typical" sequence of acquisition.

Another example, the biomechanical frame of reference, explains techniques and strategies to improve range of motion, muscle strength, and endurance. OT practitioners using this approach seek to promote participation in occupations by improving a client's ability to move through the range with ample muscle strength and endurance to complete a desired occupation. This same frame of reference can be used by physical therapists, athletic trainers, and coaches, with a different emphasis.

Selecting a Frame of Reference

Frames of reference are created to explain theory, principles, strategies, and techniques used to facilitate change for specific populations. The OT practitioner uses therapeutic reasoning to select the frame of reference that best addresses the client's goals. Figure 3.2 provides an overview of this process whereby the OT practitioner adjusts and modifies steps as they gain new information (as depicted by the arrows in the figure). The process is not necessarily sequential as the practitioner often revisits steps for selecting a frame of reference (described in Box 3.2) as they gather new information.

The process of selecting a frame of reference begins with identifying the client's occupational performance strengths and challenges. OT practitioners often use an occupation-based model of practice to structure the initial session and generate questions and gather data. They collect data and identify the client's strengths and challenges which leads to several hypotheses regarding what is interfering with or supporting the client's participation in desired activities.

Once the practitioner has gained data from the occupational profile, observation of the client, and conducted the initial evaluation, they identify possible frames of reference that are suitable for the client population, occupational needs, and underlying factors that may be influencing occupational performance. They use knowledge from the frame of reference to prioritize and address the client's occupational challenges. For example, they identify frames of reference that address the specific client factors identified as interfering with occupational performance while considering the client's age, condition, and occupational needs.

The OT practitioner examines current evidence to support use of the principles and strategies outlined in the frame of reference (see Chapter 6). They use knowledge of neuroscience, psychology, kinesiology, and health and wellness when

TABLE 3.2   Frames of Reference

Frame of Reference	Description	Guiding Principles (not inclusive)
Developmental	Identifies the client's current performance level for motor (gross, fine, oral), social, emotional, and cognitive skills and targets intervention to help the client advance.	• Repetitive practice of developmental skills as the client masters them provides experiences that promote brain plasticity and learning. • Practice of skills in a developmental sequence at the level just above where the client is functioning (Llorens, 1982).
Biomechanical	Based on concepts of kinesiology, this FOR evaluates and intervenes regarding ROM, strength, and endurance. This approach focuses on the physical limitations that interfere with the child's ability to engage in occupation	• Joint range of motion influences movement. The ability to move in directions within certain degrees of motion is due to the bony structure and the integrity of the surrounding tissues (Radomski & Latham, 2008). • Increasing strength can promote stability and balance for successful engagement in activity. • Energy is needed for a person to produce the required intensity or rate of effort over time for an activity or exercise. • To increase endurance, submaximal exertion will require adaptation to stress, resulting in hypertrophy and hyperplasia of oxidative type I slow-twitch muscle fibers and increased function in the cardiorespiratory systems (Rybski, 2012). • Decreasing pain enables clients to engage in occupations. Every pain has a source, and the intervention must be directed toward and influence that source.
Contemporary motor control and motor learning	Motor control examines how one directs and regulates movement, whereas motor learning theory describes how children learn movements. This approach is based on dynamic system theory that many factors influence movement and must be considered in intervention (O'Brien et al., 2020a).	• Motor performance results from an interaction between adaptable and flexible systems. • Dysfunction occurs when movement patterns lack sufficient adaptability to accommodate task demands and environmental constraints. • Because task characteristics influence motor requirements, practitioners modify and adapt the requirements and affordances of tasks to help children succeed. • Children develop improved neural pathways when they repeat meaningful, whole (occupation), tasks in the natural environment. • Motor learning occurs as children repeat motor tasks that are intrinsically motivating, meaningful, and for which they can problem-solve.
Ayres Sensory Integration®	The organization of sensory input to produce an adaptive response; a theoretical process and intervention approach; addresses the processing of sensory information from the body and the environment; includes modulating, discriminating, and integrating sensory information to produce meaningful adaptive responses (Parham & Mailloux, 2020).	• Sensory input can be incorporated into activities systematically to elicit an adaptive response. • Registration of meaningful sensory input is necessary before an adaptive response can be made. • An adaptive response contributes to the development of sensory integration. • Better organization of adaptive responses enhances the child's general behavioral organization. • More mature and complex patterns of behavior emerge from consolidation of simpler behaviors. • The more inner-directed a child's activities are, the greater the potential for the activities to improve the neural organization.
Behavioral	Behavior is reinforced with a reward.	• Positive reinforcement increases the likelihood that a behavior will be repeated. • Clients will stop behaviors that are ignored or receive negative reinforcement. • Stimulus in the environment results in a response (behavior).
Cognitive	Emphasizes assisting the client to identify, develop and use cognitive strategies to perform daily occupations effectively. Based on Bandura's (1996) work on the importance of self-efficacy and establishing goals to motivate clients to achieve.	• Improved performance results from the dynamic interaction of the client's skills with the parameters of the task in the context in which it needs to be performed (Missiuna et al., 2001). • Client learns strategies to use in multiple situations and feels empowered that he/she has developed solutions, thereby likely to repeat the strategy.

Adapted from O'Brien, J. & Kuhaneck, H. (2020). Using occupational therapy models and frames of reference. In J. O'Brien & H. Kuhaneck (Eds.). *Case-Smith's Occupational Therapy for Children and Adolescents* (8th ed., p. 33–36). Elsevier.

critiquing the suitability of a frame of reference for a specific client. They examine principles, strategies, techniques, and the role of the therapist to evaluate the suitability of the frame of reference in addressing the client's needs. They synthesize information from research, clinical experience, and knowledge of the specific client to determine if the frame of reference is suitable for the specific client.

The OT practitioner explores the pragmatics of using the strategies and techniques of the frame of reference in practice. They identify required training, materials, supplies, time, and

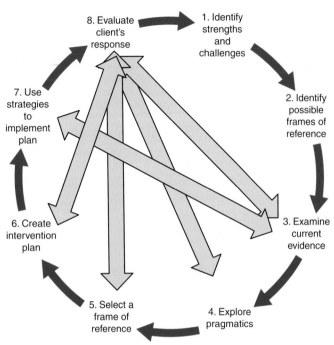

Fig. 3.2 Process for Selecting a Frame of Reference

BOX 3.2   Steps in Selecting a Frame of Reference

1. Use questions and assessments derived from the model of practice to identify the client's occupational performance strengths and challenges to indicate factors interfering with engagement in occupation.
2. Identify possible frames of reference that address factors (e.g., condition, age, client factors, occupational needs, environment) influencing the client's occupational performance.
3. Examine current evidence.
   a. According to the research evidence, what are the specific client conditions or factors addressed by this FOR?
   b. Is evidence current? What is the level of evidence? (see Chapter 6).
   c. Does evidence make sense with current theory?
   d. Is the FOR compatible with occupation-based practice?
   e. Does the evidence indicate that the frame of reference addresses the client's needs?
4. Explore pragmatics of using frame of reference in practice. Determine training, materials, supplies, time, and space needed to implement strategies and techniques of the frame of reference in practice.
5. Select a frame of reference by examining principles, strategies, techniques, and the role of the therapist.
6. Create an intervention plan based on the principles, strategies and techniques outlined in the frame of reference.
7. Implement the plan using strategies and concepts from the frame of reference.
8. Evaluate client's responses and outcomes to intervention.

---

space needed to implement strategies and techniques in practice. The OT practitioner evaluates information gathered from occupational history, client's strengths and challenges, current evidence, in combination with information gained from interacting with the client, knowledge of condition, experience, and practical contextual knowledge to select a frame of reference.

OT practitioners evaluate the principles of the frame of reference, strategies, techniques, and the role of the therapist when selecting a frame of reference to address the client's unique needs. They create an intervention plan based upon principles of both the occupation-based model of practice and the selected frame of reference. They implement the strategies and techniques in practice and reflect upon the sessions and the client's outcomes. The therapist closely monitors client responses and adjusts the intervention strategies and techniques as needed throughout the intervention process. If the client is not making desired progress, the OT practitioner may revisit the frame of reference, adjust strategies and techniques, or select another frame of reference to address the client's goals. The following case illustrates how one practitioner used an occupation-based model of practice with a frame of reference.

Case Application: Occupation-Based Model of Practice with Biomechanical Frame of Reference

Jaquin, a new OT practitioner is unsure of his role in the acute care setting. A colleague informs Jaquin that the previous therapist performed upper extremity evaluations and worked mostly on maintaining range of motion for functional activities and providing the medical team with recommendations regarding discharge home, to the rehabilitation unit, or to long-term care. Jaquin wants to address occupation more fully and create an intervention plan to address client goals.

He decides to use the Person-Environment-Occupation-Performance (PEOP) model (Baum et al., 2015) to structure his evaluation. The PEOP model emphasizes the interaction between the person factors (e.g., physical, cognitive, emotional, social, biological), environment (e.g., physical, social, political support and hindrances to engagement in occupation) and the client's past and present occupations and performance. Figure 3.3 provides a schematic of the PEOP process.

Jaquin structures the OT evaluation to examine the person factors (i.e., cognition, psychological, physiological, sensory/perceptual, motor, spirituality/meaning) that may interfere with a client's ability to do those things they wish to do (i.e., occupations, activities, tasks, roles) as well as the impact on the client's ability to return home safely. Jaquin generates specific questions to ask the client about the client's environment (including social, physical, natural, cultural) and examines how the person's strengths and limitations influence safe completion of desired activities and occupations. Jaquin gathers data on the client's cognition, motor, and social–emotional abilities to determine their influence on occupational performance.

As Jaquin gathers data from the client he decides to use knowledge from the biomechanical frame of reference to further address the client's physical limitations. The biomechanical frame of reference emphasizes the role of range of motion, muscle strength, and endurance on movement. Jaquin plans to conduct a complete range of motion (ROM) assessment, manual muscle test (MMT), and examine endurance. The principles of the biomechanical frame of reference suggest that increasing a client's range of motion, muscle strength, and endurance through repetitive activities improves motor performance.

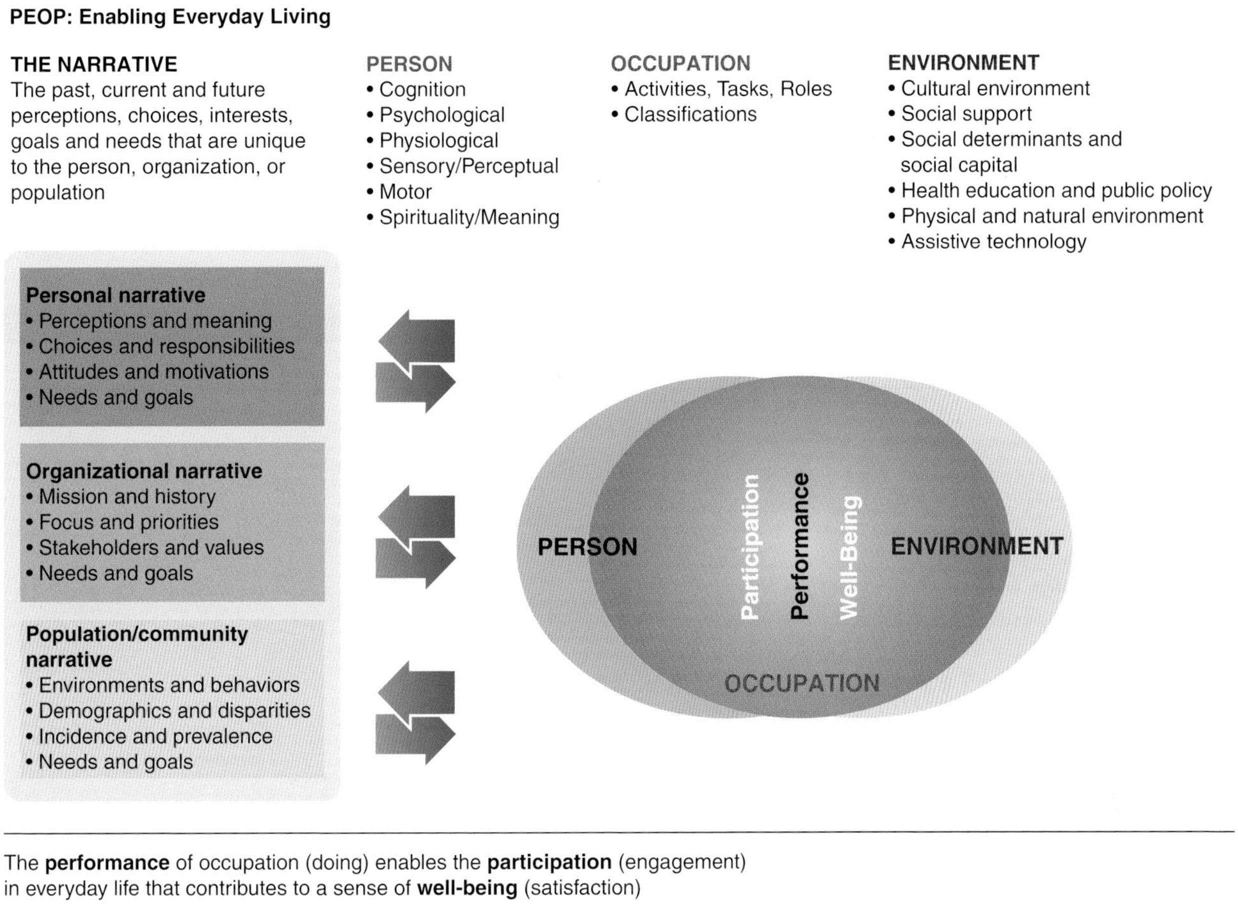

PEOP: Enabling Everyday Living

THE NARRATIVE
The past, current and future perceptions, choices, interests, goals and needs that are unique to the person, organization, or population

PERSON
- Cognition
- Psychological
- Physiological
- Sensory/Perceptual
- Motor
- Spirituality/Meaning

OCCUPATION
- Activities, Tasks, Roles
- Classifications

ENVIRONMENT
- Cultural environment
- Social support
- Social determinants and social capital
- Health education and public policy
- Physical and natural environment
- Assistive technology

Personal narrative
- Perceptions and meaning
- Choices and responsibilities
- Attitudes and motivations
- Needs and goals

Organizational narrative
- Mission and history
- Focus and priorities
- Stakeholders and values
- Needs and goals

Population/community narrative
- Environments and behaviors
- Demographics and disparities
- Incidence and prevalence
- Needs and goals

PERSON — Participation Performance Well-Being — ENVIRONMENT

OCCUPATION

The **performance** of occupation (doing) enables the **participation** (engagement) in everyday life that contributes to a sense of **well-being** (satisfaction)

Fig. 3.3 Person-Environment-Occupation-Performance Model (Baum, C. M., Christiansen, C. H. & Bass, J. D. (2015). The Person-Environment-Occupation-Performance (PEOP) Model. In C. H. Christiansen, C. M. Baum, & J.D. Bass (Eds.), *Occupational Therapy: Performance, Participation, and Well-Being* (4th ed., pp. 49–55). SLACK.)

Jaquin can address the biomechanical limitations if needed or make adaptations to promote success through compensation.

Using PEOP concepts, Jacquin acknowledges that clients will engage in activities that are meaningful to them and support their past and future interests and goals (as learned through the person's narrative) when supported by the environment (including social and physical supports). The PEOP model suggests that performing one's occupations is important for participation, engagement, and well-being. Therefore, Jaquin realizes that he must do more than improve range of motion, strength, or endurance through repetitive activities. He must engage the client in meaningful activities to support the client's unique goals and future interests. Therefore, each intervention will vary depending upon the client. Jaquin combines knowledge of the client as a person (gained by using PEOP concepts) with biomechanical principles to create a client-centered intervention plan targeting the client's desired activities.

Jaquin provides comprehensive information to the treatment team regarding numerous factors in the client's life that may impact function at discharge ensuring the patient has adequate assistance or functional ability to return home. Using the PEOP broadens the therapist's view of the client's situation and allows the therapist to address occupational performance during intervention.

Using Multiple Frames of Reference: Eclecticism

Ikiugu, Plastow, and van Niekerk (2019) use the term *eclecticism* to describe the therapist's use of multiple models in practices. Ikiugu (2007) developed a framework for combining practice models (which includes both occupation-based models and frames of reference). OT practitioners combine models to address the complex needs of clients within a variety of settings (Ikiugu, 2007; Ikiugu et al., 2009). To assist OT practitioners with combining models carefully, Ikiugu (2007) developed a Conceptual Framework for Combining Theoretical Conceptual Practice Models. The framework includes use of an organizing model of practice to address the initial evaluation of occupational performance issues and complementary models as needed. The models may shift throughout the OT process as the practitioner focuses on different goals and priorities.

It is important that OT practitioners evaluate the effectiveness of the approaches and understand if they are being used as intended. For example, using a sensory integration frame of reference requires the client lead the session and engage in a variety of challenging sensory activities (Parham & Mailloux, 2020). This approach does not mesh well with a behavioral approach where the client must follow the practitioner's set up routine.

Sensory integration theory also does not support using sensory stimuli as the "behavioral reward" (Parham & Malloux, 2020). Carefully reflecting on the frames of reference and examining how they work together is essential for sound therapeutic reasoning. The Theory Application Assessment Instrument (TIAA; Ikiugu & Smallfield, 2010) was created to help OT students and practitioners learn how to combine practice models and reflect upon practice. The Learning Activity following the case includes sample questions from the instrument.

The following case, Chris, provides an example using the Model of Human Occupation, contemporary motor control and motor learning, and psychosocial approaches. The practitioner also uses terminology from the Occupational Therapy Practice Framework -IV (AOTA, 2020) to describe intervention approaches.

CASE STUDY

Chris by Jarrett Wolske, OTD, OTR/L

Client History

Chris is a 13-year-old male preparing to transition into his first year of high school. Chris lives in a multi-generational suburban home with his maternal grandmother, parents, and two younger siblings. Chris has a diagnosis of spastic cerebral palsy with a presentation of spastic hemiplegia affecting his right side. Chris ambulates independently with an ataxic gait. Chris has a history of intensive therapy starting with early intervention. Over time, therapy transitioned to episodic outpatient care and monthly direct minutes within the elementary and middle schools.

Chris and his family sought outpatient occupational therapy due to his upcoming transition into high school. Per the parental report, "It became difficult to afford the outside therapies and we wanted Chris to have some sort of normal childhood."

Client Occupational Profile and Evaluation

To gain a better understanding of the needs of Chris and his family, the occupational therapy practitioner utilized theory-driven questions based on the Model of Human Occupation (Forsyth, 2017). These included questions about Chris's interests, hobbies, roles, and the family's concerns.

Parents: "We are worried about his coordination to do daily things. They have shorter passing periods, and we want to make sure he has enough time to change in the locker room for gym class and gather all his books. In general, we want him to be more active and involved. He spends a lot of time online and we worry that if he is not more active, he will lose what abilities he does have."

To obtain more concrete information from Chris's perspective, the practitioner utilized the Child Occupational Self-Assessment (COSA) (Keller et al., 2006). Based on Chris's diagnosis, concerns, needs, presentation, and information gathered through the MOHO, the therapist chose the contemporary motor control frame of reference to further guide the therapeutic reasoning process (O'Brien et al., 2020a). The practitioner chose subtests of the Bruininks–Oseretsky Test of Motor Proficiency Second Edition (BOT-2) (Bruininks & Bruininks, 2005). Data from the COSA and BOT-2 were combined to create a better picture of Chris's situation.

Assessment Findings

Child Occupational Self-Assessment (COSA)

Question	Perceived Competency	Importance	Child's Comments
Watch TV or a video	I am really good at doing this	Important	
Keep my body clean	I have a little problem doing this	Really important	"Shaving and cutting my own nails can be difficult."

Question	Perceived Competency	Importance	Child's Comments
Dress myself	I have a little problem doing this	Important	
Eat my meals without any help	I do this ok	Really important	"Cutting food is sometimes hard."
Buy something myself	I do this ok	Not really important	
Get my chores done	I have a little problem doing this	Not really important	
Get enough sleep	I am really good at doing this	Most important	
Have enough time to do the things I like	I have a little problem doing this	Really important	"It takes me a while to do some things, so I don't have as much time to do what I want."
Take care of my things	I have a little problem doing this	Really important	
Get around from one place to another	I have a little problem doing this	Important	
Choose things that I want to do	I am really good at doing this	Really important	
Keep my mind on what I'm doing	I do this ok	Important	
Do things with my family	I do this ok	Really important	

CASE STUDY—cont'd

Question	Perceived Competency	Importance	Child's Comments
Do things with my friends	I have a little problem doing this	Most important	"It's hard to play sports with them. Right now, all we do is watch football together."
Do things with my classmates	I do this ok	Not really important	
Follow classroom rules	I do this ok	Not really important	
Finish my work in class on time	I do this ok	Not really important	
Get my homework done	I do this ok	Not really important	
Ask my teacher questions when I need to	I am really good at doing this	Not really important	
Make others understand my ideas	I do this ok	Most important	
Think of ways to do things when I have a problem	I do this ok	Important	
Keep working on something even when it gets hard	I have a little problem doing this	Important	
Calm myself down when I get upset	I do this ok	Important	
Make my body do what I want it to	I have a big problem doing this	Most important	
Use my hands to work with things	I have a big problem doing this	Most important	
Finish what I'm doing without getting tired	I have a little problem doing this	Important	

What are two other things you are really good at that we did not talk about today?

"I'm good at making people laugh and dealing with occupational therapists like you."

What are two other things you have a big problem with that we did not talk about today?

"We talked about everything."

Is there anything else that is important to you that we did not get to talk about? Would you like to tell me?

"I don't want to be the weird kid, or the kid people feel bad for. I know I have CP, but I just want to do things like everyone else."

Bruininks–Oseretsky Test of Motor Performance (BOT-2)

Subtest	Raw Score	Scaled Score	Age Equivalency	Interpretation
Manual Dexterity	18	4	5.8–5.9	Well Below Average
Upper Limb Coordination	20	5	6.3–6.5	Well Below Average

Interpretation

Chris is a witty 13-year-old male who enjoys spending time with his family and friends, watching sports, and playing online games. He presented for an occupational therapy evaluation secondary to concerns about transitioning into high school and the activities of daily living that transition involves. Chris was assessed with the Child Occupational Self-Assessment (COSA). This is a self-report rating on the ease or difficulty in participating in occupations (daily meaningful activities) and their importance to the client. The BOT-2 is a standardized assessment to understand skill deficits in motor performance. The manual dexterity and upper limb coordination subtests were administered.

Based on assessment results, Chris has difficulties in manual dexterity and upper extremity coordination. These difficulties are negatively impacting his ability to participate in his occupations independently and safely, as reported in the COSA. This includes engagement in ADLs (dressing, grooming), peer sports, and leisure activities. These deficits are present across home and school environments.

Intervention

The practitioner focused on three self-identified areas based on the COSA: ADL, IADL, and sport participation with friends. These areas also reflected the wishes of Chris and his family.

Utilizing the contemporary motor control frame of reference, the practitioner first engaged Chris in occupations utilizing a task-oriented approach (O'Brien et al., 2020b). This allowed the practitioner to understand Chris's baseline performance. The practitioner used concepts from psychosocial frames of reference to reinforce positive experiences to promote self-efficacy and self-determination.

The practitioner then used establish and modify approaches as necessary (AOTA, 2020). The establish approach was informed by motor learning strategies. This approach was used because there were certain occupations that Chris had never performed. Environmental modifications were guided by the environmental conceptualization in the Model of Human Occupation (Fisher et al., 2017). Mindful of Chris being a teenager and his self-report of "wanting to do things like everyone else," the practitioner focused on discrete physical modifications. The practitioner also coached Chris on how to pace his activity levels and use self-advocacy techniques to communicate with his friends.

COMBINING MODELS WITH TREATMENT PROTOCOLS

Treatment protocols are created from theory designed to outline strategies and techniques to provide intervention in a uniform manner. Protocols may arise from frames of reference (such as protocols to address surgically repaired tendon lacerations based on a biomechanical frame of reference, or constraint-induced movement therapy protocols based on contemporary motor control). These protocols are based on the same theory that guides the specific frame of reference. The frame of reference provides details and evidence explaining how the intervention strategies and approaches facilitate change, whereas the protocol identifies the specific "how to" do the intervention. To make therapeutic decisions in practice, it is important to understand the basis for the protocol (which can be found in the frame of reference).

Manualized occupational therapy such as Lifestyle Redesign® protocols for diabetes management (Pyatak et al., 2015) and pressure ulcer prevention (Blanche et al., 2011) provide a structured process for improving healthy living among at-risk populations. It is important for OT practitioners to understand the rationale and reasoning for the protocol, so that they can make practice decisions for a variety of clients. The OT practitioner uses knowledge of science with information from the client's narrative to guide treatment (Blanche et al., 2011). OT practitioners use insight from a preferred model of practice to understand how a patient's roles, habits, routines, occupations, and environment influence intervention delivery to complement the protocol. The following case example illustrates how OT practitioners use a variety of practice models when following treatment protocols.

Case Example: Combining Theoretical Models

Pooja is an occupational therapist working in a pediatric outpatient clinic that provides constraint-induced movement therapy (CIMT). The treatment protocol adopted by the department includes having children wear a continuous cast, receive 3 hours of occupational therapy intervention daily for 15 treatment days, followed by 5 days of intensive bimanual focused therapy. The protocol includes weekly parent training sessions and weekend home exercise programs using a specified template guide.

Pooja uses a variety of practice models to better understand the CIMT protocol and create effective occupational therapy intervention. Figure 3.4 provides a description of the theoretical models used in the case.

Constraint-induced movement therapy is a rehabilitation approach influenced by contemporary motor control and motor learning, biomechanical, and behavioral frames of references. This information informs Pooja's decisions throughout the process. Rehabilitation approaches emphasize regaining skills and

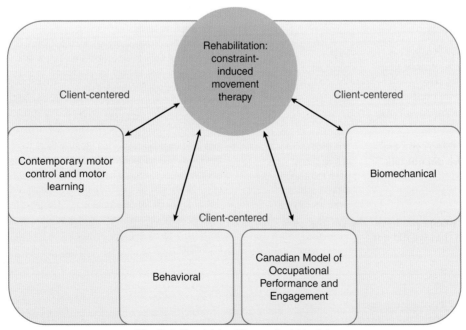

Fig. 3.4 Combining Theoretical Models

abilities (such as using the affected hand in two-handed tasks to regain motor control) rather than focusing on compensatory techniques.

Contemporary motor control and motor learning supports completing whole meaningful activities in one's natural environment (O'Brien et al., 2020a). This approach uses evidence-based motor learning strategies, including repetitive practice of meaningful movements that require children to problem-solve, while progressively increasing the challenge of motor tasks (i.e., scaffolding) to improve the child's performance (O'Brien et al., 2020a).

Pooja knows from clinical experiences and parent interviews that many of the school-aged children who attend the clinic program are independent for most activities of daily living (ADLs) by using their dominant hand only or by utilizing hemi-specific compensatory techniques. She also knows from clinical experience that the child's frustration the first week of casting can impact the child's self-efficacy, motivation, and participation in preferred activities. She decides it is important to integrate positive behavioral support strategies from the behavioral approach into the intervention plan. These support strategies encourage the child to continue with the activities, promote problem-solving, and allow the child to feel a sense of success and belief in their abilities.

To further develop the intervention plan, Pooja draws on the Canadian Model of Occupational Performance and Engagement (CMOP-E) (CAOT, 1997) to prioritize and identify activities of daily living (ADL) that are easily achievable for the children that also build skills in the affected hand. Pooja collaborates with the child and family to find ways for the child to complete as much of the ADL task as possible with the affected hand, while still engaging in the family's routine. For example, she may suggest the child squeeze toothpaste onto a toothbrush that is placed on the counter using her affected hand to encourage independence and to work on improving grip strength. When brushing teeth, a universal cuff or built-up handle is a temporary adaptation during the casted phase of the protocol that allows the child to control toothbrushing. During the bimanual phase, Pooja will discontinue adaptive equipment and using motor learning strategies to enable the child to hold the toothbrush with the affected hand and coordinate putting toothpaste on the toothbrush in the movement pattern that encourages maximal use of the affected hand and greatest efficiency with the child's morning routine. These therapeutic decisions are guided by the child's need for success and mastery while still aligning with the CIMT protocol to improve hand skills for bimanual performance.

Pooja uses knowledge of the biomechanical frame of reference to understand the client's range of motion, strength, and endurance. She grades activities using this information and positions objects with knowledge of the child's active range of motion and strength.

The practitioner in this case example uses a constraint-induced movement therapy protocol-based model, which is a rehabilitation approach, as the *organizing* model and she uses contemporary motor control and learning, biomechanical, behavioral, and CMOP-E as *complementary* models as

illustrated in Figure 3.4. This dynamic use of multiple models allows the OT practitioner to follow an evidence-based protocol, while addressing the unique needs of the client and family.

LEARNING ACTIVITY: THEORY APPLICATION ASSESSMENT INSTRUMENT

Use the case example provided above and complete the Theory Application Assessment Instrument (TAAI; Ikiugu & Smallfield, 2010, pp. 259–260).
- Discuss your findings with your peers.

STEPS OF THERAPEUTIC REASONING: USE OF PRACTICE MODELS

OT practitioners use knowledge of models of practice and frames of reference when making decisions at each stage of the therapeutic reasoning process (Wong & Fisher, 2015). The purpose of therapeutic reasoning is to gain a deep understanding of the client, contexts and issues interfering with occupational performance to provide a sound basis for intervention. It is concerned with the specific details of the person, their lives, including their illness or disability (Hutchinson et al., 2002). Therapeutic reasoning is not a linear process and involves inquiry, collaboration with the client, observation, and reflection of both client and of oneself as a practitioner (see Chapter 10). The OT practitioner may return to previous steps as they gather information or observe the client engage in activities. As they gather information during the initial interview, the OT practitioner makes decisions to explore areas or issues that arise. They reflect on the data, including assessment, interactions, and information on the client's story, experiences, and background to make decisions regarding occupational therapy intervention. Practitioners rely on knowledge of practice models to make decisions at each step of the therapeutic reasoning process.

Using Theory to Generate Questions

The first step in therapeutic reasoning involves using theory to generate questions about the client. The OT practitioner's curiosity about the client's unique situation and story, including past experiences, initiates the therapeutic reasoning process. The practitioner may have questions about the client's diagnosis, healing process, intervention approaches, and underlying factors that influence the client's performance. They may have questions about medical procedures or protocols. This information follows a medical model and primarily uses *scientific reasoning*. OT practitioners are interested in understanding the factors (such as person, environment, and tasks) that influence occupational performance. Therefore, they begin the therapeutic reasoning process using *scientific* and *narrative* reasoning to ask questions about many facets of the client's life.

Using theory to generate questions allows practitioners to fully prepare for each stage of the occupational therapy process. For example, prior to engaging a client in a semi-structured interview, authors of occupation-based models of practice suggest questions that address aspects defined in the model to provide a full picture of the client's occupational needs. The occupation-based

TABLE 3.3 Questions to Address Model of Human Occupation Components

Model	Components	Questions
Model of Human Occupation	Volition	What is important to you? (values) What is your favorite thing to do? (interests) How well do you think you do those things that you want to do? (perceived competence)
	Habituation	How do you spend your day? What are your typical roles (for example, mom)? What are the things you do in the morning?
	Performance capacity	What things are you good at doing? What is it like being you? (subjective experience)
	Environment	Where do you live? What is your home like? Where do you spend your days?

model of practice and frame of reference guide the questions and information used to create the occupational profile and further direct assessment. Table 3.3 provides sample questions based on Model of Human Occupation.

LEARNING ACTIVITY: CREATING QUESTIONS FROM THEORY

Complete Worksheet 3.6. Select an occupation-based model of practice and create questions to inform each component or element of the model.

Gather Data

The authors of occupation-based models of practice and frames of reference provide direction regarding what type of data to collect and how to gather it to understand the client's occupational performance needs. They explain the factors and concepts that influence a person's engagement in everyday living activities. The authors of models of practice and frames of reference include assessments and tools to measure the components to help OT practitioners apply concepts to practice.

For example, the Canadian Occupational Performance Measure (COPM) (Law et al., 2005) is a client-centered semi-structured interview that addresses the person's core beliefs, satisfaction with performance, and goals, which are central concepts of the Canadian Model of Occupational Performance and Engagement (CMOP-E). The Person-Environment-Occupation-Participation (PEOP) model suggests that OT practitioners use the Activity Card Sort (ACS) (Baum & Edwards, 2008) to understand the occupations for which a person engages. To measure other aspects of this model, the authors recommend that practitioners use assessments available that measure the person or environmental factors in need of further evaluation. Many assessments have been created to

specifically measure the concepts or components of the Model of Human Occupation (MOHO). The assessments are available on the MOHO clearinghouse website (www.moho.uic.edu). See Chapter 6 on selecting, choosing, and using assessments.

OT practitioners also collect data through observation and interactions with clients to understand the client's personality, lived experience, motivations, interests, and abilities. Learning about the client informs decision-making, problem-solving, and informs all aspects of the occupational therapy process.

Identify Occupational Strengths and Challenges

OT practitioners gather information based on concepts from the model and frame of reference to identify the client's strengths and challenges. They use conditional reasoning to synthesize information from a variety of sources to determine the factors influencing a person's ability to engage in desired activities.

They examine the principles of desired models and frames of reference to explain the relationships between factors and facilitate change. They use the principles associated with the occupation-based model of practice and frame of reference to make hypotheses regarding the client's occupational performance. The hypotheses generated may differ depending upon the model or frame of reference selected.

Create Intervention Plan

The practitioner uses the principles outlined in the model of practice to make decisions and address occupational challenges. Principles are the underlying assumptions regarding how systems and factors interact and result in the outcome being examined. The OT practitioner creates an intervention plan after carefully considering the client's occupational strengths and challenges. The practitioner and client collaborate to create goals for occupational therapy sessions. See Chapter 9 for specifics on creating intervention plans.

Implement the Intervention Plan

The OT practitioner implements the plan, paying careful attention to the client's responses to intervention and adjusting as needed throughout. The practitioner engages the client in creative activities to address their goals. This stage of the process involves *interactive* reasoning as the practitioner provides feedback, responds, observes, and adjusts intervention as needed. The practitioner uses *scientific reasoning* by examining and following strategies based on the principles of the model of practice and frames of reference. The art of practice involves using conditional reasoning to engage in scientific, narrative, and pragmatic reasoning, while also engaging in ethical reasoning to design intervention. Throughout the intervention stage, OT practitioners use therapeutic reasoning to make decisions, problem-solve, and consider contexts (personal and environmental).

Measure Outcomes

The outcomes of the intervention are measured throughout and may indicate the need to revise the intervention plan. OT practitioners use the outcome data to re-visit the model which may provide additional information to adjust the plan. Returning to the model and investigating the interactions more deeply may provide further insight. OT practitioners may adjust the plan after revisiting the frames of reference or select a different frame of reference. The practitioner reflects upon all aspects of the occupational therapy process to adjust intervention strategies and techniques throughout to maximize the client's progress in occupational therapy. This process includes subjective (i.e., client's satisfaction, qualitative data, lived experience) and objective measurements (standardized measures, qualitative scales, observational data).

SUMMARY

Occupation-based models of practice and frames of reference guide one's therapeutic reasoning by explaining processes and concepts of occupational performance. Using an occupation-based model of practice as one's organizing model helps OT practitioners incorporate occupational therapy theory and philosophy in practice. Frames of reference provide evidence to address underlying client factors that may be interfering with participation in one's daily occupations. Principles are statements which explain the relationships between factors based on theory. Understanding the principles of the occupation-based model of practice or frame of reference allows practitioners to use the strategies and techniques with multiple clients. OT practitioners engage in therapeutic reasoning as they consider multiple models and frames of reference to address the client's occupational performance.

REFERENCES

American Occupational Therapy Association (AOTA). (2020). Occupational therapy practice framework: domain and process (4th ed.). *American Journal of Occupational Therapy*, 74(Suppl. 2), 7412410010.

Baron, K., Kielhofner, G., Iyenger, A., Goldhammer, V., & Wolenski, J. (2006). *The Occupational Self-Assessment (OSA) (Version 2.2.)*. Chicago: Model of Human Occupation Clearinghouse, Department of Occupational Therapy, College of Applied Health Sciences, University of Illinois at Chicago.

Bass, J. D., Baum, C., & Christiansen, C. (2017). Person-environment-occupation-performance models. In J. Hinojosa, P. Kramer, & C. B. Royeen (Eds.). *Perspectives in human occupation: Theories underlying practice* (2nd ed.). Philadelphia, PA: FA Davis.

Baum, C. M., Christiansen, C. H., & Bass, J. D. (2015). Person-Environment-Occupation-Performance (PEOP) Model. In C. H. Christiansen, C. M. Baum, & J. D. Bass (Eds.), *Occupational therapy: Performance, participation, well-being* (4th ed., pp. 49–55). Thorofare, NJ: Slack.

Baum, C. M., & Edwards, D. F. (2008). *Activity card sort (ACS): test manual* (2nd ed.). North Bethesda, MD: AOTA Press.

Blanche, E. I., Fogelberg, D., Diaz, J., Carlson, M., & Clark, F. (2011). Manualization of occupational therapy interventions: Illustrations from the pressure ulcer prevention research program. *American Journal of Occupational Therapy*, 65(6), 711–719.

Bruininks, R., & Bruininks, B. (2005). *Bruininks-Oseretsky Test of Motor Proficiency* (2nd ed.). NCS Pearson.

Canadian Association of Occupational Therapists (CAOT). (1997). *Enabling occupation: An occupational therapy perspective*. Ottawa, ON: CAOT Publications ACE.

Christiansen, C. H., Baum, C. M., & Bass, J. D. (Eds.). (2015). *Occupational therapy: Performance, participation, well-being* (4th ed.). Thorofare, NJ: Slack.

Fisher, G., Parkinson, S., & Haglund, L. (2017). The environment and human occupation. In R. Taylor (Ed.), *Kielhofner's model of human occupation: Theory and application* (5th ed., pp. 91–106). Philadelphia, PA: Wolters Kluwer.

Forsyth, K. (2017). Therapeutic reasoning: Planning, implementing, and evaluating the outcomes of therapy. In R. Taylor (Ed.), *Kielhofner's model of human occupation: Theory and application* (5th ed., pp. 159–172). Philadelphia, PA: Wolters Kluwer.

Gillen, G. (2014). Motor function and occupational performance. In B. A. Boyt-Schell, G. Gillen, E. Scaffa, & E. S. Cohn (Eds.), *Willard & Spackman's occupational therapy* (12th ed., pp. 693–708). Philadelphia, PA: Wolters Kluwer.

Grajo, L. C. (2017). Occupational adaptation. In J. Hinojosa, P. Kramer, & C. B. Royeen (Eds.), *Perspectives in human occupation: Theories underlying practice* (2nd ed.). Philadelphia, PA: FA Davis.

Hutchinson, S. L., LeBlanc, A., & Booth, R. (2002). "Perceptual problem solving": An ethnographic study of clinical reasoning in a therapeutic recreation setting. *Therapeutic Recreation Journal*, 36, 18–34.

Ikiugu, M. N. (2007). *Psychosocial conceptual practice models in occupational therapy: Building adaptive capability*. St. Louis, MO: Mosby.

Ikiugu, M. N., Plastow, N. A., & van Niekerk, L. (2019). Eclectic Application of Theoretical Models in Occupational Therapy: Impact on Therapeutic Reasoning. *Occupational Therapy in Health Care*, 33(3), 286–305.

Ikiugu, M. N., Smallfield, S., & Condit, C. (2009). A framework for combining theoretical conceptual practice models in occupational therapy practice. *Canadian Journal of Occupational Therapy*, 76(3), 162–170.

Ikiugu, M. N., & Smallfield, S. (2010). Interrater, intra-rater and internal consistency reliablity of the Theory Application Assessment Instrument. *Australian Journal of Occupational Therapy*, 57, 253–260.

Iwama, M. (2006). *The Kawa Model: Culturally Relevant Occupational Therapy*. Edinburgh: Churchill Livingstone-Elsevier Press.

Keller, J., Kafkes, A., Basu, S., Federico, J., & Kielhofner, G. (2006). *Child Occupational Self Assessment (COSA) v2.1*. Model of Human Occupation Clearinghouse, Department of Occupational Therapy, University of Illinois at Chicago.

Kielhofner, G. (2004). The organization and use of knowledge. In *Conceptual foundations of occupational therapy* (pp. 10–26) (3rd ed.). Philadelphia, PA: FA Davis.

Kielhofner, G. (2008). *Model of human occupation: Theory and application* (4th ed.). Philadelphia, PA: Lippincott, Williams & Wilkins.

Kielhofner, G. & Neville, A. (1983). The Modified Interest Checklist. Unpublished manuscript. Model of Human Occupation Clearinghouse. Department of Occupational Therapy, University of Illinois at Chicago.

Law, M., Baptiste, S., Carswell, A., McColl, M. A., Polatajko, H., & Pollock, N. (2005). *Canadian occupational performance measure* (4th ed.). CAOT Publications ACE.

Llorens, L. A. (1982). *Application of developmental theory for health and rehabilitation.* Bethesda, MD: AOTA Press.

Missiuna, C., et al. (2001). Cognitive orientation to daily occupational performance (CO-OP): Part 1: Theoretical foundations. *Physical and Occupational Therapy in Pediatrics, 20*(2–3), 69–81.

O'Brien, J. C. (2018). Models of practice and frames of reference: *Introduction to occupational therapy* (pp. 138–148) (5th ed.). St. Louis, MO: Elsevier.

O'Brien, J., & Kielhofner, G. (2017). The dynamics of human occupation. In R. Taylor (Ed.), *Kielhofner's model of human occupation* (5th ed., pp. 24–37). Philadelphia, PA: Wolters Kluwer.

O'Brien, J., & Kuhaneck, H. (2020). Using occupational therapy models and frames of reference. In J. C. O'Brien & H. Kuhaneck (Eds.), *Case Smiths' occupational therapy for children and adolescents* (8th ed., p. 23; pp. 33–36). St. Louis, MO: Elsevier.

O'Brien, J. C., Coker-Bolt, P. C., & Dimitropoulou, K. (2020a). Application of motor control and motor learning. In J. C. O'Brien & H. Kuhaneck (Eds.), *Case Smiths' occupational therapy for children and adolescents* (8th ed., pp. 395–411). St. Louis, MO: Elsevier.

O'Brien, J., Stoffel, A., Fisher, G., & Iwami, M. (2020b). Occupational-centered models of practice. In N. Carson (Ed.). *Psychosocial occupational therapy* (pp. 47–75). Philadelphia, PA: Elsevier.

Parham, L. D., & Mailloux, Z. (2020). Sensory integration. In J. C. O'Brien & H. Kuhaneck (Eds.), *Case Smiths' occupational therapy for children and adolescents* (8th ed.). St. Louis, MO: Elsevier.

Polatajko, H. J., Townsend, E. A., & Craik, J. (2007). Canadian Model of Occupational Performance and Engagement (CMOP-E). In E. A. Townsend & H. J. Polatajko (Eds.), *Enabling occupation II: Advancing an occupational therapy vision of health, well-being, & justice through occupation* (pp. 22–36). Ottawa, ON: CAOT Publications ACE.

Pyatak, E. A., Carandang, K., & Davis, S. (2015). Developing a manualized occupational therapy diabetes management intervention: Resilient, Empowered, Active Living with Diabetes. *OTJR: Occupation, Participation and Health, 35*(3), 187–194.

Radomski, M. V., & Latham Trombly, C. A. (2008). *Occupational therapy for physical dysfunction.* Philadelphia, PA: Lippincott Williams & Wilkin.

Rybski, M. (2012). Biomechanical intervention approach. In *Kinesiology for occupational therapy* (pp. 309–354). Thorofare, NJ: SLACK, Inc.

Schkade, J. K., & Schultz, S. (2003). Occupational adaptation. In P. Kramer, J. Hinojosa, & C. B. Royeen (Eds.), *Perspectives in human occupation: Participation in life* (pp. 181–221). Philadelphia, PA: Lippincott Williams & Wilkins.

Taylor, R. (2017). *Kielhofner's model of human occupation: Theory and application* (5th ed.). Philadelphia, PA: Wolters Kluwer.

Turpin, M. J., & Iwama, M. K. (2011). *Using Occupational therapy models in practice: A fieldguide.* London: Elsevier Health Sciences.

Wong, S., & Fisher, G. (2015). Comparing and using occupation-focused models. *Occupational therapy in health care, 29*(3), 297–315.

WORKSHEET 3.1: GENERATING QUESTIONS

List questions you have regarding one or more of the following case scenarios. Then categorize similar questions. Return to this exercise after reading the chapter and add questions by referring to an occupation-based model of practice. Reflect on how the occupation-based model of practice provided additional structure and depth to the questions.

- A new therapist working in a school setting receives a referral to evaluate a 7-year-old child who is having trouble in school.
- A therapist working in adult rehabilitation is evaluating a 70-year-old man who experienced a stroke.
- A therapist working in acute care receives a referral to evaluate the needs of a 30-year-old who experienced a traumatic brain injury.

Generating Questions
1. Case scenario:
2. List questions about the case prior to reading chapter.
3. Categorize similar questions together.
4. List questions after reading the chapter.
5. Categorize similar questions together.
6. Describe how your questions changed or did not change.
7. How did a model of practice inform your questions about the scenario?

WORKSHEET 3.2: EXAMINING THE LITERATURE

Summarize findings from a current research article that describes the use of an occupation-based model of practice in an occupational therapy setting.

- Describe the purpose of the research.
- Summarize the methodology.
- What factors or components of the model did the authors address?
- Describe the principles (if any) outlined in the study.
- What were the findings of the research?
- What did you learn about the occupation-based model of practice from this study?

Examining the Literature
Reference (APA format) for current research article that describes an occupation-based model of practice in occupational therapy setting.
Purpose of study:
Methodology:
Briefly describe the concepts or components of the model the authors address in the study.
Describe the principles of the model outlined in the study.
Findings of study.
What did you learn from the study?

WORKSHEET 3.3: COMPARING OCCUPATION-BASED MODELS OF PRACTICE

- Complete the following chart to describe how each model would examine Grace's case.

Comparing occupation-based models of practice			
	MOHO	**PEOP**	**CMOP-E**
Components of model (Provide examples from case to describe each component.)	Volition: Habituation: Performance: Environment:	Person: Environment: Occupation: Participation:	
Provide a summary of Grace's occupational performance strengths and challenges using terminology from the model.			
Describe what is interfering with Grace's occupational performance.			
List assessments you would complete to gather more information on Grace.			
Describe how you will intervene.			
1. How are the models alike and different from each other?			
2. Which model do you prefer? Why?			
3. How do the models organize or structure your therapeutic reasoning?			

WORKSHEET 3.4: FRAMES OF REFERENCE

Compare 3 different frames of reference. Describe how an OT practitioner uses the principles to promote occupational performance.
- Describe 3 different frames of reference and list 1 or 2 principles for each frame of reference.
- Create an activity that you would use in practice addressing the selected principles.

Frames of Reference		
Frame of Reference	**List 1 or 2 principles for the frame of reference**	**Describe activity to address each principle**

WORKSHEET 3.5: COMBINING PRACTICE MODELS

Analyze the use of practice models by completing the worksheet. Refer to the Theory Application Assessment Instrument (TIAA) (Ikiugu & Smallfield, 2010) for additional questions.
- Identify the practice models used in the case and provide a brief description of each.
- Describe why the practitioner chose each of the practice models listed above.
- Explain how you would use each of the models to guide client assessment and intervention planning.

Combining Practice Models			
Practice Models Used in Case	Brief Description of Practice Model	Describe Why the Practitioner Chose Model	How Would You Use Model to Guide Client Assessment and Intervention Planning?

WORKSHEET 3.6: CREATING QUESTIONS FROM THEORY

Select an occupation-based model of practice and create questions to inform each concept or component of the model.

Creating Questions from Theory	
Occupation-based model of practice:	
Brief description:	
Concept or Component of model	Questions

4

Therapeutic Use of Self

Jane O'Brien

GUIDING QUESTIONS

1. What is therapeutic use of self?
2. What factors and processes are part of the therapeutic relationship?
3. What are skills and abilities that enhance therapeutic use of self?
4. What is the Intentional Relationship Model (IRM; Taylor, 2020)?
5. How do IRM concepts inform therapeutic relationships and guide therapy?
6. How does interactive or interpersonal reasoning inform therapeutic use of self?

KEY TERMS

Emotional intelligence

Inevitable events

Intentional Relationship Model (IRM)

Interactive (or interpersonal) reasoning

Interpersonal events

Interpretive approach

Intuitive knowledge

Multimodal approach

Mode shift

Perceptual problem-solving

Sub-optimal interactions

Therapeutic modes

Therapeutic use of self

INTRODUCTION

Therapeutic use of self refers to a "practitioner's planned use of his or her personality, insights, perceptions, and judgments as part of the therapeutic process" (Punwar & Peloquin, 2000, p. 285). Taylor, Lee, Kielhofner, and Ketkar (2009) surveyed occupational therapists' attitudes toward and experiences of therapeutic use of self to examine perceived importance in therapeutic reasoning. Of 568 respondents, 87% viewed therapeutic use of self as the most important aspect of their practice, and 80% reported that therapeutic reasoning should always include use of self.

Definitions of therapeutic use of self include communication, emotional exchange, and collaboration and partnership between therapists and clients (Taylor et al., 2009). Therapeutic use of self has been viewed as important to client-centered care and the occupational therapy process (AOTA, 2020) and authors have described factors contributing to therapeutic use of self (Allison & Strong, 1994; Chaffey et al., 2012; Eklund & Hallberg, 2001; Guidetti & Tham, 2002; Jenkins et al., 1994). Taylor (2020) developed the Intentional Relationship Model (IRM) to conceptualize the process and describe the approaches OT practitioners use when engaged with clients. The IRM

provides insight into how OT practitioners can enhance their abilities to improve therapeutic interactions and results.

This chapter provides an overview of the literature examining therapeutic use of self and the therapeutic reasoning involved during the client–therapist interaction. The author describes the Intentional Relationship Model (IRM; Taylor, 2020) and its use in practice. Case examples and learning activities are interspersed throughout the chapter to illustrate the concepts.

OVERVIEW OF THERAPEUTIC USE OF SELF CONCEPTS

Therapeutic use of self involves one's conscious interactions with clients in a manner to support occupational therapy goals (Cole & McLean, 2003; Punwar & Peloquin, 2000). Therapeutic use of self is recognized as essential to the occupational therapy process (AOTA, 2020; ACOTE, 2018; Cole & McLean, 2003; Solman & Clouston, 2016; Taylor et al., 2009). Many authors have described factors and processes that influence therapeutic use of self (Allison & Strong, 1994; Baum, 1980; Cole & McLean, 2003; Fleming, 1991; Mattingly, 1994; Peloquin, 2005; Restall et al., 2003), although until recently

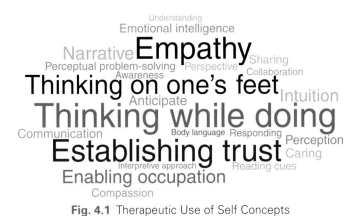

Fig. 4.1 Therapeutic Use of Self Concepts

there was no consistent organization or framework (Solman & Clouston, 2016). Figure 4.1 identifies many of the concepts described in occupational therapy literature regarding therapeutic use of self.

Therapeutic use of self includes building a relationship, establishing trust, motivating clients, and providing an enabling occupational experience (Guidetti & Tham, 2002). Communication is a key factor in creating the client–therapist relationship in occupational therapy practice (Cole & McLean, 2003). OT practitioners with good communication skills adjust their interactions to match the client (Allison & Strong, 1994; Eklund & Hallberg, 2001), which serves to keep clients motivated. Communication can facilitate a client-centered or collaborative approach to occupational therapy and support the client in reaching their goals (Cole & McLean, 2003; Sumsion, 2000). Jenkins et al. (1994) found that more experienced therapists achieved more mutual participation in the therapy session.

Empathy and caring are important in the occupational therapy process (Baum, 1980; Cole & McLean, 2003; Peloquin, 2005). Empathy refers to a "multidimensional, complex, emotional, cognitive, and movement process that emerges from an objective and subjective impression of another person's emotional state or perspective" (Davis, 1983; Decety & Batson, 2007; in Abreau, 2011, p. 624). Abreau (2011) urged OT practitioners to reflect on the empathetic process in practice. She described positive empathic interactions for practitioners as: use of creativity and imagination; use of reflection and self-regulation; willingness to enter the other's emotional state and perspective; sharing resilience stories as a source of inspiration and motivation; reading other people's actions and language patterns, variations, or prosody; and promoting other people's hope and strength (Abreu, 2011). Gahnstrom-Strandqvist and colleagues (2000) found the ability to form an empathetic relationship included learning about the client through the narrative, understanding the client's roles (past and future), and seeing the client as a person. When the therapists did not use empathy, they did not feel competent in their profession (Gahnstrom-Strandqvist et al., 2000).

To understand how therapeutic use of self is used in OT practice, researchers have examined traits in novice and expert practitioners (Akerjordet & Severinsson, 2004; Chaffey et al.,

2012; Leicht & Dickerson, 2001). More experienced therapists can understand interactions better with fewer cues, as compared to novice therapists (Leicht & Dickerson, 2001). Experienced therapists reported a preference for an intuitive cognitive style to a greater extent than novices, who preferred explicit learning (Chaffey et al., 2012). Reading and responding to cues during therapy and making decisions intuitively requires reflecting on the process, exploring one's reasons, beliefs, values, cultures, and theoretical conceptions. Intuitive knowledge refers to immediate knowledge accessed without a conscious awareness of reasoning (Chaffey et al., 2010). Intuition, which is influenced by awareness and understanding emotions, can be used as a clinical tool to build relationships with clients and contribute to decision-making (Akerjordet & Severinsson 2004). Intuition provides participants with emotional information about their practice (Akerjordet & Severinsson, 2004). Chaffey, Unsworth, and Fossey (2010) found that therapists use emotions to access intuition, trust their emotions to act upon them, and to solve problems and make decisions. Therapists with more years of experience reported being more comfortable using intuition in therapeutic reasoning than those with less experience.

Some researchers have linked emotional intelligence to therapeutic use of self (Chaffey et al., 2012; Howe, 2008). Emotional intelligence is awareness and understanding of one's own emotions (Howe, 2008). Making decisions based on the client's emotions while being self-aware allows the OT practitioner to empathize while maintaining professional boundaries and think while doing. Thinking on one's feet has been described as perceptual problem-solving, which involves observation in connection with anticipation of how a situation may possibly develop (Hutchinson et al., 2002).

OT practitioners rely on understanding the client's perspective by listening to the client's narrative (Fleming, 1991; Mattingly, 1994; Schell, 2003; Schell & Cervero, 1993). Therapeutic reasoning is both a way of thinking and interacting with clients that facilitates effective client-centered practice (Hutchinson et al., 2002; Mattingly & Fleming, 1994). Mattingly (1991) described this process as involving an interpretive approach to focus on how clients make sense of their disability and its meaning in their individual lives. This requires practitioners to anticipate future performance or responses. The Intentional Relationship Model (IRM; Taylor, 2020) provides a conceptual framework that provides practitioners with definitions, tools, and strategies to use in practice to promote therapeutic use of self.

THE INTENTIONAL RELATIONSHIP MODEL (IRM)

The Intentional Relationship Model *(IRM)* (Taylor, 2020) was created to explain the process of therapeutic use of self, which is defined as "the application of empathy and intentionality to an interpersonal knowledge base and corresponding skill set that is applied thoughtfully to resolve challenging or poignant interpersonal events in practice" (Taylor & Van Puymbrouck, 2022, p. 33). OT practitioners seek to understand clients at an

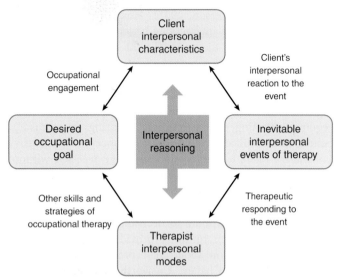

Fig. 4.2 A Model of Intentional Relationship in Occupational Therapy. (From Taylor, 2020.)

interpersonal level focusing on their communication preferences and needs (Taylor, 2020). This process involves making moment to moment decisions about how to initiate and respond to therapy and/or the therapist (Taylor, 2020). The Intentional Relationship Model (Taylor, 2020) is illustrated in Figure 4.2.

The model identifies four aspects of the therapist–client relationship:
1. Client's interpersonal characteristics
2. Inevitable interpersonal events of therapy
3. Therapist interpersonal modes
4. Desired occupational goal

OT practitioners use interactive reasoning to understand how to communicate to the client given the client's interpersonal characteristics. They make decisions regarding how they will communicate (i.e., mode use). The client's reactions to inevitable events may require the therapist to change their mode of communication to support the client's engagement in activities and achieving their occupational goal.

Client's Interpersonal Characteristics

Each person has their own personality, style, and ways of communicating based on their experiences, cultural influences, upbringing, and personality. Table 4.1 provides clinical examples of interpersonal characteristics and possible responses from the OT practitioner. These interpersonal characteristics influence the therapeutic relationship. IRM (Taylor, 2020) defines interpersonal characteristics of clients in terms of the following 14 categories:
- Communication style
- Tone of voice
- Body language
- Facial expression (affect)
- Response to change or challenge
- Level of trust
- Need for control
- Approach to asserting needs
- Predisposition to giving feedback
- Capacity to receive feedback
- Response to human diversity
- Orientation to relating
- Preference for touch
- Interpersonal reciprocity

Understanding the client's interpersonal characteristics informs the therapist's intervention decisions and mode use. For example, clients who need a high degree of control will respond better when provided choices. Knowing that a client is an introspective learner allows the therapist to provide reflective exercises and avoid "small talk" that other clients may enjoy. Understanding how a client asserts their needs allows the therapist to encourage the client to communicate. Listening to feedback or watching for feedback from the client allows the therapist to best match their style with the client to make therapeutic gains. The therapeutic relationship is about creating a positive relationship with the client, so the client achieves their goals. Knowing the client's interpersonal characteristics allows the therapist to make decisions quickly and understand therapy situations more clearly so that adjustments can be made to promote therapy goals.

> ### LEARNING ACTIVITY: INTERPERSONAL CHARACTERISTICS EXAMPLES
>
> Provide examples describing the interpersonal characteristics (listed in Worksheet 4.1) of a close family member or friend.
> - Describe how a person meeting them for the first time should approach them.
> - Describe an activity that the person might enjoy.
> - Describe how their interpersonal characteristics influence your activity choice.

Inevitable Interpersonal Events

In every therapeutic relationship, there are circumstances or situations that occur in therapy that may evoke strong emotions (positive or negative). Knowing how to anticipate them and respond to them therapeutically takes practice. According to IRM, an interpersonal event is "a naturally occurring communication, reaction, process, task, or general circumstance that occurs during therapy and that has the potential to detract from or strengthen the therapeutic relationship" (Taylor, 2020, p. 59.). Table 4.2 provides a description and example of each category of inevitable interpersonal events. When an event occurs, the OT practitioner must address it in a way to foster the therapeutic relationship. Inevitable events should not be ignored or taken lightly as that can threaten the client's occupational therapy intervention progress. However, when the OT practitioner responds optimally to these events, it provides opportunities for change. Inevitable events occur during the therapy process and are unavoidable. OT practitioners anticipate and notice these events, so they are prepared to address them therapeutically. Role playing can be an effective way to try out strategies for practice.

TABLE 4.1 Examples of Interpersonal Characteristics (based on the Intentional Relationship Model; Taylor, 2020).

Interpersonal Characteristic	Clinical Example	Possible Responses from Therapist
Communication style	Trey is aggressive and negative when questioned during the initial interview. He is unhappy about his recent accident and does not want to talk to the therapist. He answers questions briefly, providing limited explanation. His wife confirms her husband is "not a talker."	Engage Trey in an activity at which he can be successful to learn about him. Allow him to initiate conversation.
Tone of voice	Marli asks questions in a loud demanding tone. She responds to questions in this same tone.	Begin session with relaxation techniques (Marli may be anxious). Engage in role play activities to allow Marli to express feelings.
Body language	Aisha turns away and avoids eye contact when the therapist enters the room. He shrugs his shoulders when the therapist says hello. Aisha is reluctant to engage in therapy.	Begin the session with short simple activities and find goals that are meaningful to the client. Provide a different setting for therapy (walk outside) or include a peer.
Level of trust	Skylar, a 10-year-old boy with coordination problems, is afraid of having his feet off the ground and does not want to engage in activities on the swing despite encouragement from the therapist.	Provide movement activities that Skylar can control where he does not have to lift his feet off the ground and follow through with expectations so Skylar can develop a level of trust.
Need for control	Marvin sits in the same seat every session. He starts the session with a cup of tea. One day he attends and someone else is in his seat and he becomes very upset.	Begin the session with a cup of tea as always. Start with another familiar activity until Marvin begins to relax and engage. Have Marvin appraise his ability to be flexible.
Approach to asserting needs	Collin is unable to take the top off a container but refuses to ask for help from the therapist. He would rather "do without."	Ask Collin if he needs help. Role play situations to illustrate the benefits in asserting one's needs. Discuss how other people feel when helping him.
Response to change and challenge	Praya becomes visibly upset when transitioning to different classes at school.	Role play transitions. Provide clear schedules. Reinforce coping strategies.
Affect	Aline vacillates from giddy and silly to angry and mad quickly, depending upon the intervention activity.	Reinforce coping strategies, role play emotions and managing one's affect.
Predisposition to giving feedback	Cory provides harsh and negative feedback to the OT practitioner every session.	The OT practitioner hypothesizes that Cory is also critical of his own performance and may not be progressing as he hopes. The practitioner provides a chart for him to plot his progress each session. The form includes questions to promote positive feedback as well.
Capacity to receive feedback	Rich becomes irritable when the therapist provides feedback that he should pay more attention to others when maneuvering his new wheelchair in the community. He ignores the therapist and continues to get close to others and objects.	The therapist decides that Rich's capacity to receive feedback may interfere with his progression towards goals, prompting a discussion. In a quiet setting, the therapist brings up the scenario and reviews Rich's strengths, asks him for feedback, and works with him to address this together.
Response to human diversity	Lucille, an 85-year-old woman, becomes unpleasant and shows an aversion to the student therapist who speaks with an accent. Lucille tells the supervisor that she does not want to work with the student because "she's not from here."	The supervisor may assign the student to other clients. The supervisor may have a conversation with Lucille to encourage her to be open to the creativity and knowledge the student may bring.
Orientation toward relating	Hisah displays his nurturing relationship through hugging, holding hands, and close contact with friends and family in public.	The OT practitioner is aware that Hisah displays his emotions through physical acts. To keep the professional boundaries, she lets Hisah know when she needs to get close to support him.
Preference for touch	Caleb does not like to be touched by people who are not family.	The therapist lets Caleb know when she needs to touch him and keeps this to a minimum if possible.
Interpersonal reciprocity	Sarah quickly realizes the therapist also has children and frequently inquires about the therapist's children, issues around parenting, and provides advice to the therapist.	The therapist relates to Sarah and responds to her questions, but is careful to maintain professional boundaries.

LEARNING ACTIVITY: ROLE PLAY INEVITABLE EVENTS

Use Worksheet 4.2 to describe your findings. In pairs, select an interpersonal event category from Table 4.2. Role play a scenario illustrating a negative or positive event based on this category. Have one partner play the "therapist" and the other the "client".
- How did the therapist handle the event?
- What might have triggered the client's response?
- Describe your emotions during the role play (as therapist and client).
- Did the therapist facilitate communication?
- What other things could the therapist have done?
- How might the client and therapist learn from this experience?

Therapeutic Interpersonal Modes

A therapeutic mode is a specific way of relating to a client. The IRM identifies six **therapeutic modes** as illustrated in Figure 4.3.

See Table 4.3 for a brief description of each mode. OT practitioners have natural modes that they prefer. However, one's preferred mode may not always match with a client's interpersonal characteristics and needs. Since OT practitioners work with a variety of clients, it is best to learn how to use all modes flexibly and comfortably. The **multimodal** interpersonal style allows the therapist to match the client's preferred mode and

TABLE 4.2 Inevitable Interpersonal Events (based on Taylor, 2020; Taylor & Van Puymbrouck, 2022)

Interpersonal Event	Definition	Clinical Example
Expression of strong emotion	External displays of internal feelings are shown with a high level of intensity beyond usual cultural norms for interaction. Can be positive or negative expressions.	Macy (2-year-old) bursts into tears when it is time to leave the OT play group.
Intimate self-disclosures	Statements or stories reveal something unobservable, private, or sensitive about the person making a disclosure. These can be stories about oneself or about close others.	Jake reveals in an OT group session that he knows several clients on the mental health unit who used drugs when off campus.
Power dilemmas	Tensions arise in the therapeutic relationship because of the client's innate feelings about issues of power, the inherent situation of therapy, the therapist's behavior, or other circumstances that underscore the client's lack or loss of power over aspects of their lives.	Buddy, a 75-year-old man who experienced a recent stroke refuses to go to a rehabilitation unit and insists he goes home (despite his wife and the team's advice).
Nonverbal cues	Communications do not involve the use of formal language. Some examples of these are facial expressions, movement patterns, body posture, and eye contact.	Becca smirks and sighs when asked to make a sandwich as part of the evaluation. She handles the ingredients forcefully and makes little eye contact with the therapist. She works quickly.
Verbal innuendos	Communications in which the client says something illusive or oblique that is meant to serve as a hint about a more direct communication.	Marcus makes comments about the quality of the projects he completes in OT, stating things such as: "Wow, now I can build cabinets at home." "This picture frame looks like my daughter made it." "Maybe I can get a job painting after this."
Crisis points	Unanticipated, stressful events cause clients to become distracted or temporarily interfere with a client's ability for occupational engagement.	Jasmine sustained a head injury requiring she engage in an inpatient rehabilitation program. However, since she is unemployed, she learned she may lose her apartment and have no place to live upon discharge.
Resistance and reluctance	Resistance is a client's passive or active refusal to participate in some or all aspects of therapy for reasons linked to the therapeutic relationship. Reluctance is disinclination toward some aspect of therapy for reasons outside the therapeutic relationship.	Karl refuses to participate in group "mealtime sessions" because he does not want someone to "feed him" or others to see he is "messy now." Karl is reluctant to try adaptive equipment because he does not want to "look different" among his friends.
Boundary testing	A client's behavior violates or asks the therapist to act in ways outside the defined therapeutic relationship.	A young adult receiving day treatment mental health services asks an OT practitioner (close in age) to go to the movies.
Empathic breaks	The therapist fails to notice or understand a communication from a client, or communication or behavior initiated by the therapist is perceived by the client as hurtful or insensitive.	A client becomes quiet when the therapist states "finally, you did it!" Later that day, the client avoids eye contact with the therapist. The therapist approaches the client and the client explains that he has been working hard, not feeling like he was making adequate progress, and the comment "finally, you did it!" sounded to him like the therapist was also frustrated in his progress. The client perceived it as hurtful.
Emotionally charged therapy tasks or situations	Activities or circumstances can lead clients to become overwhelmed or experience uncomfortable emotional reactions such as embarrassment, humiliation, or shame.	Payxon is unable to remember her family members' names although she recognizes their faces. She bursts into tears.
Limitations of therapy	There are restrictions on the available or possible services, time, resources, or therapist actions.	Agnes and the OT practitioner planned to take a walk outside along a trail, but the therapy team is short-staffed and they cannot leave the intervention room.
Contextual inconsistencies	Any aspect of a client's interpersonal or physical environment changes during the course of therapy.	The OT kitchen is being renovated for 2 weeks.

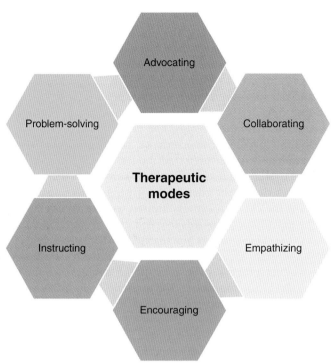

Fig. 4.3 Therapeutic Modes

shift to other modes when needed. The use of a mode and any *mode shifts* (conscious change in mode) are based on the interpersonal events of the session and the client. For example, a client may perceive that the therapist using encouragement is too cheerful and is not listening to their concerns regarding progress towards goals. The therapist may decide to switch from encouraging to empathizing mode to better listen and understand the client's viewpoint to modify the intervention for better therapeutic results.

LEARNING ACTIVITY: SELF-ASSESSMENT OF MODES

Worksheet 4.3: Complete the Self-Assessment of Modes Questionnaire (Taylor, et al., 2013; Taylor & Popova, 2019) and identify your preferred modes of communication.
- Describe your thoughts regarding your mode assessment. Is this what you expected?
- How do these modes support therapeutic relationships?
- In what situations might these modes not work?
- How might you develop skills in your less preferred modes?

TABLE 4.3 The Six Therapeutic Modes based on the Intentional Relationship Model (Taylor, 2020; Taylor & Van Puymbrouck, 2022)

Mode	Definition	Therapy Example
Advocating	The therapist ensures that the client's rights are enforced and resources are secured. May require the therapist to serve as a mediator, facilitator, negotiator, enforcer, or other type of advocate with external persons and agencies.	The medical team recommends the client go to rehabilitation but the client wants to go home with home health services. The OT practitioner completes a home evaluation and secures adaptive equipment.
Collaborating	The therapist expects the client to be an active and equal participant in therapy, and ensures choice, freedom, and autonomy to the greatest extent possible.	Using a family-centered approach, the OT practitioner collaborates with the parents to create intervention whereby the child is active and has choices and the parents are involved in decisions along the way.
Empathizing	The therapist continually strives to understand the client's thoughts, feelings, and behaviors while suspending any judgment. The therapist ensures that the client verifies and experiences the therapist's understanding as truthful and validating.	The OT practitioner working in a school setting asks Gavin how he feels about school. The practitioner validates Gavin's concerns and uses this information to make decisions. For example, Gavin feels he misses out on some of the fun lunchtime talk because he goes to the OT room for lunch. The OT understands how social times are important and together they decide that Gavin will eat foods he can handle on his own (i.e., finger foods, easily unwrapped and not messy) so he can sit with peers.
Encouraging	The therapist seizes the opportunity to instill hope in a client and celebrate a client's thinking or behavior through positive reinforcement. The therapist conveys an attitude of joyfulness, playfulness, and confidence.	Margie reaches her goal of making a simple lunch for herself and a friend. The OT practitioner claps and enthusiastically reinforces the accomplishment.
Instructing	The therapist carefully structures therapy activities and is explicit with clients about the plan, sequence, and events of therapy. The therapist provides clear instruction and feedback about performance and sets limits on a client's requests or behavior.	The OT practitioner teaches 10-year-old Alice to jump rope by carefully reviewing the steps and providing clear directions with demonstration. The practitioner provides feedback about how Alice performed and reinforces key concepts.
Problem-solving	The therapist facilitates pragmatic thinking and solving dilemmas by outlining choices, posing strategic questions, and providing opportunities for comparative or analytic thinking.	The OT practitioner engages Max in an activity to figure out and problem-solve how to use public transportation to participate in interesting local events. The practitioner poses specific questions to structure the session. In the end, Max chooses the event and describes the bus that he needs to take to get there (and times).

Interpersonal Reasoning

Interactive reasoning refers to the process of determining how to therapeutically engage with clients, including reading and providing cues, adjusting one's interactions, and promoting a relationship that benefits the client. Taylor (2020) uses the term **interpersonal reasoning** to describe the IRM process "by which a therapist decides what to say, do, or express in reaction to the occurrence of an interpersonal dilemma in therapy" (p. 66). While both terms describe the reasoning involved during therapeutic interactions, the authors of this textbook will use interactive reasoning unless specifically referring to the IRM model.

See Table 4.4 for definitions of each step of the interpersonal reasoning process as defined in IRM (Taylor, 2020). The first step involves using observational skills and information about the client to anticipate the client's interpersonal characteristics and what events may occur. The anticipatory step relies on knowledge, observational skills, and experience. It involves awareness of an intuitive sense of the person's personality traits and communication style. It may be influenced by culture, upbringing, and setting. In this sense, practitioners keep an open mind that things may not always be what one thinks at the start of a session. For example, the OT practitioner may anticipate that the client will be impatient with the recovery process given the client's "type A" personality (as stated by his wife), need to succeed, and competitive nature (as observed by the practitioner), which may result in frustration during therapy.

Knowing this about the client, the OT practitioner pays attention when the client suggests in a frustrating tone that a more qualified therapist might be better at addressing his goals. The OT practitioner identifies this interaction as an interpersonal event that can be defined as "power struggle." The practitioner takes a deep breath and reminds herself not to take it personally. This is an important step in the reasoning process as it allows the therapist to make the event about the client and view it as an opportunity for client growth.

The next step in the process is to determine if a mode shift is required. Being aware of the situations that may arise and carefully working through them by examining different modes strengthens the therapeutic relationship. Using *mode shifts* to change the direction of the therapy session changes the dynamics and can strengthen the therapeutic relationship. The practitioner considers modes that are suitable for addressing the client's frustration in therapy. She uses knowledge about the client's interpersonal characteristics, the interpersonal event, and awareness of her preferred modes. The OT practitioner decides to shift modes from problem-solving (as that was the mode that caused the client to be frustrated) to empathizing to allow the client to express himself without feeling judged by the practitioner. Towards that end, the OT practitioner sits next to the client and asks him to explain what he is feeling and why. They have a frank conversation about the frustrations of not making progress. The practitioner avoids encouraging and problem-solving modes. She uses knowledge of interview techniques to listen and respond (such as paraphrasing, asking questions, listening).

It is important to gather feedback from the client to understand their perception of the experience. The practitioner ends the session by asking the client if it was helpful to discuss his frustrations and progress. This example illustrates the interpersonal reasoning process. Therapeutic relationships build over time as one gets to know clients and understand their motives for behaviors.

Inevitable interpersonal events occur during occupational therapy intervention and may be turning points in the relationship and, consequently, the client's progress towards goals. Therefore, it is important for OT practitioners to thoughtfully work through those events.

Understanding the interpersonal reasoning process provides a structure for OT practitioners to examine multiple aspects of the situation. For example, OT practitioners may find that

TABLE 4.4	The Six Steps of the Interpersonal Reasoning Process (from: Taylor & Van Puymbrouck, 2022, p. 40)
Step of Interpersonal Reasoning	**Definition**
Anticipate	Use observational skills, information from others who have interacted with the client, and your direct experience interacting with the client to anticipate the likely interpersonal events that may occur during therapy, given your knowledge of the client's interpersonal characteristics.
Identify and cope	Use IRM language to label a difficult client characteristic or interpersonal event when it occurs. Do what it takes to collect yourself and get emotional perspective on the situation. Remind yourself not to take it personally.
Determine if a mode shift is required	Ask yourself the following questions to determine whether a mode shift is required: • What mode am I currently using with this client, if any? • What are the effects of the mode on the client? • Would another mode better serve the interpersonal needs of this client at this moment?
Choose a response mode or mode sequence	Interact within the mode or modes that you think the client prefers or needs at this moment. Think about a sequence of modes that you might use to accommodate changes in what the client might need from moment to moment.
Draw on any relevant interpersonal skills associated with the modes	Think about other communication, rapport-building, and conflict resolution skills that you might draw on in association with your mode use.
Gather feedback	Gather nonverbal or verbal feedback from the client as to whether he or she feels comfortable with the way you approached the event or difficulty.

a client is "non-compliant, resistant, and unwilling to engage in the intervention activities." They might attribute reasons for this behavior by believing the client "is passive-aggressive, unrealistic in their expectations, unmotivated, or invested in being in the patient role." If the practitioner does not work collaboratively with the client to understand and address the circumstances creating non-compliance and resistance, the client may not reach their goals. Conversely, once the OT practitioner learns the client's motives for the behavior, the practitioner may be able to address those barriers with the client leading to positive therapy outcomes.

OT practitioners have many anecdotal stories of changing the course of therapy, addressing a concern, and re-establishing the therapeutic relationship (Mattingly & Fleming, 1994). For example, there was an older woman who did not want to go to the rehabilitation gym for occupational therapy. By trying to understand the situation more clearly, the OT practitioner learned that the woman was concerned about her appearance in public since her stroke because she could not adequately put makeup on or comb her hair. She explained to the practitioner that she was raised that women do not leave the house without being "properly" groomed. The OT practitioner embraced this new information and created intervention to address morning grooming activities in the client's room. Once the client was "ready", she gladly went to the rehabilitation gym. The client received compliments from others, who also held her beliefs and they asked for assistance to learn to complete their morning grooming activities. The OT practitioner created a "Make-over" group. Group members used assistive devices and adapted materials to perform their morning routines. The group sessions addressed postural control, reaching, bilateral hand skills, fine motor skills, problem-solving, timing and sequencing, and social participation. This group became a unique part of the rehabilitation gym and eventually members completed a "runway" walk as part of their physical therapy gait training. This example shows the importance of the therapeutic relationship and understanding circumstances from multiple perspectives.

LEARNING ACTIVITY: INTERPERSONAL REASONING

Worksheet 4.4: Select one example of an inevitable interpersonal event (outlined in Table 4.2). Describe the interpersonal reasoning steps (see Table 4.4) that may provide insight into the event.
- What additional questions surfaced from doing this exercise?
- How does imagining and practicing the interpersonal reasoning process enhance one's therapeutic use of self?

LEARNING ACTIVITY: EXPLORING INEVITABLE EVENTS

Worksheet 4.5: Contact an OT practitioner to identify and describe inevitable events that they experience in practice.
- How can using the interpersonal reasoning process inform the event?

MEASUREMENTS OF MODE USE

The IRM acknowledges that OT practitioners have natural preferred communication styles. Thus, understanding your preferred mode use and acknowledging situations where these modes may support the therapeutic relationship is a good starting point. For example, when working with children using the encouraging mode of being playful, exuberant, and positive may help children challenge themselves and feel proud when they succeed. However, it may not work for an adult client in acute care who is discouraged and wondering how she will now take care of her children after a traumatic injury. Understanding when to use a different mode allows practitioners to work effectively with a variety of clients. OT practitioners who carefully match their mode use to the client's situation create strong therapeutic relationships.

A variety of assessments have been developed based on the IRM to provide information to understand mode use in practice settings. These assessments are available on the IRM Clearinghouse website (https://irm.ahs.uic.edu/). See Chapter 10 for descriptions of the assessments.

APPLICATION OF IRM IN PRACTICE

The IRM provides a structure to understand therapeutic relationships and to develop skills and abilities to promote enhanced interactions to benefit clients in occupational therapy. The following case example shows how concepts from IRM may be applied in practice. Figure 4.4 illustrates the shifts in modes.

Fiona is a 3-year-old girl with right hemiplegic cerebral palsy, visual field cut, cognitive and language delays. She recently received botulinum toxin injections to her right bicep. The physiatrist referred her to occupational therapy to assess right arm range of motion, fabricate a right elbow extension splint, and provide a home exercise program to maximize the benefit of the injection to improve Fiona's ability to use her right arm for daily activities and play.

Prior to the appointment, the OT (Isabella) performed a chart review. The OT evaluation from Early Intervention a year ago reported that Fiona was hypersensitive to touch based on clinical observations and findings from the Infant/Toddler Sensory Profile (Dunn, 2002). The evaluation indicated delayed cognition in the context of play and delayed bimanual skills. Additionally, the neuropsychology report from last month stated that Fiona is functioning at approximately the 20-month level.

The therapist uses the information to anticipate how Fiona and her parents may present so that she may adjust her mode to best relate to them. Isabella considers the parents are traveling an hour after school to come to the therapy session and may be busy. Isabella decides she wants to maximize the therapy time and collaborate with the parent, while quickly assessing Fiona's needs.

The mother arrives on time with Fiona and her 5-year-old brother. The mother is tense and attentive to the children and surroundings. Fiona is rubbing her eyes upon arrival and eating crackers from a bag her brother is holding for her. After observing these behaviors, Isabella uses *pragmatic reasoning* and decides to start with the parent interview since she believes

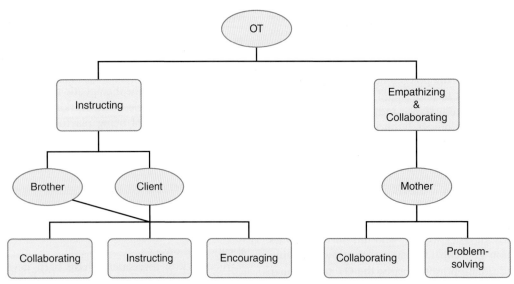

Fig. 4.4 Use of Therapeutic Modes in Case Example

that Fiona prefers to finish her snack. In her experience, she knows that children rubbing their eyes indicates fatigue or that it is nearly nap time. Isabella wants to engage Fiona in the evaluation activities before she becomes sleepy.

Isabella decides that she will use instructing and encouraging modes during the session and she will include the big brother. She will instruct Fiona and her brother on movement activities that are fun and playful. She will use encouraging words and actions during the session. Isabella anticipates that Fiona may be tired, leading Isabella to consider the pace of the activities and ways to modify activities as needed.

Isabella starts with the parent interview to give Fiona time to become comfortable in the new setting and finish her snack. She notices the mother is tense and has her arms crossed as she stands behind Fiona's stroller. The mother responds to questions with short answers and does not engage in small talk with the therapist.

Isabella hypothesizes that the mother may be tense because she is worried about her child or feeling overwhelmed from daily expectations. This is an assumption, so she keeps an open mind. She decides to use *empathizing* mode to connect with the mother and better understand the family. This will help her design a successful home exercise program for Fiona. Isabella has an energetic personality and likes to get things done; she can be "bossy" or "pushy" at times. Her preferred modes are encouraging and problem-solving. Isabella soon realizes that in this encounter a calm, more soothing tone, and use of empathizing and collaborating modes might be more effective.

During the interview, Isabella is attentive, makes eye contact, and listens to the mother. She asks follow-up questions and engages in a conversation, so the mother feels comfortable. Occasionally, Isabella validates the mother's concerns and asks for clarification. These skills are all part of empathizing with clients. Isabella avoids making judgement, providing solutions, and advising the mother. She provides opportunities for questions throughout the interview.

She gathers information about Fiona's family, interests, routines and habits, environment, and current level of function. Fiona requires assistance for most self-care except eating finger foods. She has shown some recent interest in donning a shirt but requires maximum assistance especially with her right sleeve.

After the interview is complete, Isabella asks the mother if she could put away Fiona's snack. Isabella wants to build rapport with Fiona and does not want her first interaction to be taking something away from her. As Isabella brings out the goniometer to measure range of motion, Fiona cries out, refuses to participate, and holds her right arm close to her body and yells. This represents an inevitable interpersonal event in the session signaling that Isabella needs to change her mode of interacting with Fiona (away from instructing). She stops and takes a deep breath (and is careful not to take it personally). She decides to move towards a *collaborating mode*, whereby Fiona has some say in the activity and plays with her brother.

Isabella invites Fiona's brother to play a game with Fiona. She hands Fiona a round squishy ball to hold in her left hand and grab as many stickers (one at a time) from her brother, who is holding them at different positions (requiring Fiona to reach with her right upper extremity). This allows the OT to assess active range of motion of her right upper extremity. Isabella then asks Fiona's mother if she can have her brother join in on a "game" to help communicate that passive range of motion will not hurt. Isabella plays a "game" to see how far her brother's arm can move. This allows the therapist to assess passive range of motion in a playful way. Fiona wants to copy her brother and cooperates with the game.

Feeling confident, the occupational therapist continues with the assessment and presents Fiona with a developmentally appropriate toy to assess cognitive skills and play. Fiona refuses, throws the toy, and starts to cry. Isabella realizes she used instructing more than collaborating, may have been too pushy, and tried to do too many activities too quickly without encouraging the client and praising her for all that she has done willingly.

She returns to the crackers since the client showed interest in them. She places them farther away encouraging Fiona to get out of the stroller and onto the floor mat where other toys are also available. Isabella does her best to measure arm movements with a goniometer without touching Fiona. In a few minutes Fiona begins to engage with a light-up, musical toy. Isabella assesses her natural spontaneous use of her right hand in bimanual tasks to manipulate toys. She also takes video of Fiona as she moves, eats, and plays to document the approximate range of motion at her elbow and shoulder as she moves around. The video captures her resting posture which she can document later. If she is unable to get precise measurements during this assessment, she will have some data for baseline performance.

Based on today's session she decides to schedule a second appointment for splinting. Fiona's mother is agreeable to returning and the two of them brainstorm ways to help her be more comfortable when she fabricates the splint such as putting on a preferred movie or TV show to distract her. Her mother reports Fiona is most alert and cooperative first thing in the morning so Isabella schedules her for an 8 am appointment.

The OT reasons that a splint made with fiberglass casting material that does not need hands-on pressure to form or a prefabricated adjustable elbow extension splint might work better for Fiona due to her sensory sensitivities and aversion to touch. She will consult with the physiatrist about Fiona's plan of care.

Isabella collaborates with Fiona's mother to create a home exercise program that fits into their daily routine activities. Together, they agree that it would be easier and result in more opportunities for Fiona to naturally use both hands if the exercises are part of their routines. Isabella uses *collaborating* and *problem-solving modes* to work with Fiona's mother to find the most efficient and effective ways to incorporate active range of motion during the day.

Fiona eats 3 meals plus 2 snacks each day. Isabella suggests that since Fiona has active spontaneous right gross grasp of larger items she could work on stabilizing bowls, containers, or sippy cups during preferred snacks. To increase the challenge and encourage elbow extension, her mother might move the objects progressively farther away on the tabletop. They also decided together that stretching could be completed during dressing, bathing, and post-bath lotion application since Fiona's mother already had her hands on the child.

Fiona's mother states that she enjoys fingerplays and nursery songs and they sing songs every day. The therapist suggested doing 2–3 of these paired with arm movements before naps and bedtime to get additional stretching and active range of motion embedded in her routine. In addition, the occupational therapist suggests the mother encourage Fiona to reach for and extend her elbow to point to pictures in books with both hands. The OT practitioner creates a one-page handout of the home recommendations. She asks the mother for feedback on how the session went and if she felt like Fiona responded to her interaction styles positively. The practitioner asks the mother if she felt her needs were adequately addressed and if she has any suggestions for the next session.

The occupational therapist used various modes of interacting in a one-hour session. Her ability to respond to the child (who at times was resistant) and family quickly and in the moment resulted in an effective occupational therapy session.

SUMMARY

Therapeutic use of self refers to how practitioners use their own personality, style, insights, perceptions, and judgments to interact and facilitate the occupational therapy process (Punwar & Peloquin, 2000). It includes how practitioners empathize, collaborate, communicate, manage their emotions, perceive interactions, respond to and read cues, think on their feet, adjust their style, anticipate and interpret events. OT practitioners develop skills and abilities through experience, and reflection. The Intentional Relationship Model (IRM; Taylor, 2020) was created to conceptualize and provide terms to describe the process. IRM suggests that practitioners use 6 modes of communication in practice: advocating, collaborating, encouraging, empathizing, instructing, and problem-solving. Practitioners have natural preferred modes for interactions. However, the therapeutic relationship is about meeting the client's occupational goals and therefore, practitioners may have to use other modes in practice. The IRM provides measurements to help practitioners define skills and abilities in each mode and reflect upon one's use of the modes in practice. IRM defines inevitable interpersonal events that occur during therapy and outlines an interpersonal reasoning process that allows OT practitioners to determine if a mode shift may facilitate the therapeutic process.

REFERENCES

Abreu, B. C. (2011). Accentuate the positive: reflections on empathic interpersonal interactions (Eleanor Clarke Slagle Lecture). *American Journal of Occupational Therapy, 65*, 623–634.

Accreditation Council of Occupational Therapy Educators (ACOTE). (2018). *Standards and Interpretive Guide.* Retrieved from: https://acoteonline.org/accreditation-explained/standards/

Akerjordet, K., & Severinsson, E. (2004). Emotional intelligence in mental health nurses talign about practice. *International Journal of Mental Health Nursing, 13*, 164–170.

Allison, H., & Strong, J. (1994). Verbal strategies used by occupational therapists in direct client encounters. *Journal of Research, 14*, 122–129.

American Occupational Therapy Association (AOTA). (2020). Occupational therapy practice framework: Domain and process (4th ed.). *American Journal of Occupational Therapy, 74*(Suppl. 2), S1–S87.

Baum, C. V. M. (1980). Occupational therapist put care in the health system. *American Journal of Occupational Therapy, 34*, 505–516.

Chaffey, L., Unsworth, C. A., & Fossey, E. (2010). A grounded theory of initiation among occupational therapists in mental health practice. *British Journal of Occupational Therapy, 73*, 300–308.

Chaffey, L., Unsworth, C. A., & Fossey, E. (2012). Relationship between intuition and emotional intelligence in occupational therapists in mental health practice. *American Journal of Occupational Therapy, 66*, 88–96.

Cole, B., & McLean, V. (2003). Therapeutic relationships, redefined. *Occupational Therapy in Mental Health, 19*(2), 33–56.

Davis, M. H. (1983). Measuring individual differences in empathy: Evidence for a multidimensional approach. *Journal of Personality and Social Psychology, 44*, 113–126.

Decety, J., & Batson, C. D. (2007). Social neuroscience approaches to interpersonal sensitivity. *Social Neuroscience, 32*, 257–267.

Dunn, W. (2002). *Infant/Toddler Sensory Profile. User's Manual.* San Antonio, TX: The Psychological Corporation.

Eklund, M., & Hallberg, I. (2001). Psychiatric occupational therapists' verbal interaction with their clients. *Occupational Therapy International, 8*(1), 1–16.

Fleming, M. H. (1991). The therapists with the three-track mind. *American Journal of Occupational Therapy, 45*, 1007–1014.

Gahnstrom-Strandqvist, K., Tham, K., Josephsson, S., & Borell, L. (2000). Actions of competence in occupational therapy practice. *Scandinavian Journal of Occupational Therapy, 7*, 15–25.

Guidetti, S., & Tham, K. (2002). Therapeutic strategies used by occupational therapists in self care training: A qualitative study. *Occupational Therapy International, 9*, 257–276.

Howe, D. (2008). *The emotionally intelligent social worker.* Basingstoke: Palgrave Macmillan.

Hutchinson, S. L., LeBlanc, A., & Booth, R. (2002). "Perceptual problem-solving": An ethnographic study of clinical reasoning in a therapeutic recreation setting. *Therapeutic Recreation Journal, 36*, 18–34.

Jenkins, Z. M., Mallett, J., O'Neill, C., McFadden, M., & Baird, H. (1994). Insights into "practice" communication: An interactional approach. *British Journal of Occupational Therapy, 70*(4), 154–160.

Leicht, S. B., & Dickerson, A. (2001). Clinical reasoning: Looking back. *Occupational Therapy in Health Care, 14*(3/4), 105–130.

Mattingly, C. (1991). What is clinical reasoning? *American Journal of Occupational Therapy, 45*, 979–986.

Mattingly, C. (1994). The narrative nature of clinical reasoning. In C. Mattingly & M. H. Fleming (Eds.). *Clinical Reasoning: Forms of Inquiry in a Therapeutic Practice* (pp. 239–269). Philadelphia, PA: FA Davis.

Mattingly, C., & Fleming, M. H. (Eds.). (1994). *Clinical Reasoning: Forms of Inquiry in a Therapeutic Practice.* Philadelphia, PA: FA Davis.

Peloquin, S. M. (2005). Eleanor Clarke Slagle lecture – Embracing our ethos, reclaiming our heart. *American Journal of Occupational Therapy, 59*, 611–625.

Punwar, J., & Peloquin, M. (2000). *Occupational therapy: Principles and practice.* Philadelphia: Lippincott.

Restall, G., Ripat, J., & Stern, M. (2003). A framework of strategies for client-centered practice. *Canadian Journal of Occupational Therapy, 70*, 103–112.

Schell, B. A. (2003). Clinical reasoning: The basis of practice. In E. B. Crepeau, E. S. Cohn, & B. A. Schell (Eds.). *Willard and Spackman's occupational therapy* (10th ed., pp. 131–152). Philadelphia, PA: Lippincott Williams & Wilkins.

Schell, B. A., & Cervero, R. M. (1993). Clinical reasoning in occupational therapy: An integration review. *American Journal of Occupational Therapy, 47*, 605–610.

Solman, B., & Clouston, T. (2016). Occupational therapy and the therapeutic use of self. *British Journal of Occupational Therapy, 79*(8), 514–516.

Sumsion, T. (2000). A revised occupational therapy definition of client-centered practice. *British Journal of Occupational Therapy, 63*, 304–309.

Taylor, R. (2020). *The intentional relationship model* (2nd ed.). Philadelphia, PA: FA Davis.

Taylor, R. R., Lee, S. W., Kielhofner, G., & Ketkar, M. (2009). Therapeutic use of self: A nationwide survey of practitioners' attitudes and experiences. *American Journal of Occupational Therapy, 63*, 198–207.

Taylor, R., & Van Puymbrouck, L. (2022). Therapeutic use of self: Applying the intentional relationship model in group therapy. In J. OBrien & J. Solomon (Eds.). *Occupational analysis and group process* (2nd ed., pp. 33–48). St. Louis, MO: Elsevier.

Taylor, R. R., Ivey, C., Shepherd, J., Simons, D., Brown, J., Huddle, M., et al. (2013). *Self-assessment of Modes Questionnaire – version II.* Chicago, IL: University of Illinois at Chicago.

Taylor, R. R., & Popova, E. (2019). *Self-Assessment of Modes Questionnaire.* Chicago, IL: University of Illinois at Chicago.

WORKSHEET 4.1: INTERPERSONAL CHARACTERISTICS EXAMPLES

Provide examples describing the interpersonal characteristics (listed in Worksheet 4.1) of a close family member or friend.
- Describe how a person meeting them for the first time should approach them.
- Describe an activity that the person might enjoy.
- Describe how their interpersonal characteristics influence your activity choice.

Interpersonal Characteristics Examples	
Family member or friend:	
Interpersonal Characteristic	**Example**
Communication style	
Tone of voice	
Body language	
Facial expression (affect)	
Response to change and challenge	
Level of trust	
Need for control	
Approach to asserting needs	
Predisposition to giving feedback	
Capacity to receive feedback	
Response to human diversity	
Orientation toward relating	
Preference for touch	
Interpersonal reciprocity	
How should a person meeting them for the first time approach them?	
Describe an activity the person may enjoy.	
How did their interpersonal characteristics influence activity choice?	

WORKSHEET 4.2: ROLE PLAY INEVITABLE EVENTS

In pairs, select an interpersonal event category (see Table 4.2). Role play a scenario illustrating a negative or positive event based on this category. Have one partner play the "therapist" and the other the "client." Reflect upon the role play by responding to questions on worksheet.

Role Play Inevitable Events
Describe the event:
How did the therapist handle the event?
What might have triggered the client's response?
Describe your emotions during the role play (as therapist and client).
Did the therapist facilitate communication?
What other things could the therapist have done?
How might the client and therapist learn from this experience?
Other comments:

WORKSHEET 4.3: SELF-ASSESSMENT OF MODES

Complete the Self-Assessment of Modes Questionnaire (Taylor et al., 2013; Taylor & Popova, 2019) and identify your preferred modes of communication.

Self-Assessment of Modes
Name:
Date:
Preferred Modes:
Describe your thoughts regarding your mode assessment. Is this what you expected?
How do these modes support therapeutic relationships?
In what situations might these modes not work?
How might you develop skills in your less preferred modes?
Other comments:

WORKSHEET 4.4: INTERPERSONAL REASONING

Select one example of an inevitable interpersonal event (outlined in Table 4.2). Describe the interpersonal reasoning steps (See Table 4.4) that may provide insight into the event.
- What additional questions surfaced from doing this exercise?
- How does imagining and practicing the interpersonal reasoning process enhance one's therapeutic use of self?

Interpersonal Reasoning	
Name:	
Example of inevitable event:	
Step of Interpersonal Reasoning	Description
Anticipate	
Identify and cope	
Determine if a mode shift is required	
Choose a response mode or mode sequence	
Draw on any relevant interpersonal skills associated with the modes	
Gather feedback	
What additional questions surfaced from doing this exercise?	
How does imagining and practicing the interpersonal reasoning process enhance one's therapeutic use of self?	
Other comments:	

WORKSHEET 4.5: EXPLORING INEVITABLE EVENTS

Contact an OT practitioner to identify and describe inevitable events that they experience in practice.
- How can using the interpersonal reasoning process inform the event.?

Exploring Inevitable Events	
Name:	
Practitioner's name:	
Description of practice setting:	
Description of inevitable events in practice:	
How can using the interpersonal reasoning process inform the event?	
Step of Interpersonal Reasoning	Description
Anticipate	
Identify and cope	
Determine if a mode shift is required	
Choose a response mode or mode sequence	
Draw on any relevant interpersonal skills associated with the modes	
Gather feedback	

5

Using Evidence to Support Therapeutic Reasoning

Teressa Garcia Reidy and Nicole Whiston Andrejow

GUIDING QUESTIONS

1. What is evidence-based practice?
2. Why use evidence to support occupational therapy intervention?
3. How do OT practitioners use evidence to inform therapeutic reasoning?
4. What practical tips, tools, and habits can OT practitioners use to ensure therapeutic reasoning is guided by the best available evidence?

KEY TERMS

Case–control study

Case series

Case report

Cohort study

Descriptive study

Evidence-based intervention

Evidence-based practice

Level of evidence

Meta-analysis

Peer-reviewed

Pretest/posttest

Randomized control trials

Single-subject design

Systematic review

INTRODUCTION

Evidence-based practice requires that OT practitioners synthesize knowledge from the best available research as well as clinical experience, and the client's situation, environment, and priorities. This process requires that OT practitioners develop skills in critically analyzing research, theory, and information from a variety of sources. They examine research findings while considering the unique needs and priorities of the client and the setting for which occupational therapy services are being provided (Thomas & Law, 2013).

OT practitioners examine research regarding occupational therapy, human development, neuroscience, psychology, cognition, assessments, and other related topics. They may explore research describing cultures, policies, advocacy, and occupational justice. Examining program development, opportunities, and creative intervention plans based on sound theoretical models may inspire innovative and effective programming and promote decision-making. Being able to critically examine and synthesize research from a variety of disciplines provides evidence for practice decisions and strengthens one's ability to articulate the rationale for choices. Research evidence provides the foundation for therapeutic reasoning. Using current evidence in practice requires that OT practitioners develop skills to locate, review, and critically analyze the quality and suitability of the research. They examine and synthesize information

from research, clinical experiences, and their clients' life histories to create and implement effective occupational therapy intervention.

This chapter describes the therapeutic reasoning process to find, analyze, and use the best available evidence in practice. The authors explain the types and levels of evidence used to support practice decisions. They describe how to search for and evaluate evidence. They provide practical tips, tools, and suggestions to support the use of evidence to inform therapeutic reasoning in practice. Case examples and learning activities are interspersed throughout the chapter to illustrate concepts.

EVIDENCE-BASED PRACTICE TO ENHANCE THERAPEUTIC REASONING

Therapeutic reasoning is a cognitive process whereby OT practitioners analyze, decide, prioritize, synthesize, and anticipate outcomes based upon the best available data or information for every step of the OT process. Figure 5.1 provides a schematic of the processes involved in engaging in evidence-based practice. OT practitioners seek to base decisions on the best possible research evidence. This requires that they search for the evidence, critically analyze it, thoughtfully determine if the evidence is valuable, and determine the appropriateness of the evidence based on their clinical experience and the client's situation and priorities. They may also seek input from experts or

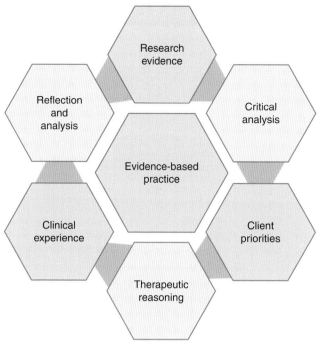

Fig. 5.1 Evidence-Based Practice Process

While OT practitioners may find engaging in evidence-based practice time consuming, the knowledge gained may improve effectiveness, result in better client outcomes, and inspire effective and creative occupational therapy intervention. OT practitioners use the evidence to justify and articulate their decisions throughout the OT process. Understanding the evidence supporting assessments, interventions, and methods to measure occupational outcomes requires dedication to engaging in scholarly inquiry.

THE CYCLE OF EVIDENCE-BASED PRACTICE

Evidence-based practice refers to the "conscientious, explicit, and judicious use of current best evidence in making decisions about the care of individual patients" (Sackett, Rosenberg, Gray, Haynes, & Richardson, 1996, p. 71). OT practitioners use evidence to support practice decisions at each step of the therapeutic reasoning process. Box 5.1 provides examples from practice and descriptions of evidence that may inform each step in the process. Research informs one's thinking, interpretations, choices, and decisions at each stage. Engaging in evidenced-based practice allows practitioners to:

- Update practice knowledge over time
- Articulate what is being done and why
- Provide quality care
- Support practice decisions
- Achieve better results
- Make better clinical decisions, and
- Enhance therapeutic reasoning

Create a Question

The cycle involved in engaging in evidence-based practice is shown in Figure 5.2. The first step of evidence-based practice is to create a question of which you would like to learn. For example, OT students may want to learn the role of OT with children with autism or how pet therapy helps college students.

colleagues with more experience to decide to apply the concepts in practice. Importantly, they measure outcomes and reflect on their decisions throughout the process. OT practitioners adjust and adapt procedures, strategies, techniques, and assessment measures as they gain new information or find that the evidence suggests different approaches. As OT practitioners synthesize the evidence and problem-solve how it informs practice, they engage in therapeutic reasoning. They use the evidence and their analysis of how it informs practice to make decisions and prioritize occupational therapy evaluation, intervention, and reflection on outcomes.

BOX 5.1 Evidence at Each Stage of the Therapeutic Reasoning Process

Step in Therapeutic Reasoning Process	Evidence	Practice Example
Generate questions based on theory	• Evidence on model of practice with client population • Evidence (often scientific, but may also be on lived experience) on client condition, progression, medical management (population based)	• Examine the factors that influence occupational performance. • Review occupation-based models of practice to create questions to examine human performance. • Explore current information regarding the client's condition to better direct questions.
Gather data	• Research on assessment tools (purpose, reliability, and validity)	• Explore reliability, validity, and sensitivity of measurements. • Examine research on performance-based assessments. • Determine methods to elicit the client's narrative.
Create conceptualization	• Research describing principles of frames of reference that may be appropriate for the client.	• Synthesize information from multiple sources to create a hypothesis of what is interfering with the client's ability to engage in desired occupations. • Synthesize information using evidence to determine how occupational therapy intervention can influence a client's performance. • Use evidence from multiple sources to determine intervention focus and priorities.

Continued

BOX 5.1   Evidence at Each Stage of the Therapeutic Reasoning Process–cont'd

Step in Therapeutic Reasoning Process	Evidence	Practice Example
Create an intervention plan	• Research on frame of reference (e.g., principles, strategies, techniques) • Research on interventions with client population • Practice experience • Peer consultations	• Determine frame of reference that addresses client's priorities and is based on current evidence. • Use strategies and techniques as outlined in the frame of reference to guide practice decisions. • Examine the principles of change as outlined in the frame of reference to create client-centered activities. • Incorporate peer consultation and professional experiences along with research evidence into intervention planning.
Implement intervention	• Research on role of OT using frame of reference. • Research on therapeutic use of self • Peer consultation • Techniques to engage in reflection	• Implement intervention being mindful of one's therapeutic use of self. • Adapt and modify intervention as needed. • Use peer consultation for feedback on intervention approaches as needed. • Use evidence to facilitate reflection regarding all aspects of the intervention process.
Evaluate outcomes	• Research on outcome measurements	• Measure outcomes of intervention using multiple tools (e.g., assessments, client satisfaction, performance on goals).

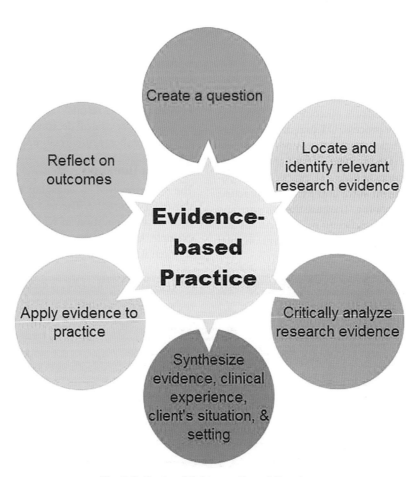

Fig. 5.2 Cycle of Evidence-Based Practice

They may wonder how they will intervene to facilitate occupational engagement for people with mental illness residing in rural communities. They may be curious about the effectiveness of creative sports programs for people with physical or mental conditions.

Being curious provides the impetus to search for research evidence to support one's therapeutic reasoning. Research questions may be related to effectiveness of intervention, usefulness of assessment, description of condition, prediction of outcome, and lived experience of the client (Brown, 2017). Table 5.1 provides

TABLE 5.1	Types of Research Questions
Type of Research Question	**Examples**
Effectiveness of intervention	What is an effective intervention to improve feeding of toddlers with sensory aversions?
Assessment	What is the validity and reliability of the Child Occupational Self-Assessment (COSA)?
Condition	What is the progression of multiple sclerosis?
Prediction of outcome	What factors predict independent living in older adults after a CVA?
Lived experience	How do veterans describe the experience of returning home after active tours of duty?

Locate and Identify Relevant Evidence

OT practitioners gather information from research (literature review), assessments, observation, interview, and experience as outlined in Figure 5.3. They identify the research evidence to inform practice decisions, which may include information on the client's condition, diagnoses, interventions, culture, occupational interests, and environment. They search for reliable and credible sources for information.

For example, OT practitioners examine the evidence to understand the reliability, validity, and sensitivity of assessments they may use to understand a client's functioning and occupational performance. They examine research evidence on the psychometric properties of assessment tools to determine if the measurement is appropriate for the specific client. They use knowledge gained from the research to decide whether to use the assessment in their practice setting.

sample research questions related to each type of question. The nature of the research question informs the research design and methodology. For example, studies evaluating the effectiveness of interventions often use experimental designs, such as randomized control trials with large sample sizes. Research examining the lived experiences of clients may involve qualitative data using small sample sizes. This may involve focus group sessions or semi-structured interviews to learn about the client's interests, habits, routines, and discuss their attributes and desires.

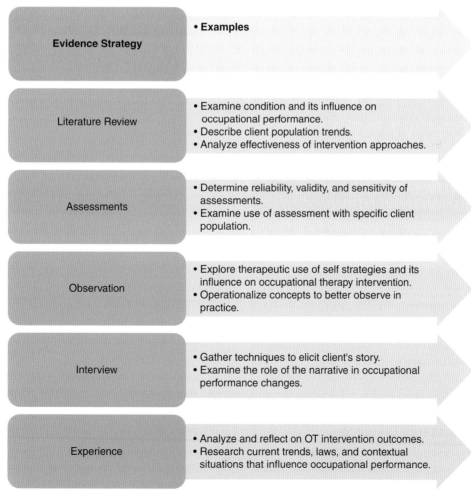

Fig. 5.3 Strategies to Gather Evidence

Evidence Strategy
• **Examples**

Literature Review
• Examine condition and its influence on occupational performance.
• Describe client population trends.
• Analyze effectiveness of intervention approaches.

Assessments
• Determine reliability, validity, and sensitivity of assessments.
• Examine use of assessment with specific client population.

Observation
• Explore therapeutic use of self strategies and its influence on occupational therapy intervention.
• Operationalize concepts to better observe in practice.

Interview
• Gather techniques to elicit client's story.
• Examine the role of the narrative in occupational performance changes.

Experience
• Analyze and reflect on OT intervention outcomes.
• Research current trends, laws, and contextual situations that influence occupational performance.

Since OT practitioners are interested in occupational performance, researchers (Gillen, 2013; Velozo, 2021) suggest they examine performance-based assessments (such as, Executive Function Performance Test [EFPT; Baum, Morrison, Hahn, & Edwards, 2003], Assessment of Motor and Process Skills [AMPS; Fisher & Bray Jones, 2012], and Multiple Errands Test [MET; Morrison et al., 2013]). Performance-based assessments provide data on how the client engages in daily activities. See Chapter 6 for more information on selecting assessments.

LEARNING ACTIVITY: EVIDENCE ON PERFORMANCE-BASED ASSESSMENTS

Use the template provided in Worksheet 5.2 to summarize the findings of a current research article examining a performance-based assessment.
- How do the findings inform occupational therapy practice?
- What are the advantages of using a performance-based assessment?

OT practitioners also examine research supporting the principles of intervention outlined in models of practice and frames of reference (see Chapter 3). For example, rather than basing one's intervention on the word of a colleague, OT practitioners evaluate the principles for using that approach. Understanding the underlying principles allows the OT practitioner to identify if the approach is suitable for a specific person or population and allows the practitioner to adapt and modify evaluation or intervention as needed. The evidence strengthens one's decisions and allows OT practitioners to adjust, modify, and adapt activities to meet the client's needs. The art of therapy involves using one's therapeutic reasoning to create and implement intervention tailored for each client based on information from multiple sources.

Once the OT practitioner identifies the question or area of interest, and locates research evidence, they critically analyze the research to make inferences as related to the specific client and practice setting.

LEARNING ACTIVITY: EVIDENCE FOR PRINCIPLES OF OT INTERVENTION

Use Worksheet 5.3 to complete a research note summarizing the findings from a peer-reviewed study that supports one of the following principles of OT intervention.
- People engage in meaningful activities for longer periods of time or with better quality of movement.
- Repetitive practice of developmental skills provides experiences that promote brain plasticity.
- To increase strength, the muscle must be overloaded to the point of fatigue, which recruits more muscle units and causes hypertrophy and hyperplasia of glycolytic type II fast twitch muscle fibers (Rybski, 2012).
- Motor learning occurs as clients repeat motor tasks that are intrinsically motivating, meaningful, and for which they can problem-solve.

Critically Analyze Research Evidence

OT practitioners are trained to evaluate current evidence so they can make decisions on how the research applies to their clients and practice. Critically analyzing research requires knowledge of research design, statistics, and a review of the strengths and limitations of the methods. A variety of formats exist to review research (e.g., American Occupational Therapy Association AOTA, 2021b; Law et al., 1998). Box 5.2 provides a sample form for a critical review.

Practitioners begin by reviewing the abstract of the study to decide if the study is relevant to their question. They review the background and literature to determine if the reason for the research is founded on current concepts. Next they examine the purpose of the study or the hypotheses that will be examined.

OT practitioners analyze the quality, strengths, and limitations of the research. They consider current OT theory and concepts in relation to the research findings to determine how the findings fit into OT practice. The practitioner also considers the client's situation, previous experience, and the practice setting. They use pragmatic reasoning to explore the suitability of the intervention in context. As they examine the research, OT practitioners engage in scientific reasoning by analyzing the methods, hypotheses, experimental conditions, findings, and results.

Qualitative studies may provide research on the client's experiences and perspectives. OT practitioners use narrative reasoning to apply these findings to clients within their practice setting, realizing that some concepts of the findings may apply to their clients while others do not. The process of prioritizing, reflecting, and making decisions involves therapeutic reasoning.

BOX 5.2   Critical Review

Name:

Citation (APA format):

Purpose or hypothesis:

Background or need:

Research design:
- Type of study
- Level of evidence
- Number of subjects
- Inclusion/exclusion criteria

Methodology
- Intervention and control groups

Outcome measures
- Were measures valid and reliable?

Results
- What results were statistically significant?
- Were differences clinically meaningful?
- Do the findings support the author's claims?

Limitations

Conclusions/implications for practice
- What type of clients may benefit from this approach?
- Would you use this approach in practice? Why or why not?

Types And Levels Of Evidence

OT practitioners identify the type of research design (see Table 5.2) to determine the level of evidence provided by the research. The level of evidence provides an indication of the quality of the research design and is related to the type of research being conducted. There are different evidence hierarchies (Arbesman, Scheer, & Lieverman, 2008; OCEBM Levels of Evidence Working Group, 2011; Sackett, Straus, & Richardson, 2000). Box 5.3 outlines the AOTA hierarchy (Arbesman et al., 2008), which is an adaptation of the Sackett and colleagues' (2000) hierarchy. OT practitioners critically appraise the evidence available to find sources that both support and describe limitations of interventions to ensure they are using evidence-based interventions. AOTA offers summaries of current research on the Evidence Exchange website (American Occupational Therapy Association AOTA, 2021a).

Level I. Findings from systematic reviews provide a strong level of evidence (level I) to support practice decisions. A systematic review involves review of numerous research publications on a topic of interest. The authors gather multiple peer-reviewed research articles on a specific topic and provide a critique of the strengths and limitations of each study and level of evidence. The authors of systematic reviews analyze the quality of research articles and summarize the state of the science for that topic. They provide areas for future research and recommendations for practice based on the current state of research. For example, Case-Smith, Weaver, and Fristad (2015) conducted a systematic review on the effectiveness of sensory processing interventions for children on the autism spectrum. A systematic review of randomized controlled trials provides high quality evidence. Randomized control trials are studies that include a control and intervention group with objective measurements. Randomized control trials provide evidence on the effectiveness of an intervention. OT practitioners must determine how the

research conducted relates to the individual client since many factors influence occupational therapy outcomes.

A meta-analysis is similar to a systematic review, but the authors gather the results of a specific construct or measure from quantitative studies and statistically analyze the data. This allows the researchers to compare differences between studies.

Level II. Research that is not randomized but involves two groups (for example, a control group and intervention group) may inform therapeutic reasoning. Cohort studies, for example, include groups over time and may add to the strength of the study by increasing the number of participants. For example, a cohort study may include first grade children for 2 years. Case–control studies use retrospective observational data to answer questions about risk factors that predict a condition (Brown, 2017).

Level III. OT practitioners may examine research that is not randomized and includes one group, such as pretest/posttest

BOX 5.3   Levels of Evidence (Arbesman et al., 2008)

Levels of Evidence	Definitions
I	Systematic reviews, meta-analysis, randomized control trials
II	Two groups, nonrandomized studies (e.g., cohort, case–control)
III	One group, nonrandomized (e.g., before and after, pretest and posttest)
IV	Descriptive studies that include analysis of outcomes (single-subject design, case series)
V	Case reports and expert opinions that include narrative literature reviews and consensus statements

Note: Based on Sackett *et al.* (2000)

TABLE 5.2   Types of Research Studies

Type	Description
Systematic Review	A study that uses a specific protocol to review all currently published peer-reviewed papers on this topic.
Meta-analyses	A study that provides a statistical analysis examining multiple studies addressing the same question.
Randomized Control Trial	Experimental study that compares treatment group to control group to determine cause and effect relationship with random allocation of subjects and blinding of researchers, subjects, and therapists.
Cohort Study	Exploratory longitudinal study that follows a cohort (group of subjects that share similar characteristics) that is exposed to treatment or diagnosis and compares effects to a comparison group not exposed to treatment to describe potential relationships.
Case–Control Study	Exploratory study that compares two groups of people: those with the disease or condition under study (cases) and a very similar group of people who do not have the disease or condition (controls).
Pretest and Posttest	A study that measures outcomes in participants before and after the implementation of an intervention. May also include treatment and control groups.
Case Series	A case series is a type of study that tracks subjects who have received a similar treatment or examines their medical records for exposure and outcome.
Single Subject Design	Experimental study consists of one subject or a small set of subjects where the subject serves as its own control in study design by alternating between baseline and intervention phases and observing target behavior to determine cause and effect relationship.
Descriptive Study	Observes a group of interest at a specific time point to classify and document characteristics, explore factors that influenced an outcome, and define patterns.
Case Reports	A retrospective in-depth analysis describing an individual, single group, or event.

studies. These studies typically address a specific condition or population. The researchers measure desired factors before and after the intervention to determine the effectiveness of the intervention. Studies with more than 30 subjects are generally considered stronger statistically, although OT practitioners also examine the study design. OT practitioners using the research findings for decision-making also examine the suitability of the measurements to occupational performance outcomes.

Level IV. Case series provide additional information that may support practice decisions. Since a case series has no control group and is based on a small sample, it does not provide the strongest of evidence. OT practitioners carefully analyze the findings and view the results cautiously when using concepts from the study in practice. A case series may provide the OT practitioner with ideas of how to create an intervention plan for a specific client population, however not all aspects of the case may transfer to another client. Single-subject designs involve the subject serving as their own control, rather than comparing the findings to another person or group. Research using a single-subject design includes establishing a baseline that includes a period of time where the researcher measures the client's performance without intervention, providing intervention and measuring outcomes, and then returning to a period where the subject does not receive intervention, but outcomes are again measured.

Level V. Case reports and expert opinions are often used with new approaches. They represent the weakest level of evidence for decision-making. However, they can serve to highlight approaches that are emerging and have potential in practice. When examining this research, OT practitioners carefully examine the rationale for decisions. Finally, descriptive studies describe a phenomenon and may provide insight that supports assessment or intervention planning. Descriptive studies are often used to describe the properties of assessments (such as validity and reliability studies). They may also describe intervention approaches and strategies that may be used in practice. Descriptive studies may provide ideas for activity selection or indicate strategies to work with clients who have rare conditions.

Synthesize Evidence with Clinical Experience, Client's Situation, and Practice Setting

With the increasing availability of sources of evidence, OT students and practitioners examine the rigor and suitability of a study's findings to inform therapeutic reasoning. Evidence-based practice requires synthesizing information from one's own experience, best available current evidence, the client's specific condition and situation and the client's response to the intervention. OT practitioners may seek new information throughout the occupational therapy process and revise hypotheses and strategies to ensure best practice. Box 5.4 provides a list of questions to consider when reviewing evidence to make therapeutic decisions.

OT practitioners synthesize all available information to prioritize goals, make decisions, and select approaches to address the client's needs within the practice setting. Figure 5.4 provides examples of the therapeutic reasoning used during the OT process. For example, OT practitioners rely on conditional reasoning to integrate research evidence for practice with information regarding a specific client. This requires that they

---

BOX 5.4   Exploring Intervention Approaches

- What is the approach, strategy, or technique that is working in practice?
- What is the theory that informs this approach?
- What are the principles explaining change when using this approach?
- Is this approach based on occupational therapy philosophy?
- Does the approach address occupational therapy's scope of practice?
- Is the approach client-centered?
- How does the approach address occupation?
- What type of client or population benefits from this approach?
- Is it safe? Harmful?
- What are some contraindications for using this approach?
- Do clients like the approach?
- Does it require additional training? Materials?
- How is change measured using this approach?

---

combine many forms of therapeutic reasoning when deciding how to proceed. They must understand the research evidence (e.g., levels of evidence, design, methodology, and findings), which requires scientific reasoning. They use narrative reasoning to understand the client's story to prioritize goals and create occupation-based intervention in consideration of the research evidence. They collaborate with clients using knowledge of the client's story and rely on interactive reasoning to read the client's responses and maintain a therapeutic relationship as they implement concepts in practice. They use information from research, clinical experience, and the client to adjust and modify approaches. They use pragmatic reasoning to decide how all the information may be applied in practice given the practice setting. OT practitioners engage in ethical decision-making when they contemplate the effectiveness of intervention with clients, considering costs, evidence, practice standards, and the client's rights. They refer to the evidence throughout the process as they reflect on their role, the client's responses, and the information gained from evidence (e.g., research, clinical experience, and client).

Apply Evidence and Reflect on Outcomes

The OT practitioner reflects on each step of the OT process revisiting research evidence to adjust as needed. They may explore research to uncover additional intervention strategies or techniques to facilitate occupational performance. They may revise intervention based on new knowledge gained from examining research. They may select new assessments to measure outcomes. They may gain new insights as they reflect upon the outcomes based on current evidence. The reflective process helps the OT practitioner learn, improve performance, and facilitates therapeutic reasoning.

For example, the outcomes of occupational therapy intervention can be measured by examining intervention outcomes (goal attainment, assessment changes), client satisfaction, or program evaluation. Since measuring outcomes is essential for evaluating intervention success, OT practitioners use research evidence to select assessment tools they will use to address client changes over time. Patient surveys may indicate satisfaction with intervention and may support program evaluation.

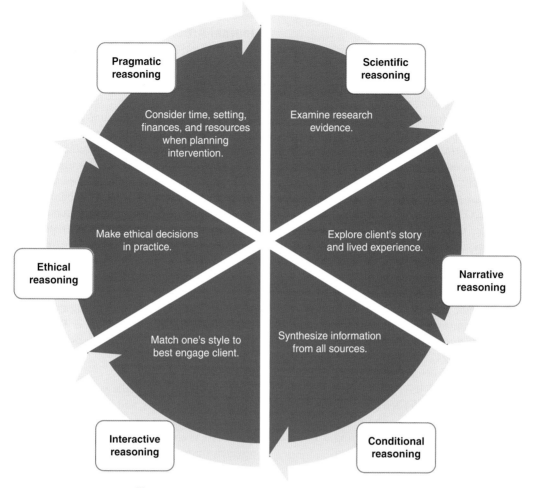

Fig. 5.4 Types of Reasoning Used to Find Evidence

LEARNING ACTIVITY: EXAMINING EVIDENCE FROM SEVERAL SOURCES

Use Worksheet 5.4 to describe evidence from several sources (e.g., website, research article, blog, news article, YouTube video) regarding a specific condition or topic of interest.
• Which source is most reliable and provides the best evidence?
• How do you decide which source is most reliable and provides the best evidence?

LEARNING ACTIVITY: RESEARCH EXCHANGE

Visit the Research Exchange on the AOTA website (https://www.aota.org/Practice/Researchers/Evidence-Exchange.aspx). Find the critically appraised paper (CAP) worksheet and submission guidelines. Find a suitable intervention study and complete a CAP.
• What resources did you find on the website that may be helpful in practice?

Finding evidence to support the theory and principles underlying changes in performance may require conducting a literature review, consulting with colleagues, and creating hypotheses and testing them in practice. Box 5.5 provides a list of questions

practitioners may consider to critically examine research to determine if the findings should inform current practice.

Using Protocols In Practice

Protocols supported by research evidence and used with occupation-centered care and evaluation of the client's response to treatment may guide occupational therapy. Protocols are guides designed to "reduce reasoning errors and the potentially biasing

BOX 5.5   Reviewing Research Evidence

• Is the practitioner's client population similar enough to the study cohort?
• Are the outcome tools used in this study sufficient to capture changes made by the intervention?
• What level of evidence is this research? Is it strong enough to change current practice approaches with the patient population?
• Is this research emerging and should the practitioner continue to read evidence on the topic before implementing it into clinical practice?
• Are there systematic reviews available about this topic that can summarize multiple studies and demonstrate whether it is efficacious?
• Are the methods of this study translatable to a clinical setting? Will the practitioner be able to carry out the assessment or intervention in the manner described in the study to get similar results?

effects that can arise from clinical opinions" (Turpin & Higgs, 2017, p. 396). For example, health professionals can overemphasize the effectiveness of their own interventions because they might only see the short-term effects of the intervention. In addition, they might be overly influenced by situations and outcomes that they have access to, while potentially being unaware of or undervaluing other possibilities (such as interventions offered by other health professionals) (Turpin & Higgs, 2017). Clinical protocols and guidelines are developed from information from a broad range of sources, including frames of reference, research evidence, broader trends in patient outcomes or statistics about adverse incidents, epidemiological trends in population health, and patients' opinions and experiences (Turpin & Higgs, 2017). OT practitioners use therapeutic reasoning to determine how to best use a protocol while engaging in client-centered occupation-based practice. They observe the client's reactions, progress, and responses so they can adjust activities or requirements in real time if needed.

For example, when working in a home setting with clients who recently had orthopedic surgery a practitioner relied on a treatment protocol based on current evidence that outlines the selection and sequence of interventions to guide the progression of functional training. The OT practitioner used therapeutic reasoning skills to blend this evidence with evidence gained through observations of the client's level of fatigue, edema, pain, and endurance. The practitioner adjusted the protocol based on the client's responses and progress. The OT practitioner included meaningful occupations, such as playing a favorite game or preparing a meal for family, into the session.

LEARNING ACTIVITY: JUSTIFYING OT INTERVENTIONS TO COLLEAGUES

A physiatrist at an outpatient pediatric neurorehabilitation clinic is hesitant to write an order for occupational therapy to make a long arm cast for a trial of constraint induced movement therapy (CIMT) for a child who has hemiplegic cerebral palsy. The physiatrist is concerned that the child will lose hand function in her less affected hand while casted.
- Describe how you would approach the physician about your intervention plan.
- Find at least 2 peer-reviewed studies that support the position that CIMT will improve both unimanual and bimanual function (one of them should be a randomized control trial).
- Find one research article that addresses the physician's concerns about loss of skill.

SEARCHING FOR AND EVALUATING RESEARCH EVIDENCE

LEARNING ACTIVITY: EXAMINING INTERVENTION APPROACHES

Use Worksheet 5.5 (based on Box 5.4) to evaluate the evidence provided in a chosen research study examining the effectiveness of an intervention approach.
- Describe the strengths and limitations of the findings.
- Discuss your recommendation and rationale for using this intervention in practice.

SOURCES OF EVIDENCE

Journal Articles

Peer-reviewed journal articles have been evaluated by objective reviewers who examine the background, methodology, findings, results, and conclusions of a research study prior to publication. This provides an extra layer of support for the research. However, OT practitioners and students still must carefully examine research findings to determine the validity of the findings in one's practice and with specific clients.

Readers also may consider the journal's impact factor, which indicates the journal's rigor, reputation, and readership. It correlates with how often the journal's publications are cited in other research and work. A higher impact score indicates a larger readership, stronger journal credibility and reputation, which suggests the strength of the publication. For example, *American Journal of Occupational Therapy* (AJOT) is the highest-rated OT journal with an impact factor of 2.25 (2-year) (Clarivate Analytics, 2021). Some journals appeal to readers from a variety of disciplines and health professions, especially medical journals. For example, *The Journal of the American Medical Association* (JAMA) has an impact factor of 56.3 (Clarivate Analytics, 2021).

Textbooks

Textbooks provide a synthesis of research and theory to assist students, practitioners, and faculty in making therapeutic decisions but should not be considered the only source of information. Readers are encouraged to review primary sources, such as research studies.

Continuing Education

OT practitioners and students may receive additional information and creative ideas for evaluation and intervention through continuing education and workshops. Participants should evaluate the course materials and consider the quality of the material provided before applying it to practice. For example, speakers proposing new intervention approaches should provide research to support its use in practice that is consistent with occupational therapy theory and philosophy. References supporting content should include a variety of research studies in peer-reviewed publications describing principles of the approach or assessment, strategies, and methods. Participants should be careful of statements that promise too much if there is little research to support them. They also should view anecdotal evidence from the speaker cautiously if it is not supported by research. The speaker should clearly describe the approach along with rationale that is supported by research evidence. Participants evaluate the risk for performing an intervention that may be based on limited evidence. Importantly, practitioners critically analyze content from workshops and continuing education presentations before applying it in practice. See Box 5.6 for questions to consider when evaluating workshops and continuing education information.

Practice Experience

Another important source of information that contributes to one's therapeutic reasoning is one's own practice and

BOX 5.6 Evaluating Continuing Education and Workshops

- Are references current?
  - What type of references are being used to support the material? (Case studies, personal examples, or research evidence)
- Is there current research to support this?
  - Speakers should be able to articulate theory and research.
  - Where does the research come from?
  - Why is there limited (or no) research to support this?
- Is the material based on current theory?
- Does the material make sense?
- Is the material occupation focused?
- Is the author following occupational therapy principles?
- How would this information translate into clinical practice?
- Does the approach require additional resources? Training?
- What are the cultural implications of this approach?

collaboration with clients and colleagues. OT practitioners frequently use evidence from their own practice to support decision-making. They carefully document intervention approaches that work well in practice and their rationale for using the approaches strengthens their therapeutic reasoning skills.

Taking the time to reflect on what works well with specific clients (and why) allows the OT practitioner to learn from each client and session. Problem-solving with colleagues and clients can explain, clarify, or validate reasoning which may lead to additional solutions and hypotheses important to the therapeutic reasoning process. Being able to ask questions, listen to feedback, identify challenges, and seek out solutions is an essential feature of reasoning. Seeking mentorship within one's work setting, professional organizations (e.g., state organizations, AOTA), or through networking fosters therapeutic reasoning and professional growth. Practitioners benefit from discussing professional issues, reflecting on practice, and engaging in conversations to provide best practice.

Networking

Community of practice groups, journal clubs, in-service training, and online discussion groups provide practitioners with opportunities to access research and may save time. The Research Exchange link through AOTA provides summaries of current research. OT practitioners may decide to partner with faculty at local universities to engage OT students in seeking evidence for practice.

LEARNING ACTIVITY: CRITICAL REVIEW

Use Worksheet 5.6 to critically review a research article to inform occupational therapy practice.

Case Application: Using Evidence in Practice

This case example illustrates how one therapist gathered evidence from a variety of sources to guide therapeutic reasoning in practice. Joseph works as a school-based therapist and many of his clients are adolescents on the Autism Spectrum who are transitioning from school to vocational placements. Joseph would like to find an appropriate assessment to complete with his clients that assesses a variety of functional skills to inform effective job placements.

The school district provides him access to a library of testing materials that he can sign out and he has some funds budgeted for new assessments. Furthermore, he supervises fieldwork students from a local university and is a member of the pediatric occupational therapy group as part of the state occupational therapy association and a member of the American Occupational Therapy Association (AOTA).

- What steps can Joseph take to find a good measure to assess his clients?
- How will he know if the assessment fits his population or is a well-developed test?

He begins by sending an email to occupational therapists in the district and those in the state pediatric occupational therapy group for ideas on possible assessments. He also reaches out to a co-worker who is considered an expert in the field of vocational placement and transition to identify assessments that might be suitable.

He uses a scholarly search engine (that he has access to from the school for which he serves as a fieldwork supervisor) using key terms "occupational therapy vocational assessments" and "autism spectrum disorder," "vocational assessments" and "transition." He signs up for email alerts within the search engine website to send him articles published on this topic. He also explores the AOTA website for information on assessments.

He identifies possible assessments and searches for peer-reviewed articles through the university library. He uses his AOTA membership to explore publications in the *American Journal of Occupational Therapy* (AJOT) and the critically appraised topic (CAT) reviews. He looks for assessments that address vocational transitions for teens who have autism.

He finds the Vocational Fit Assessment (Persch, Gugiu, Onate, & Cleary, 2015) that was created to assess a client's abilities while considering the demands of the job. The assessment gathers information on the pros and cons of each possible job match and areas for potential intervention (Persch et al., 2015). Joseph explores the psychometrics of this test and finds that Persch and colleagues (2017) conducted a study to examine the inter-consistency and test–retest reliability of the Vocational Fit Assessment and reported it is a reliable tool to match people with disabilities to potential vocational placements. The Vocational Fit Assessment (Persch et al., 2015) is a tool to help job coaches, teachers, and supervisors match clients to jobs by looking at the individual worker abilities along with the job demands. It is also within his budget and does not require additional training.

Joseph decides he will use this assessment on a trial basis. He will monitor the results of the assessment over time to determine if students are being appropriately placed. He will request feedback on each student's performance from the job coaches using a brief survey with questions requiring a response on a 10-point Likert scale (so that he can measure the program over time). He creates a one-page overview of the assessment with the list of current references and sends it to his colleagues to thank them for their help.

Joseph used research evidence to find an assessment to better address his clients' needs. The assessment has been used with other populations and exhibits good inter-rater reliability. He monitors clients' progress with transitions to work by getting additional feedback from the job coaches to see if the assessment findings allow him to match them to jobs more accurately.

LEARNING ACTIVITY: COMMUNICATING FINDINGS TO CLIENTS

A patient arrives in the clinic with an internet search of interventions related to his condition. He has evidence from social media group threads, research articles, and websites. The client would like you to incorporate some of these interventions into his plan of care.

- While maintaining a client-centered approach, address his search and explain to him the benefits of choosing interventions based on credible evidence. The explanation should be clear to someone not in health professions. Do not use professional jargon.

TIPS TO IMPLEMENT EVIDENCE-BASED APPROACHES IN PRACTICE

Gathering quality evidence to support therapeutic reasoning for evaluation, intervention, and outcome planning is essential to providing quality occupational therapy services to clients. Implementing evidence-based approaches into practice occurs slowly (Bayley et al., 2012; Crausaz, Kelly, & Lee, 2011). In fact, for OT practitioners, clinical experiences are a strong predictor of the degree of implementation of evidence-based practice (Thomas & Law, 2013). Crausaz and colleagues (2011) found that changing clinical behavior is one of the most challenging barriers to using research evidence to support occupational therapy practice.

Fortunately, there are strategies to engage in evidence-based practice within existing organizational structures. Creating habits and routines to incorporate evidence-based practice into one's professional routines supports and promotes therapeutic reasoning and benefits clients (Jeffery, Robertson, & Reay, 2020). Table 5.3 provides practical strategies to incorporate evidence into practice.

LEARNING ACTIVITY: CREATING PRACTICE EVIDENCE

Contact a local OT practitioner and together create a research question addressing a current concern. Design a research project that could be completed in the setting as a new therapist (and with existing resources). Use Worksheet 5.7 as your guide to describe the design, rationale, and plan. (Hint: Keep the design and topic simple.)

STRATEGIES TO ESTABLISH EVIDENCE FOR PRACTICE

OT practitioners may decide to try novel intervention strategies with limited evidence to address client goals in practice. They begin by examining the level of evidence available (such as a case report or expert opinion). Once they determine that there may be some benefit to the client in using this approach, they examine related research. This may provide insight on how theories support this type of approach. They explore the population for which the approach is designed and evaluate if the approach is consistent with current research. For example, current neuroscience research supports engaging clients in whole, meaningful activities within the natural contexts as opposed to rote exercises in controlled settings (Chan, Luo, Yan, Cai, & Peng, 2015; Hetu & Mercier, 2012; Van de Winckel et al., 2013; Wright, Hunt, & Stanley, 2005). Intervention approaches that support rote exercises should be viewed cautiously. Keeping current on published information about a new trend in therapy informs reasoning.

LEARNING ACTIVITY: USING EVIDENCE AT EACH STAGE OF THE THERAPEUTIC REASONING PROCESS

Watch the Videoclip 5.1 on the Evolve learning site. Use Worksheet 5.8 and record examples of how the OT practitioner used evidence in practice throughout the OT process.

OT practitioners synthesize information from a variety of sources to determine if it is reasonable to use an untested (or weakly supported) approach in practice. OT practitioners must be careful consumers of information and determine if it "makes sense" based on occupational theory, neuroscience, anatomy, and human behavior. OT practitioners determine if the approach promises too much or makes broad claims that cannot be supported. For example, a practitioner should be cautious when reading materials from advertisements pretending to be research or case studies that present weak findings or minimal discussion of the limitations to the study. OT practitioners also consider the safety, ethical, and psychological implications of an intervention approach. OT practitioners using novel approaches evaluate client progress through assessment and clinical observations. They set a timeframe to measure outcomes and discontinue the intervention approach if it is not working. The following case example illustrates the process of using evidence to select measures to evaluate occupational therapy outcomes.

Case Example: Evaluating Outcome Measures

An interdisciplinary rehabilitation program integrates medical, physical, and cognitive behavioral approaches to evaluate and treat adolescents with chronic pain. Adolescents attend the full day program receiving daily individual and group-based therapy for 4 weeks. The occupational therapist recognized that the intervention delivered in daily therapy was effective in helping patients to achieve their goals, however, the standardized assessments used did not show that positive change. During the development of the program, a variety of assessments were administered, but they did not adequately capture the occupational performance changes. The team classified the assessments into 3 categories:

- Measured functional outcomes but not sensitive to changes for clients in the program.

TABLE 5.3   Strategies to Implement Evidence into Practice

Strategy	Description
Use search engines to alert.	OT practitioners can use search engines to set up alerts for new research published in their practice areas. OT practitioners may set alerts for interventions, patient populations, or diagnoses they treat most often. Setting the search engine to deliver the evidence to an inbox alerts practitioners to new information as it is published.
Create a journal club.	Creating a journal club devoted to a practice area allows members to find and share resources. Members can alternate who finds, summarizes, and creates discussion questions related to a peer-reviewed article. Journal clubs are effective for teaching new practitioners to use research evidence in practice (Szucs, Benson, & Haneman, 2017). With proper documentation, journal clubs may be a low-cost method for continuing education credits making it appealing to practitioners and administrators.
Engage in training opportunities.	Most occupational therapy settings conduct regular in-service trainings. Setting up regular trainings to allow practitioners time to use search engines, critically review articles, discuss key findings of research, and describe how the findings may inform their practice may improve the quality of care provided.
Engage in case-based integration discussions.	OT practitioners enjoy discussing cases to learn more, reflect, and refine skills for practice. Engage team members in this process by presenting a case to the group; ask members to problem-solve together using evidence to support their decisions. (This may need to be a two-part meeting.) • Discuss possible solutions or strategies, using research evidence from multiple sources. • Have members reflect on the process and generate a question or area to explore for the next meeting.
Incorporate evidence-based practice as part of the organization's performance plan.	Bayley and colleagues (2012) found that structure and support at the organizational level can influence implementation of evidence-based practice. Create goals that include using research evidence to evaluate, intervene, or measure outcomes into the yearly performance plan. For example, setting a goal to increase the use of psychometrically strong assessment tools in occupational therapy evaluation and at discharge enables the department to track progress in occupational therapy over time.
Complete a practice audit of one facet of practice or day to day activities.	Select an area of practice and complete a contextual analysis of the use of best practice. For example, Radomski, Anheluk, Arulanantham, Finkelstein, and Flinn (2018) evaluated the use of occupation in home exercise programs post stroke. They found that only 1 in 24 home programs used occupation and the others focused on upper extremity exercises. The practitioners used this analysis and research findings suggesting that occupation is best for transfer of learning and carryover. Additionally this analysis served as a springboard to create a plan to incorporate occupation into home programs moving forward.
Engage in professional presentations.	Participating in professional presentations (including guest lectures, in-service training, or professional conferences) encourages speakers to review current literature, clarify concepts, and learn new information which may inform practice.

- Child Occupational Self-Assessment (Kramer et al., 2014).
- Roland Morris Disability Questionnaire (Roland & Fairbank, 2000).
- Occupational Questionnaire (Smith, Kielhofner, & Watts, 1986)

■ Sensitive to change but relied on patient effort which was highly variable day to day with this population.
  - Manual Muscle Testing (Cuthbert & Goodheart, 2007)
  - Dynamometer & Pinch Gauge (Mathiowetz, Vizenor, & Melander, 2000)

■ Sensitive to change but not relevant to occupational performance problems for clients in this program.
  - Bruininks–Oseretsky Test of Motor Proficiency (Bruininks & Bruininks, 2005)
  - Wold Sentence Copying Test (Maples, 2003)
  - Children's Kitchen Task Assessment (Rocke, Hays, Edwards, & Berg, 2008)
  - Nine Hole Peg Test (Grice et al., 2003; Smith, Hong, & Presson, 2000)

The team decided to identify standardized assessments to measure functional outcomes of adolescents with chronic pain. In the first meeting the team completed a retrospective chart review to list and code OT goals with the following categories: ADL/IADL training; activity tolerance and modifications; pain management and coping strategies; energy conservation and joint protection; school participation; social participation; executive functioning; sleep hygiene; and leisure work or volunteer participation. Team members researched available assessments to measure functional outcomes.

At the next meeting, team members presented ideas for assessments, including research on the purpose, validity, reliability, sensitivity, suitability for this population, and administration and scoring details. The OT team reviewed assessments completed by other team members to limit overlap in content and maximize the client's time and effort during evaluations. After examination and review, the OT members decided to administer the Child and Adolescent Scales of Participation (Bedell, 2009, 2011) and the Upper Extremity Functional Index (Stratford, Binkley, & Stratford, 2001) at admission and discharge for the next five patients to determine if these measures were sensitive to changes for clients in the program.

At the follow-up meeting (4 weeks later), the outcome data from the assessments showed that 4 out of 5 patients made improvements from admission to discharge on scores and they met 80% of their short-term goals (24/30 total) and 70% of their long-term goals (7/10). The occupational therapist reported positive gains in home, school, and community participation. Since the measures were sensitive enough to indicate changes, the team continued to track the data with an additional 10 clients.

LEARNING ACTIVITY: SELECTING OUTCOME MEASURES

Select two assessments that would be suitable to use as an outcomes measure for a selected practice setting and population. Find one research article describing the psychometric properties of each assessment.
- Summarize the findings and decide which assessment you would select as a possibility. Why or why not?
- Does the assessment measure the client's occupational therapy goals and priorities?

- Is the assessment reliable? Valid?
- Is the assessment sensitive enough to detect changes?
- How often can you administer the assessment?
- What is the theory supporting the assessment?
- How does the assessment inform occupational therapy practice?

SUMMARY

Using the best possible evidence in occupational therapy practice requires OT practitioners to analyze research findings to make decisions based on knowledge from available research, clinical experience, and client priorities. OT practitioners use therapeutic reasoning to synthesize information regarding the ever-changing factors that influence occupational performance. Evidence to inform and support one's therapeutic reasoning allows OT practitioners to problem-solve and create effective intervention for a diversity of clients and within a variety of settings.

Research evidence may explain the principles underlying evaluation and interventions. As OT practitioners understand the complexities of the principles of practice, they are better able to design meaningful and effective interventions that result in positive client outcomes. Evidence may help OT practitioners design creative intervention plans for individuals and groups and evidence may provide OT practitioners with guidelines for intervention.

Evidence supports therapeutic reasoning by explaining, through research, underlying principles, intervention strategies, techniques, and the role of the OT practitioner. Being able to sift through the evidence and use it in practice benefits clients. Developing strategies, habits, and routines to examine evidence fosters therapeutic reasoning and allows OT practitioners to stay current and creative, while benefiting clients. Establishing search engines and participating in journal clubs, training opportunities, case-based discussions, professional development plans, practice audits, and professional presentations are ways to integrate evidence into practice. Oftentimes questions arise in the practice setting that can be examined through research. Collaborating with faculty and students is an effective way for OT practitioners to examine these questions and to bridge the gap between theory and practice.

REFERENCES

American Occupational Therapy Association (AOTA). (2021a). AOTA Evidence Exchange. Retrieved from: https://www.aota.org/Practice/Researchers/Evidence-Exchange.aspx.

American Occupational Therapy Association (AOTA). (2021b). AOTA Evidence-Based Practice Project. CAP Worksheet. Retrieved from: https://www.aota.org/-/media/Corporate/Files/ConferenceDocs/2021/Call%20For%20Papers/2021%20CFP/04-2022_Annual_CAP_Worksheet.docx

Arbesman, M., Scheer, J., & Lieverman, D. (2008). Using SOTA's critical appraised topic (CAT) and critically appraised paper (CAP) series to link evidence t practice. *OT Practice*, *13*(5), 18–22.

Baum, C. M., Morrison, T., Hahn, M., & Edwards, D. F. (2003). *Test manual: Executive Function Performance Test*. St. Louis, MO: Washington University.

Bayley, M. T., Hurdowar, A., Richards, C. L., Korner-Bitensky, N., Wood-Dauphinee, S., Eng, J. J., & Graham, I. D. (2012). Barriers to implementation of stroke rehabilitation evidence: findings from a multi-site pilot project. *Disability and Rehabilitation*, *34*(19), 1633–1638.

Bedell, G. (2009). Further validation of the Child and Adolescent Scale of Participation (CASP). *Developmental Neurorehabilitation*, *12*, 342–351.

Bedell, G. (2011). The Child and Adolescent Scale of Participation (CASP) administration and scoring guidelines. Retrieved from: https://sites.tufts.edu/garybedell/files/2012/07/CASP-Administration-Scoring-Guidelines-8-19-11.pdf.

Brown, C. (2017). Descriptive and predictive research designs: understanding conditions and making clinical predictions: *The Evidence-Based Practitioner*. Philadelphia, PA: FA Davis.

Bruininks, R., & Bruininks, B. (2005). *Bruininks-Oseretsky Test of Motor Proficiency* (2nd ed.). Bloomington, MN: NCS Pearson.

Chan, J. S. Y., Luo, Y., Yan, J. H., Cai, L., & Peng, K. (2015). Children's age modulates the effect of part and whole practice in motor learning. *Human Movement Science*, *42*, 261–272.

Case-Smith, J., Weaver, L. L., & Fristad, M. A. (2015). A systematic review of sensory processing interventions for children with autism spectrum disorders. *Autism*, *19*(2), 133–148.

Clarivate Analytics. (2021). 2018 Journal Impact Factor. Retrieved from: http://mjl.clarivate.com/

Crausaz, J., Kelly, M., & Lee, S. (2011). Three educational approaches to enhance the evidence-based practice behaviour of Irish occupational therapists. *World Federation of Occupational Therapists Bulletin*, *64*(1), 11–17.

Cuthbert, S. C., & Goodheart, G. J. (2007). On the reliability and validity of manual muscle testing: a literature review. *Chiropractic & Osteopathy*, *15*(4), 1–23.

Fisher, A. G., & Bray Jones, K. (2012). *Assessment of Motor and Process Skills* (7th ed.). Fort Collins, CO: 3 Star Press.

Gillen, G. (2013). A fork in the road: An occupational hazard? *American Journal of Occupational Therapy*, *67*, 641–652.

Grice, K. O., Vogel, K. A., et al. (2003). Adult norms for a commercially available Nine Hole Peg Test for finger dexterity. *American Journal of Occupational Therapy*, *57*(5), 570–573.

Hetu, S., & Mercier, C. (2012). Using purposeful tasks to improve motor performance: Does object affordance matter? *British Journal of Occupational Therapy, 75*(8), 367–376.

Jeffery, H., Robertson, L., & Reay, K. L. (2020). Sources of evidence for professional decision-making in novice occupational therapy practitioners: clinicians'. perspectives. *British Journal of Occupational Therapy* 0308022620941390.

Kramer, J., Velden, M., Kafkes, A., Basu, S., Federico, J., & Kielhofner, G. (2014). *Child Occupational Self-assessment*. Model of Human Occupation Clearinghouse, Department of Occupational Therapy, College of Applied Health Sciences, University of Illinois at Chicago.

Law, M., Steward, D., Pollock, M., Letts, L., Bosch, J., & Westmorland, M. (1998). *Critical review form – quantitative studies*. McMaster University.

Maples, W. C. (2003). The Wold Sentence Copy Test of Academic Performance. *Journal of Behavioral Optometry, 14*(3), 71–76.

Mathiowetz, V., Vizenor, L., & Melander, D. (2000). Comparison of Baseline Instruments to the Jamar Dynamometer and the B&L Engineering Pinch Gauge. *The. Occupational Therapy Journal of Research, 20*(3), 147–162.

Morrison, T. M., Giles, G. M., Ryan, J. D., Baum, C. M., Dromerick, A. W., Polatajko, H. J., & Edwards, D. F. (2013). Multiple Errands Test–Revised (MET–R): A performance-based measure of executive function in people with mild cerebrovascular accident. *American Journal of Occupational Therapy, 67*, 460–468.

OCEBM Levels of Evidence Working Group. (2011). The Oxford 2011 levels of evidence. Retrieved from https://www.cebm.ox.ac.uk/resources/levels-of-evidence/ocebm-levels-of-evidence

Persch, A. C., Gugiu, P. C., Onate, J. A., & Cleary, D. S. (2015). Development and psychometric evaluation of the Vocational Fit Assessment. *American Journal of Occupational Therapy, 69*(6), 6906180080.

Persch, A., Guo, K., Case, C., & Cleary, D. (2017). Internal Consistency and Test–Retest Reliability of the Vocational Fit Assessment. *American Journal of Occupational Therapy, 71*(4_Supplement_1). 7111500041p1-7111500041p1.

Radomski, M. V., Anheluk, M., Arulanantham, C., Finkelstein, M., & Flinn, N. (2018). Implementing evidence-based practice: A context analysis to examine use of task-based approaches to upper-limb rehabilitation. *British Journal of Occupational Therapy, 81*(5), 285–289.

Rocke, K., Hays, P., Edwards, D., & Berg, C. (2008). Development of a performance assessment of executive function: The Children's Kitchen Task Assessment. *American Journal of Occupational Therapy, 62*(5), 528–537.

Roland, M., & Fairbank, J. (2000). The Roland-Morris Disability Questionnaire and the Oswestry Disability Questionnaire. *Spine, 25*(24), 3115–3124.

Rybski, M. (2012). Biomechanical intervention approach: *Kinesiology for occupational therapy* (pp. 309–354). Thorofare, NJ: Slack Inc.

Sackett, D., Straus, S. E., & Richardson, W. S. (2000). *How to Practice and Teach Evidence-Based Medicine* (2nd ed.). Edinburgh: Churchill Livingstone.

Sackett, D., Rosenberg, W. M. C., Gray, J. A. M., Haynes, R. B., & Richardson, W. S. (1996). Evidence-based medicine: What it is and what it isn't. *British Medical Journal, 312*, 71–72.

Smith, Y. A., Hong, E., & Presson, C. (2000). Normative and validation studies of the Nine-Hole Peg Test with children. *Perceptual and Motor Skills, 90*, 823–843.

Smith, N. R., Kielhofner, G., & Watts, J. H. (1986). The relationships between volition, activity pattern, and life satisfaction in the elderly. *American Journal of Occupational Therapy, 40*(4), 278–283.

Stratford, P. W., Binkley, J. M., & Stratford, D. M. (2001). Development and initial validation of the upper extremity functional index. *Physiotherapy Canada, 53*(4), 259–267.

Szucs, K. A., Benson, J. D., & Haneman, B. (2017). Using a guided journal club as a teaching strategy to enhance learning skills for evidence-based practice. *Occupational Therapy in Health Care, 31*(2), 143–149.

Thomas, A., & Law, M. (2013). Research utilization and evidence-based practice in occupational therapy: A scoping study. *American Journal of Occupational Therapy, 67*, e55–e65..

Turpin, M., & Higgs, J. (2017). Clinical reasoning and evidence-based practice. In T. Hoffmann, S. Bennett, & C. Del Mar (Eds.), *Evidence-Based Practice Across the Health Professions* (3rd ed., pp. 364–383). Chatswood, NSW: Elsevier Australia.

Van de Winckel, A., Klingels, K., Bruyninckx, F., Wenderoth, N., Peeters, R., Sunaert, S., … Feys, H. (2013). How does brain activation differ in children with unilateral cerebral palsy compared to typically developing children during active and passive movement sand tactile stimulation? An fMRI study. *Research in Developmental Disabilities, 34*, 183–197.

Velozo, C. (Host). (2021 – present). Using measurement to highlight occupational therapy's distinct value. [Video podcast]. AOTA. https://www.aota.org/Practice/Researchers/Evidence-Podcast/slagle-2021-measurement-distinct-value.aspx

Wright, M. G., Hunt, L. P., & Stanley, O. H. (2005). Object/wrist movements during manipulation in children with cerebral palsy. *Pediatric Rehabilitation, 8*(4), 263–271.

Worksheets

WORKSHEET 5.1: RESEARCH NOTE – USING EVIDENCE IN PRACTICE

Summarize the findings of one research article that may inform occupational therapy practice in an area of which you are interested.

Reference [Do not use theoretical papers, systematic reviews, or studies for non-peer-reviewed sources for this assignment.]
Overview [Synthesize information to concisely describe purpose of study and what the authors did.]
Intervention Approach: [Describe the intervention approach that the study examines.]
Findings [Describe key findings and results clearly and concisely.]
Implications for OT: [Describe how the findings influence occupational therapy practice decisions.]

WORKSHEET 5.2: RESEARCH NOTE – EVIDENCE ON PERFORMANCE-BASED ASSESSMENT

Summarize the findings of a current research article examining a performance-based assessment.

Reference: [Do not use theoretical papers, systematic reviews, or studies from non-peer-reviewed sources for this assignment.]
Overview: [Synthesize information to concisely describe the purpose of study and what the authors did.]
Description of performance-based assessment: [Provide an overview of the purpose, scoring, and administration of the assessment. Describe the population for which the assessment is designed]
Findings: [Describe key findings and results clearly and concisely.]
Implications for occupational therapy: [Describe how the findings inform occupational therapy practice decisions.]
What are the advantages of using a performance-based assessment?

WORKSHEET 5.3: RESEARCH NOTE – EVIDENCE FOR PRINCIPLES OF OT INTERVENTION

Complete a research note summarizing the findings from a peer-reviewed study that supports one of the following principles of OT intervention.
- People engage in meaningful activities for longer periods of time or with better quality of movement.
- Repetitive practice of developmental skills provides experiences that promote brain plasticity.
- To increase strength, the muscle must be overloaded to the point of fatigue, which recruits more muscle units and causes hypertrophy and hyperplasia of glycolytic type II fast twitch muscle fibers (Rybski, 2012).
- Motor learning occurs as clients repeat motor tasks that are intrinsically motivating, meaningful, and for which they can problem solve.

Reference [Do not use theoretical papers, systematic reviews, or studies for non-peer-reviewed sources for this assignment.]
Principle: [Describe the principle you are addressing.]
Overview [Synthesize information to concisely describe purpose of study and what the authors did.]
Intervention Principle: [Describe the intervention principle that the study examines.]
Findings [Describe key findings and results clearly and concisely.]
Implications for OT: [Describe how the findings influence occupational therapy practice.]

WORKSHEET 5.4: EXAMINING EVIDENCE FROM SEVERAL SOURCES

Describe evidence from several sources (e.g., website, research article, blog, news article, YouTube video) regarding a specific condition or topic of interest.

Describe question or topic of interest for which you are looking for evidence:		
Source	**Description of information**	**Evidence**
Which source is most reliable and provides the best evidence?		
How do you decide which source is most reliable and provides the best evidence?		
Summary and conclusions		

WORKSHEET 5.5: EXAMINING INTERVENTION APPROACHES

Evaluate the evidence provided in a chosen research study examining the effectiveness of an intervention approach.
- Describe the strengths and limitations of the findings.
- Discuss your recommendation and rationale for using this intervention in practice.

Citation of research study:
What is the theory that informs this approach?
Describe the approach, strategy, or technique.
Explain the principles of change when using this approach. • How is change measured using this approach?
What type of client or population benefits from this approach?
Is this approach based on occupational therapy philosophy? • Does the approach address occupational therapy's scope of practice? • How does the approach address occupation
Is the approach client-centered? • Do clients like the approach?
Describe the study design. • What was the control intervention? (if there was a control) • How long was the intervention?
Findings • Describe the findings. • Is the approach effective?
What are the strengths and limitations to the research?
Describe the intervention approach. • What are contraindications for using this approach? • Is this approach safe or harmful in any way? • Does it require additional training? Materials?
Discuss your recommendation for using this intervention in practice.

WORKSHEET 5.6: CRITICAL REVIEW

Complete a critical review of a current peer-reviewed article using the format provided.

Name:
Citation (APA format)
Purpose or hypothesis
Background or need
Research design   • Type of study   • Level of evidence   • Number of subjects   • Inclusion/exclusion criteria
Methodology   • Intervention and control groups
Outcome measures   • Were measures valid and reliable?
Results   • What results were statistically significant?   • Were differences clinically meaningful?   • Do the findings support the author's claims?
Limitations
Conclusions/implications for practice   • What type of clients may benefit from this approach?   • Would you use this approach in practice? Why or why not?

WORKSHEET 5.7: CREATING PRACTICE EVIDENCE

Contact a local OT practitioner to identify a research question of current concern. Design a research project that could be completed in the setting as a new therapist (and with existing resources).

Name of Research Project:

1. Background and need (1–2 paragraphs; use literature to support the background and need, cite recent sources; clearly articulate the purpose, aims, or question you are addressing)
   a. Purpose of study
2. Research design (include a description of the following)
   a. Type of study (e.g., qualitative, quantitative, mixed, before and after, cohort, descriptive, single-subject)
   b. Setting (describe where this will take place)
   c. Subjects (number, inclusion, and exclusion criteria)
   d. Measurements (e.g., how are you measuring the outcomes? Why did you select them?)
   e. Procedures (1-2 paragraphs describing what you will do in the study; you may list procedures).
3. Data analysis
   • Describe what you will measure and what statistics (qualitative or quantitative) you will use to determine outcomes.
   • Describe why you used these measures.
4. How will this study inform occupational therapy practice?
5. Other considerations (This is optional. Describe anything not included above that you feel is necessary for your study.)

WORKSHEET 5.8: EVIDENCE AT EACH STAGE OF THE THERAPEUTIC REASONING PROCESS

Step in Therapeutic Reasoning Process	Evidence from Videoclip Observation
Generate questions based on theory	
Gather data	
Create conceptualization	
Create an intervention plan	
Implement intervention	
Evaluate outcomes	

6

Assessment: Gathering Information and Making Hypotheses

Teressa Garcia Reidy and Nicole Whiston Andrejow

GUIDING QUESTIONS

1. What is the thought process (reasoning) that occupational therapy practitioners use to select assessments to gather pertinent information about a client?
2. How do occupational therapy practitioners use therapeutic reasoning to interpret findings from assessments?
3. How do occupational therapy practitioners synthesize the data from the assessment to create hypotheses regarding factors that are influencing a client's occupational performance?
4. What factors may influence assessment findings?

KEY TERMS

Assessment
Conditional reasoning
Ethical reasoning
Evaluation process
Interactive reasoning
Narrative reasoning
Non-standardized assessment
Occupational profile

Pragmatic reasoning
Reliability
Rehabilitation approach
Scientific reasoning
Sensitivity
Specificity
Standardized assessment
Validity

INTRODUCTION

Trey is an occupational therapy student completing his level II fieldwork in an outpatient rehabilitation unit. He is preparing to complete an evaluation on a 37-year-old man who experienced a stroke. His supervisor asks him to select assessments he will administer to better understand the client's needs.

Trey contemplates the setting, clientele, and his role as the occupational therapist working in a rehabilitation setting. In addition to evaluating the client's physical skills and abilities, Trey would like to learn about the client's interests, motivations, habits, and routines.

Trey engages in therapeutic reasoning to select assessments, prioritize the evaluation process, and make hypotheses to guide his intervention plan.

- *How will he select assessments?*
- *How will he evaluate the client's occupational performance?*
- *What factors may influence the assessment findings?*

OT practitioners gather data and create hypotheses to conceptualize factors influencing occupational performance as part of the therapeutic reasoning process. The reasoning involved requires the OT practitioner to synthesize information from multiple sources. The evaluation process is an opportunity for the therapist to discover the client's desires and life experiences to identify supports and barriers to health, well-being, and

participation in desired occupations (American Occupational Therapy Association AOTA, 2020).

During the evaluation, OT practitioners use assessments (such as clinical observations, interviews, questionnaires, standardized, and non-standardized tests) to identify a client's strengths and challenges. Assessments are specific measurement tools that help practitioners understand the client's background, client factors, performance skills, performance patterns, and personal and environmental factors that influence occupational performance (Hinojosa & Kramer, 2014). OT practitioners synthesize information gathered from assessments to hypothesize how multiple factors interfere or support the client's participation in desired occupations. OT practitioners refine or change hypotheses as they gather more data during the evaluation and intervention processes. Figure 6.1 illustrates the dynamic nature of the process.

The therapeutic reasoning process guides occupational therapy (OT) practitioners as they use information to create hypotheses about the client's occupational performance and to create goals to address the client's needs (Kramer & Grampurohit, 2020). The hypotheses (based on research evidence from models of practice and frames of reference) and goals are used to create a specific intervention plan for the client.

The authors describe the therapeutic reasoning involved in gathering data, selecting assessments, and making hypotheses

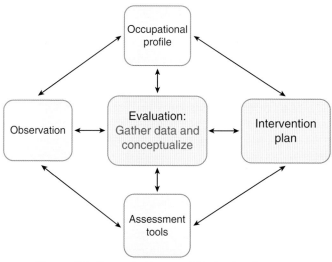

Figure 6.1 Dynamic Nature of Evaluation Process.

to guide intervention planning. They describe factors that may influence decisions on the validity of the assessment. Case examples and learning activities are interspersed throughout the chapter to illustrate concepts for practice.

GATHERING DATA

The initial evaluation provides the first opportunity to establish rapport and learn about the client and their family. OT practitioners gather information, observe and assess a client's strengths and challenges, hypothesize reasons for the client's performance difficulties, and use this information to create an intervention plan that addresses those factors interfering with the person's ability to engage in daily occupations.

Occupational therapy practitioners begin the evaluation process by gathering information through an occupational profile. The occupational profile includes information on the client's concerns about engagement in occupations, background and life history, values and interests, and priorities for treatment. AOTA's occupational profile provides a general guideline, whereas occupational profiles based on occupation-based models of practice provide specific questions that target the components of the model providing a more thorough and detailed description of the client's occupational history. Developing an occupational profile is an ongoing process that allows OT practitioners to learn about the client and discover the client's interests, goals, and motivations. The information from the occupational profile may indicate factors that support or impede participation in activities. Findings from the occupational profile guide the choice of assessments, goal setting, and intervention planning.

LEARNING ACTIVITY: OCCUPATIONAL PROFILE

Complete an occupational profile (see Worksheet 6.1) on a peer. From the profile, identify their interests and determine what you would like to observe them doing to better understand their occupational performance.

OBSERVATIONAL ASSESSMENT

OT practitioners gather important performance data by observing clients engage in a variety of activities. They observe processing skills (e.g., sequencing, problem-solving, timing, generalization skills), motor skills (e.g., movement, posture, coordination, strength, range of motion), and social–emotional skills (e.g., communication with others, range of emotions). OT practitioners carefully analyze the occupation, activity, or task to determine factors that support or interfere with the client's ability to engage in the desired activity (see Chapter 2).

They use scientific reasoning to determine how the client's condition or diagnoses manifest for the individual. For example, adults with Parkinson's disease may experience tremors interfering with mobility, while others experience intention tremors that affect fine motor skills and not mobility. OT practitioners use narrative reasoning to understand how the client's story influences activity choices and performance. For example, the OT practitioner may note that a boy (who loves painting) uses both arms more accurately when painting than when asked to complete his homework. The child may identify as the "artist" in the family, receive recognition for his creativity, and describe stories of paintings that influenced him. In this example, the OT practitioner decides that since the child identifies as a "painter," he is more motivated to engage in those activities.

OT practitioners use pragmatic reasoning to plan the evaluation session by considering the time, setting, resources, space, costs, and materials available. They consider how long each part of the evaluation takes when selecting assessment tools and examine the space and training required. For example, the assessment may require additional training or be expensive to purchase. Some assessments cost additional money to score. OT practitioners use ethical reasoning as they weigh the pros and cons of using a specific assessment tool or allow financial decisions or setting specific rules (that may not always benefit the client) to direct the evaluation process. For example, an OT practitioner may advocate for more training if a particular assessment tool requires it.

OT practitioners use interactive reasoning while engaging a client in an assessment. As OT practitioners observe clients asking questions and engaging with others, they take note of how clients indicate their needs, make eye contact with others, express emotion, and engage in group or activity expectations for behaviors. For example, an OT practitioner may decide to change one's approach if the client does not respond positively to the OT practitioner's suggestions. An OT practitioner may determine that the client's passive nature in a group is not allowing the client to work towards the stated goals. The OT practitioner may reason that the client needs more assistance in the group process to successfully engage in the task.

Conditional reasoning involves understanding the many factors that are involved in one's occupational performance. For example, the OT practitioner may observe a client successfully complete a simple meal preparation task in the outpatient treatment setting, while questioning if the client will be able to prepare meals successfully at home. Conditional reasoning may lead to seeking answers to questions, such as:

- With whom do they share space?
- What is the space like?

- What are the expectations of their performance upon discharge?
- For whom are they preparing meals?
- What are the time expectations?
- Do they have the motor, processing, and social emotional skills to handle multiple demands required upon discharge?

When engaging in conditional reasoning, OT practitioners combine narrative, scientific, ethical, interactive, and pragmatic reasoning.

LEARNING ACTIVITY: OBSERVATIONS

Observe a client and OT practitioner interaction (for example, observe Video 6.1 on the Evolve site). Using Worksheet 6.2 document the observations that inform each type of therapeutic reasoning.

Analyzing Occupations, Activities or Tasks

OT practitioners carefully observe clients as they engage in activities to identify the performance skills, patterns, client factors, and contexts that support or hinder occupational performance (see Appendix 6.1 for an example of an activity analysis). Table 6.1 describes the terms used to analyze occupations, activities, and tasks based on the Occupational Therapy Practice Framework (AOTA, 2020) and provides examples. OT practitioners use occupation, activity, or task analysis during the assessment process to better understand the client's strengths and challenges.

Performance skills include motor, process, and social-interaction actions that can be observed as one engages in an occupation. Practitioners observe clients moving, reaching, manipulating objects, figuring out how things work, sequencing tasks, and communicating verbally and nonverbally with others. By analyzing the performance skills required to complete one's daily activities, OT practitioners determine what may be interfering with the ability of clients to engage.

As a person engages in daily activities, they develop a set way of doing things, which is referred to as one's routines. Engaging in a routine provides structure to a person's life and some parts of the routine become habits, which require less attention. Routines are rituals that are performed based on cultures or beliefs, such as family dinner or family traditions. A person's routines, habits, and rituals become central to their roles (such as worker, parent, volunteer, athlete), which provide additional meaning to their life and contribute to their identity.

Client factors include values, beliefs, spirituality; body functions; and body structures (AOTA, 2020). For example, increased muscle tone (body function) in a child with hemiplegia may interfere with the child's ability to use both hands together for dressing. Understanding the performance at this level informs intervention planning. OT practitioners address occupations, while also targeting factors that impede performance.

The personal and environmental context in which an occupation occurs influences performance. Personal factors include those things unique to the person, such as age, background, history, interests (AOTA, 2020). Environmental factors include natural and human-made settings, buildings, materials and their properties, rules and expectations, societal attitudes, and policies. For example, walking along a quiet pathed parkway in mild weather requires a different skill set than walking along a crowded sidewalk during a snowstorm.

OT practitioners examine discrepancies between the client's desires and observed behaviors to determine how to intervene. They synthesize all the available information from the client and from observations of the client's performance to create a hypothesis or conceptualization of what is influencing occupational performance. At this point in the process, the OT practitioner may have created preliminary hypotheses while also deciding that a more detailed assessment is needed to further refine, support, or adjust the hypotheses.

TABLE 6.1   Terms Used to Analyze Occupations, Activities, and Tasks

Term	Definition	Examples
Performance skills (motor, process, social interaction)	"Observable, goal-directed actions that result in a client's quality of performing desired occupations" (AOTA, 2020, p. 80).	*Motor:* Moves in and out of positions with ease. *Process:* Completes each step of the project. *Social-interaction:* Makes eye contact with a peer.
Performance patterns	"Habits, routines, roles, and rituals that may be associated with different lifestyles and used in the process of engaging in occupations or activities" (AOTA, 2020, p. 80).	*Habits:* Puts coat in the same spot when returning home. *Routines:* Follows a set sequence of activities after dinner. *Roles:* Worker at local grocery store. *Rituals:* Reads a bedtime story to children every night.
Client factors (values, beliefs, spirituality; body functions; body structures)	"Specific capacities, characteristics or beliefs that reside within the person and that influence performance in occupations" (AOTA, 2020, p. 75).	*Values, belief, spirituality:* Dedicated to honest work; finds meaning in providing for family. *Body functions:* Awareness of time of day; sees small details (vision), has full upper body range of motion; moves independently. *Body structures:* Fully intact neurological system, voice and speech systems intact, no visible deficits in muscles or limbs.
Context (environmental and personal factors)	"Construct that constitutes the complete makeup of a person's life as well as the common and divergent factors that characterize groups and populations" (AOTA, 2020, p. 76).	*Environment:* Quiet, spacious room with comfortable chairs, table, and minimal decorations with soft lighting and windows to outside (with view of tree-filled park). *Personal:* 13-year-old who identifies as they and is in the 8th grade lives with family (parents and 2 younger siblings) in a city apartment. They enjoy art, music (plays guitar), and socializing with friends.

LEARNING ACTIVITY: ACTIVITY ANALYSIS

Observe a peer completing an activity. Record observations of performance skills, patterns, client factors and contexts. Use Worksheet 6.3 to analyze the components of what you observed.

SELECTING AN ASSESSMENT

OT practitioners use information from the occupational profile, clinical observations, and knowledge of occupation-based models of practice and frames of reference, to determine the assessment tool to administer. Information from the assessment provides additional data and a baseline performance level to assist the OT practitioner in creating an intervention plan. Selecting an appropriate assessment tool requires careful decision-making and knowledge of the purpose, link to theory, match with client, assessment tool properties, and pragmatics. See Box 6.1 for questions to consider when selecting an assessment. Figure 6.2 outlines a decision tree to help OT practitioners search and select the right tool.

BOX 6.1 Selecting an Assessment

Brief description of Client:
Brief description of Assessment:
Purpose: What occupations does the client want to address?

Link to theory
- Does the tool address an element or component of the model of practice or frame of reference?
- Will the findings from the assessment help understand concepts related to the model of practice or frame of reference?

Match with client
- Does the assessment provide information that is relevant to the client's identified goals?
- Does the assessment consider the influence of environment, cultural beliefs, or religious practices on the client's performance?
- Does the assessment provide an objective measure of performance that can determine if the client met the goals identified?

Assessment Tool Properties
- Does the assessment provide an objective measure of performance?
- What does the assessment really measure?
- Is there evidence to support the validity of the scores? Does the assessment measure what it says it does? What are the definitions and on what are they based?
- How do we know the information from the measure is reliable? Has it been examined with clients like mine?
- Is the measure responsive to change in the clients and context similar to my clients?

Pragmatics
- What age range and diagnoses does the assessment cover?
- What are the criteria for testing?
- How long does it take to administer the assessment?
  - Can the assessment be completed in segments and still be valid?
- What testing materials and space are needed?
- Are there any training requirements for administering and scoring the assessment?

Purpose

Throughout the evaluation process, OT practitioners use therapeutic reasoning to speculate reasons a client is not fully engaged in their occupations. They select assessment tools to provide more detailed information to inform intervention planning. They begin by examining the purpose of the assessment tool and the elements that the tool measures. They select tools that address occupations of interest or provide additional information about the client's performance. Assessments include survey, interviews, observations, or measurements (such as paper and pencil tests, performance, rating scales, self-report, or computer programs).

Assessments may measure outcomes, such as occupational performance, quality of life, or adaptive behaviors. They can be used to address specific occupations, such as play, leisure, work, activities of daily living, school, or social participation. Other assessments examine performance skills, client factors, or body functions and structures (e.g., range of motion, bilateral hand skills, emotional regulations, cognition, social skills). Assessments can provide a measure of the person's daily routines and habits and also describe the physical or social influences on human performance.

OT practitioners identify the purpose of the assessment to make sure it addresses the client's needs. They select assessments that provide a deeper understanding of the client's occupational participation. This may involve selecting assessments to better explain the underlying mechanisms influencing occupational performance. They may also select assessments that provide information on the client's subjective views of their performance and seek information to determine the client's occupational identity. Since understanding the client's needs, motivations, and occupational goals is critical to occupational therapy intervention, OT practitioners may select assessments that require clients to reflect on their decisions, actions, and occupational history.

Assessment findings are used to better understand the client's strengths and challenges. Examining a client's abilities by administering an assessment often provides details and explanations that may not be clear through direct observation. For example, the Test of Playfulness (TOP; Skard & Bundy, 2008) operationalizes playfulness so that OT practitioners may see and measure it in practice. O'Brien et al., (1999) found that administering the TOP helped students understand playfulness, observe the behaviors in practice, and write playfulness goals.

Findings from assessments may also be used to qualify clients for services, justify insurance payments, and measure progress. OT practitioners use therapeutic reasoning to make sound decisions about the types of assessments they use in practice.

Link to Theory

Frequently, OT practitioners select assessment tools that are linked to occupation-based practice models and frames of reference. Box 6.2 provides examples of assessments created to examine concepts of occupation-based models of practice. Using the assessments designed along with the model allows

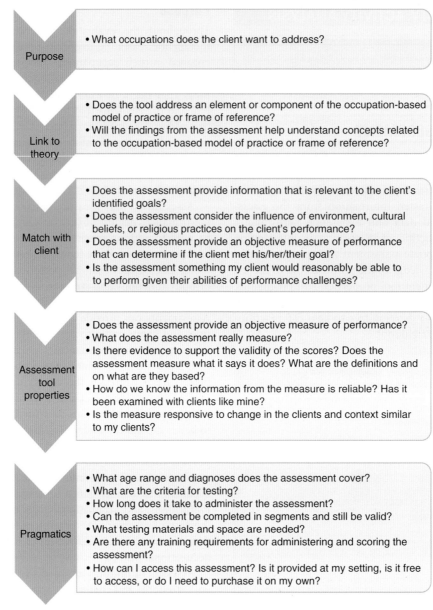

Figure 6.2 Selecting the Right Assessment.

OT practitioners to observe and measure the concepts from the model to better understand the client's needs.

OT practitioners select assessments that are aligned with that occupation-based model. For example, if the OT practitioner uses the Performance-Environment-Occupation-Performance Model (PEOP; Baum, Bass, & Christiansen, 2015), it is reasonable that they would also use the Activity Card Sort (Baum & Edwards, 2008), or Kitchen Task Assessment (Baum & Edwards, 1993; Rocke etal., 2008) to assess the client's occupational performance as these were developed specifically to address concepts for this model. These assessments provide information about the client's occupational performance to guide intervention planning. Conversely, if an OT practitioner uses the Model of Human Occupation (Taylor, 2017), it makes sense to administer the Model of Human Occupation Screening Tool (MOHOST) (Parkinson et al., 2006) designed specifically to measure a client's occupational performance as related to MOHO concepts (i.e., volition, habituation, performance capacity, and environment).

Occupation-based models of practice provide details and depth regarding occupational performance. Therefore, OT practitioners do not have to use two occupation-based models of practice (although they may use multiple frames of reference). Chapter 3 provides more information on occupation-based models of practice and frames of reference.

Assessments may also measure the performance skills based on frames of reference. For example, the Evaluation in Ayres Sensory Integration (EASI) (Mailloux et al., 2018) examines a client's sensory functioning based on concepts from Ayres Sensory Integration® (Ayres, 2004). When using assessments based on frames of references, OT practitioners use the principles of the frame of reference to direct the intervention. Therefore, it is important that OT practitioners understand the purpose of the assessment and its theoretical base. OT practitioners carefully select assessments that measure concepts from the model of practice or frame of reference that best address a client's occupational performance challenges.

BOX 6.2   Assessments Linked to Theory

Model of Practice	Assessment	Description of concept
Model of Human Occupation	Volitional Questionnaire (De las Heras, C., Geist, R., Kielhofner, G., & Li, Y, 2007) Pediatric Volitional Questionnaire (Basu, Kafkes, Schatz, Kiraly, & Kielhofner, 2008)	Volition: Interests (those things they do), values (what is important) and perceived efficacy (how well they feel they do it)
	Occupational Self-Assessment (Baron, Kielhofner, Iyneger, Golhammer, & Wolenksi, 2006): Child Occupational Self-Assessment (Kramer et al., 2014)	Subjective view of importance (value) and person's efficacy (how well they feel they complete activities).
	Model of Human Occupation Screening Tool (Parkinson et al., 2006)	Screening tool to examine motivation for occupation, pattern of occupation, communication and interaction skills, process skills, motor skills, and environment.
Canadian Model of Performance and Engagement.	Canadian Occupational Performance Measure (Law et al., 2005)	Detect change in a client's self-perception of occupational performance over time in self-care, productivity, and leisure. Client describes occupations normally performed and identifies satisfaction and performance problems.

LEARNING ACTIVITY: IDENTIFYING ASSESSMENTS

Complete Worksheet 6.4 to identify assessments that measure aspects of each of the models of practice or frames of reference listed.

Match with Client

It is important to find an assessment that addresses the client's identified goals and needs. OT practitioners determine if the assessment is suitable for the client based on age, condition, skills and requirements, environment, and purpose of the assessment. See Box 6.3 for factors to consider when selecting assessments suitable for clients. OT practitioners examine the assessment tool to determine if it has been normed on the specific population of interest, and if the items or tasks are culturally appropriate for a specific client. If the client feels uncomfortable with the assessment objects, they may not perform well, resulting in an unrealistic representation of their abilities. OT practitioners consider the influence of the client's environment, cultural beliefs, or religious practices on test performance.

OT practitioners carefully examine the skills and abilities required to complete the assessment, including the requirements for attention, cognition, social interaction, and motor performance. For example, some motor assessments for children require attention or cognitive skills to complete. If the OT practitioner is interested in evaluating a child's motor skill, they may select an assessment that does not require the child to attend for long periods of time or respond to multi-step directions. The goal of the assessment is to provide a realistic measure of the client's performance to inform intervention planning and to determine if the client has met their goal. OT practitioners analyze the administration directions and procedures to anticipate if the client will be able to complete the assessment. They note if accommodations are available and decide how accommodations may alter the findings to determine the suitability and usefulness of the assessment.

BOX 6.3   Matching Assessments for Clients

Client Characteristics
Age of client:
Characteristics or needs of client to be evaluated:
What do you hope to learn about the client from this assessment?
Assessment Characteristics
Purpose of Assessment (What does the assessment measure?)
Age range:
What are the skills (motor, processing, social) and requirements for completing the assessment?
Pragmatics
Time to administer and score:
Setting:
Materials needed:
Training:
Costs associated with assessment:
Summary
Does the assessment provide additional information to inform occupational therapy intervention planning?
Can the client complete the assessment as required?
Do you anticipate any difficulties in completing the assessment?

Assessment Tool Properties

The OT practitioner seeks to provide an objective measure of performance to inform intervention planning and to measure goal attainment.. By examining the information presented in the assessment manual, OT practitioners decide if the authors have clearly defined the measures and determine if the assessment measures the concept of interest. They must decide if the assessment is a valid (i.e., true) measure of the stated construct. Content validity refers to evidence that the assessment adequately covers the relevant domains of the construct (Coster, 2006).

It is also important to know that the information gained from the assessment is trustworthy (or reliable). Reliability refers to knowing that the information gained at one point in time or from one source is likely to be replicated on another occasion (test–retest) or when provided by a different source (inter-rater) (Coster, 2006).

Sensitivity and specificity refer to the ability of the measure to detect changes. Sensitivity is the ability of the assessment to detect the condition when it is present, whereas specificity refers to the ability to rule out the condition when it is not present (Asher, 2014). OT practitioners use assessment data to measure changes in client performance over time. Therefore, they must examine if the measure is responsive to changes within their client population. They review research evidence that examines if the measure is sensitive enough to detect changes in performance over time and if these changes are clinically meaningful (Coster, 2006). For example, some tests require at least 6 months before re-testing. Next they determine if their client population is likely to show similar changes.

OT practitioners also examine the reliability of administering a subtest or section of an assessment to determine if the scores or findings are meaningful. They consider cultural and environmental influences by reading the research evidence and acknowledging the item development. For example, some tests may include items that require English as one's first language and include items that do not translate well to other cultures. Some assessments have been validated in multiple languages.

Pragmatics

OT practitioners consider the practical aspects involved in administering, scoring, and interpreting assessments. All information regarding the assessment is available in the administration manual. Tests may be designed for specific age groups and diagnoses. OT practitioners examine the inclusion and exclusion criteria to determine if the assessment is appropriate for their client. They consider the cost of the assessment, including test materials, scoring forms, and training. The time to complete the assessment may require that it be completed in two sittings. The manual should state whether this affects the test validity or reliability. Testing space and equipment requirements must be considered as well.

LEARNING ACTIVITY: SELECTING AN ASSESSMENT

Select an assessment to administer in 30 minutes on a client (age and diagnosis to be determined by you) and document your considerations by following Worksheet 6.5.

TYPES OF ASSESSMENTS

Assessment tools are used to understand performance skills, performance patterns, client factors, contexts (i.e., personal and environmental factors) and activity demands that influence occupational performance (Hinojosa & Kramer, 2014). OT practitioners use interviews, questionnaires, written tests, physical measurements (such as ROM), and performance tests to describe clients' performance. Asher (2014) provides an index of occupational therapy assessment tools.

Non-standardized Assessments

OT practitioners use non-standardized assessments (such as observation, interview, or questionnaires) to identify a client's strengths and challenges. While non-standardized assessments provide guidelines for administration and scoring (if part of the assessment), they do not require the practitioner to administer them using specific wording, time, or procedures. Non-standardized assessments can measure progress, but they do not compare measures to a group of same-age peers. The assessments may be structured but because they are not standardized, the OT practitioner can adapt and modify tasks for the individual. Non-standardized assessments may provide qualitative or quantitative data.

When using a non-standardized assessment to measure progress over time, the OT practitioner documents how the client performed the task and the context in which the task was performed. For example, a client who could not make himself a sandwich may have this for a goal at the end of 2 weeks' time. The OT practitioner who conducted the initial assessment documents where and how the client performed meal preparation, type of directions provided, and assistance provided. At the end of 2 weeks, the OT practitioner uses the same instructions and setting to determine if the client has made changes in performance.

Standardized Assessments

Standardized assessments offer a "systematic procedure for observing behavior and describing it with the aid of a numerical scale or fixed categories" (Chronbach, 1990, p. 3 in Asher, 2014, p. 10). Standardized assessments provide a structured way to measure a client's performance in comparison to the general population. Standardized assessments often provide a numerical score that can assist with measuring changes in a client. Standardized assessments must be administered in a specific way. The test manual provides specific wording and administration procedures. When used with a large population of clients, standardized assessments can identify trends in needs of a given population and the efficacy of intervention within that population.

Developing clinical competency

Administering an assessment requires practice and competency. Each examiner must review the administration manual, observe others administering and scoring the test, and seek and receive feedback. Some publishers of assessments offer online tools, trainings, and video examples of administration and scoring to help OT practitioners become proficient in administering and scoring the tool. An OT practitioner may develop competency by working with a supervisor to ensure accuracy in using the correct procedures. They can videotape themself completing the assessment and re-score to compare their own reliability. Some assessments require additional training to ensure standardized administration. Practitioners may have to attend a course, score assessments, and work with trainers to complete a checklist to establish inter-rater reliability. It is the professional responsibility of each OT practitioner to establish competency in administering and scoring both standardized and non-standardized assessments.

The following case example describes the therapeutic reasoning used to select assessments that address the client's priorities, align with an occupation-based model of practice, and meet institutional requirements.

CASE EXAMPLE: SALLY

Sally is an OT practitioner working in an outpatient neurorehabilitation day program. She is scheduled to evaluate Tim, a teen who had a brain injury while skiing. She completed her chart review and gathered information regarding his course of therapy and medical intervention during her pretreatment preparation time. She noted he had a left femur fracture with an order for toe touch weight-bearing status. He continues to be disoriented to place and time. He has headaches that he rated as 5/10 during previous sessions.

Prior to his appointment, Sally made a checklist of what she would prioritize to assess in her 60-minute session. She planned to administer the Canadian Occupational Performance Measure (COPM) to assess his self-care, productivity, and leisure. The COPM provides information on current performance and satisfaction in these areas and is based on the Canadian Model of Occupational Performance and Engagement (CMOP-E).

Tim's mother may answer questions that might be difficult for him (due to his cognitive impairments as a result of the brain injury). The OT practitioner hopes to gain information about Tim's insight into his injuries and current abilities, interests, and goals. Sally evaluates Tim's physical abilities by completing range of motion and manual muscle testing. She also observes fine motor control, motor planning, bimanual coordination, sequencing, and visual motor coordination as Tim puts on and takes off a button-down shirt.

When Tim arrives at the clinic, he is holding his head and wearing sunglasses as his mother pushes his manual wheelchair into the clinic's gym. Tim states his headaches continue to bother him. He reports his current level of pain as 6/10 and that he has double vision and difficulty writing. Sally uses *interactive reasoning* to wait for a response, speak softly, make eye contact, and smile at him, while asking Tim to complete assessments (COPM, range of motion, and manual muscle testing, dressing task) that are not overwhelming at this point.

Sally uses scientific reasoning as she makes observations related to Tim's performance. She decides to further examine his vision and visual perceptual skills. She starts with a button-down shirt activity. During the activity, she observes his performance skills and movement functions, including: external rotation of

his shoulders, elbow flexion and extension, dynamic sitting balance and trunk strength, pinch strength, and coordination. She also observes his functional vision skills. Sally observes his eyes converging when he looks down at his buttons. He has a tremor in his left hand when attempting to button but completes 4/5 buttons before he reports his hands are getting tired.

Tim transfers from his wheelchair to a table mat with supervision, maintaining his toe touch weight-bearing (TTWB) precautions. Sally makes a note that he has sufficient upper body strength to transfer himself. He does not lose his balance, so she rates his static sitting balance "good" in the electronic health record. He then puts the shirt on independently while sitting on the edge of the mat. Sally rates this "good" for dynamic sitting balance on the evaluation template. He doffs his sunglasses independently and puts them in an eyeglass case. He does not align the buttons correctly and she notices that he keeps one eye closed when trying to button. Tim reports he has double vision and light sensitivity. He also mentions that he has been meeting with a virtual tutor to start addressing his missed classwork but looking at the computer screen hurts his eyes.

Using *pragmatic reasoning*, Sally realizes Tim's pain and fatigue impact how much of the assessment Tim will complete in the allotted time, Sally hoped to gain information about Tim's current performance level by using a standardized performance test. However, she decides to gather information on Tim's ADL skills and participation by allowing Tim's mother to complete the Pediatric Evaluation of Disability Computer Adaptive Test (Haley, Coster, Dumas, Fragala-Pinkham, & Mood, 2012).

Next, Sally completes a brief visual screen to assess convergence, tracking, saccades, reading close and at a distance. When she is done with her assessment she sends a referral to neuro-ophthalmology and alerts the physiatrist in team rounds that Tim's vision is impacting his ability to engage in daily activities. Sally decides to ask Tim to complete the upper body dressing subtest of the self-care portion of the Wee Functional Independence Measure (WeeFIM; Granger et al., 1998) which is a required outcome tool in her facility used to track the client's progress across the rehabilitation continuum.

This case study highlights the flexibility needed when evaluating clients in a clinical setting. Sally evaluated all domains of functioning by prioritizing the assessment tasks and setting up the tasks to assess multiple domains (e.g., motor, process, and social-interaction skills; client factors; environmental and personal factors). See Box 6.4 for the list of assessments used in this example. She did not complete a formal range of motion test or manual muscle test, rather she observed his skills during the dressing task. She gathered enough information to identify how his impairments influenced his participation level in ADLs and schoolwork. The next step in the process is to synthesize all the available data and create hypotheses or conceptualization of what is interfering with the client's occupational performance.

INTERPRETING ASSESSMENT DATA AND CREATING HYPOTHESES

Therapeutic reasoning involves synthesizing information obtained during the evaluation process (i.e., occupational profile, observation, and assessment) and creating hypotheses to explain factors interfering with occupational performance. OT practitioners make judgments about the quality of the assessment findings. For example, the client may have difficulty following directions (due to medications) influencing findings. A

child may be tired after a busy school day and not perform to their potential. OT practitioners note the client's behaviors and make statements on the validity of the findings. They compile all the data to hypothesize how to intervene to support the client's occupational performance.

Box 6.5 outlines the steps in this process.

Score and Interpret Findings

After completing the occupational profile, observations, and assessment, the practitioner scores and interprets the findings. The practitioner often reviews the manual to determine what the specific scores mean, but it is important to view the results along with all available data.

- *Standard scores* are used to compare a client's results to the population. Standard scores are useful when determining changes over time. They are based upon the population and age expectations.
- *Raw scores* are based on the assessment and provide little information as they differ between tests. Furthermore, raw scores do not consider age or the population score. For example, knowing that a client received the raw score of 30 does not provide any information if one does not know the possible total points available or what is considered an acceptable score. Raw scores generally do not provide accurate measurements of change. The administration manual

---

BOX 6.4   Assessments Selected for Case Example: Sally

Assessment	Description	Area(s) addressed
Canadian Occupational Performance Measure (Law et al., 2005)	Client-centered interview that measures client's satisfaction and performance.	Self-care, productivity (such as school performance), and leisure
WeeFIM (Child Functional Independence Measure; Uniform Data System for Medical Rehabilitation, 2004)	Provides measure of severity of disability in performing self-care, communication, and cognitive tasks.	Only the self-care (ADL) section was completed. Examined independence in self-care with regards to physical and cognitive
PEDI-Cat (Pediatric Evaluation of Disability Inventory – Computer Adaptive Test; Haley et al., 2012)	PEDI uses observation, interview, and judgment of professionals familiar with the child to assess self-care, mobility, and social function.	Items are rated on functional skills, caregiver assistance and level of adaptions and assistance required for performance.
Clinical observations	Eye convergence and movements during dressing task. Range of motion and manual muscle testing; balance and upper body strength while transferring. Fine motor skills for dressing and sequencing. General problem-solving and communication skills.	Functional vision examined during activities. Functional range of motion, muscle strength, and coordination. The OT practitioner observed Tim problem-solve, sequence, and use his hands during dressing task. He communicated with her throughout the assessment.
Pain scale	Self-report of pain on scale of 0 (no pain) to 10 (extreme pain)	Pain level

---

BOX 6.5   Steps to Interpreting Findings and Creating Hypotheses

1. Complete occupational profile, observations, and assessment.
2. Score and interpret findings:
   i.   Calculate assessment scores and compare to normative sample.
   ii. Determine behaviors or factors that may have interfered with assessment findings.
   iii. Interpret assessment findings.
3. Summarize findings considering information from occupational profile, observations, and assessments.
   i. Identify client's strengths and challenges.
   ii. Decide what is interfering with the client's ability to do those things they want to do.
4. Create hypotheses that explain the interactions between factors influencing the client's occupational performance challenges.
   i.   Identify reasons why the client is experiencing challenges.
   ii. Use principles from models of practice and frames of reference to explain relationships between factors.
   iii. Identify data that supports the hypotheses.
5. Create measurable goals specific to client.
   i. Prioritize goals using available information.

may indicate clinically meaningful changes in raw scores based on research findings. For example, an increase of 2 points on a raw score of the COPM is considered clinically significant (Law, Baptiste et al., 2005).

- *Age equivalent scores* provide age level performance, but they are not as accurate as the standard score. Clients may achieve maximum performance early (for example, tests of visual performance) and receive an age equivalent score that does not provide valuable data. The OT practitioner uses clinical judgment to balance how much to weight the information gained from standardized assessments with findings from observation, self-assessment, or interviews.

Interpreting the findings involves analyzing the scores on the assessment in light of the client's performance. OT practitioners use their judgment and knowledge of the context of the testing

session and clinical experience to interpret the findings. The assessment manual provides information on how to interpret scores. OT practitioners examine the scores in light of available information from client interview, observation, and assessment findings to make hypotheses regarding the client's strengths and challenges.

Behaviors Influencing Findings

OT practitioners consider behaviors or factors that may have interfered with the assessment findings. Personal factors, such as a client not feeling well, or meeting the OT practitioner for the first time, or having a difficult day emotionally may interfere with performance on a standardized test. Practitioners also evaluate their performance in administering the test to consider if they may have influenced the findings. This may be the first time administering the test, or the testing was disrupted, or administration errors were made, including providing too many directions or assisting the client too much. The practitioner notes on the evaluation report factors that may have influenced the findings and makes a statement about the accuracy or truthfulness (i.e., validity) of the findings.

For example, a child who refuses to pick up any blocks scores very low on a fine motor test. However, the OT practitioner observes the child pick up markers and draw, button his coat, and pick up small candy using a pincer grasp. The child plays with playdoh and makes a tower. He swipes away the blocks even when playing. In this case, the OT practitioner documents his score on the test and indicates that the child's dislike of blocks contributed to his low score on the assessment, but the child demonstrated sufficient fine motor skills.

Interpret Assessment Findings

OT practitioners interpret assessment findings by considering factors that may influence the person's performance on the assessment (such as behaviors, contexts, testing time, and location). They synthesize information from multiple sources to determine how the client's strengths and challenges may have influenced assessment findings. They may examine the assessment subtest or items to determine patterns of performance. Interpreting assessment findings requires therapists to use therapeutic reasoning and requires practice and reflection.

SUMMARIZE FINDING AND IDENTIFY STRENGTHS AND CHALLENGES

OT practitioners evaluate information gained during the occupational profile, and through observation of the client's approach to activities during the assessment and assessment findings to identify the client's occupational strengths and challenges. They often complete an occupation, activity, or task analysis to determine how the client's strengths and challenges influence their abilities to engage in desired activities. They summarize the findings by determining the factors interfering with the client's participation in desired activities. This becomes the basis for developing hypotheses and creating goals for intervention.

CREATING HYPOTHESES

OT practitioners summarize the findings of the evaluation and create a list of the client's strengths and occupational performance challenges or problems. Using professional knowledge, information from models of practice and frames of reference, and evaluation findings, the practitioner identifies reasons why the client is not able to engage in desired activities.

They begin by brainstorming possible reasons why the client is experiencing challenges and analyzing what is interfering with the client's performance. They create hypotheses using information gained from the assessment, interview and observation of client, activity analysis, and knowledge of the client's condition along with their professional experience.

OT practitioners make decisions on what is interfering with the client's ability to engage in desired activities and may further explore research evidence, models of practice and frames

of reference to create hypotheses to explain occupational challenges. At this stage, the OT practitioner seeks to define how the challenges a client experiences interfere with occupational performance. They make their hypotheses based on available data. Furthermore, the OT practitioner examines principles of change as related to the client's challenges. (See Table 6.2.)

CREATE MEASURABLE GOALS

OT practitioners use knowledge of the client's current level of functioning to create goals that are important to the client's identity. Together, the OT practitioner and client create meaningful goals that can be achieved in the allotted intervention times or number of sessions. They prioritize goals to match the client's needs and challenges. OT practitioners seek to understand the client's lived experience so they can create client-centered goals.

The following case example illustrates the therapeutic reasoning process to develop and create goals and hypotheses.

Case Example

A 58-year-old man who experienced a stroke is no longer able to use his right side. He is a self-employed plumber who must complete work using both hands. His first question is "When can I get back to work?" The OT practitioner created the following strengths and challenges and developed a hypothesis for organizing the intervention plan using the Model of Human Occupation (Taylor, 2017) and contemporary motor control/motor learning.

Strengths:
- Client verbally expressed desire to return to work.
- Client attempted to move his right UE to complete tasks.
- Client slightly moved fingers and wrist (R UE).
- Client responded to all requests.

Challenges:
- Client is unable to move his R UE at shoulder and elbow.
- Client speech was slurred.

Model of Practice/ Frame of Reference	Hypothesis	Data to support	Possible solutions
Biomechanical	ROM deficits in bilateral hands interfere with client's fine motor skills resulting in difficulty performing self-care tasks.	Limited PROM and AROM in B UEs secondary to contractures from arthritis. Client does not have full range of motion in either hand (ulnar deviated, contractions at PIP/DIPs). She is not able to get herself bathed or dressed in the morning without assistance.	Adaptations to clothing, built-up handles, compensatory techniques.
Model of Human Occupation	Client's occupational identity as athlete has been altered since physical injury, resulting in low self-efficacy leading to limited occupational engagement.	Client's habits have changed since injury whereas he does not want to engage in social activities with friends. He spends his time alone at home. His performance abilities have changed (i.e., poor mobility, coordination, and balance) and he does not feel he can adapt (perceived efficacy).	Address performance skills through rehabilitation activities. Adapt activities so he can feel achievement and participate at his level. Create changes in his habits, by identifying group programs for athletes with disabilities (e.g., adapted basketball). Work collaboratively with client to promote self-efficacy.

TABLE 6.2 **Creating Hypotheses Based on Models of Practice/Frame of Reference**

ROM – range of motion; PROM – passive range of motion; AROM – active range of motion; B UEs – bilateral upper extremities; PIP – proximal interphalangeal; DIP – distal interphalangeal.

• Client leans to left when sitting.

Hypotheses: Client's inability to use his right side (performance capacity) interferes with his ability to complete morning ADL activities and work (occupations). Engaging in work is essential to the client's occupational identity. He may experience skill deficits for which he will have to adapt (occupational adaption). He is experiencing a disruption in his habits and roles (habituation) which may impact his belief in his skills and abilities (perceived efficacy).

The OT practitioner reasoned that the client is motivated to return to work (volition) and will use this goal to address his physical challenges. Since the client is highly motivated, the practitioner will provide exercise programs and engage the client in the planning process. The practitioner hypothesizes that engaging the client in the problem-solving process will facilitate cognition and empower the client to make necessary adaptations during the recovery process. The OT practitioner uses motor control/motor learning concepts to design intervention to promote recovery through whole meaningful activities, while also attending to the client's motivation and self-efficacy.

Models of practice and frames of reference explain interactions between multiple systems based on research and theory (see Chapter 3). This allows the practitioner to use the principles outlined in the practice model to explain reasons for the client's difficulties. Since occupation-focused models of practice explain human performance, they can explain the interactions between factors influencing occupational performance. Table 6.2 provides examples of hypotheses based on the biomechanical frame of reference and the Model of Human Occupation (MOHO), data to support hypotheses, and possible occupational therapy intervention solutions.

The following case study illustrates the process involved in generating hypotheses leading to creating goals for intervention.

TELEHEALTH CONSIDERATIONS FOR ASSESSMENTS

There are additional considerations when administering a standardized assessment via telehealth (Table 6.3). The first priority is the safety of the client. The practitioner determines if the client is aware of safety issues and determines the level of assistance required for the client to be safe. It is possible that a caregiver may need to be present during the telehealth assessment.

OT practitioners completing an assessment via telehealth must be compliant with Health Insurance Portability and Accountability Act (HIPAA) by determining if their professional licensure allows for telehealth services and identifying how the client's personal information is protected. When sending materials to clients, the OT practitioner follows copyright law and guidelines established on using the assessment in telepractice. Many standardized assessments have specific testing materials or instructions that must be used for the findings to be considered valid and reliable, making it difficult to complete via telehealth. Some computer methods and scoring platforms

CASE STUDY

During his initial evaluation with Sally, Tim reported that one of his prioritized Occupational Performance Problems on the COPM was "Focusing and typing his assignments for school." He rated his Current Performance as a 2 and Satisfaction as a 1. (Clients rate their performance and satisfaction on a scale of 1 (not able to perform/not satisfied at all) to 10 (able to perform extremely well/extremely satisfied)). Additionally, he reported pain as 5/10 and stated he experienced headaches, light sensitivity, and double vision. The OT practitioner verified through observations that Tim had trouble with fine motor skills (difficulty buttoning) and lining up the buttons. He made limited eye contact and stated it was difficult to remain on the computer for school. He also said that he was "bored" because he did not do as much with his friends since he needs to use a wheelchair.

Creating hypotheses (Conceptualization): Sally hypothesized that Tim's pain, vision difficulties, and fine motor skills interfere with Tim's school and ADL performance. Furthermore, his current system of working on the computer for long periods of time is more stressful on his vision, resulting in more pain and less performance. While the school is supportive of Tim's situation, he does not get frequent rest breaks from the computer or social breaks with friends. Sally hypothesized that Tim may be feeling a loss of his identity (as a friend) since the ski accident and working primarily online. He expressed frustration that he cannot do the things he used to do, which interferes with his self-efficacy (belief in his skills and abilities).

Sally and Tim collaborate to create the following goals:
1. Tim will use 2 strategies to decrease visual fatigue and headache pain so he can participate in 30 minute virtual school sessions.
2. To engage in schoolwork, Tim will complete homework assignments using a laptop with blue screen (to reduce glare and light) for 10 consecutive minutes without complaints of pain or feeling fatigue.
3. To develop a sense of efficacy for his occupational identity and quality of life, Tim will engage in 1 new social activity (in the community, not virtually) with a peer ×1 hour weekly.

The OT practitioner collaborates with the neuro-ophthalmologist to identify visual impairment issues and strategies to ameliorate or cope with these deficits to help Tim reach his goals. Sally decides that she will use a **rehabilitation approach** to support Tim's progress so that he can begin to participate in daily activities while improving his ability to attend to school (through meaningful repetition and practice) and regain his strength, endurance, and skills as he is engaging. Box 6.6 outlines the principles of the rehabilitation approach.

Description of Therapeutic Reasoning

In creating her hypotheses regarding Tim's occupational performance, Sally used *narrative reasoning* as she incorporated information from Tim's story about "hanging out with friends" prior to the accident and how it felt so different now that he needed to use a wheelchair for longer distances. Tim told Sally stories of skiing with friends and how he missed being outside. As Tim spoke, Sally watched his reactions and the look on his face when he had difficulty buttoning his shirt. Tim looked frustrated and became quiet. He often sighed and stated, "I'm done, my head hurts." She used *interactive reasoning* to suggest that Tim was feeling inadequate and frustrated with his abilities and was upset that he could not do the things he wanted to do. This was keeping him from socializing with friends and he was losing his occupational identity. Sally used *pragmatic reasoning* as she considered how long Tim would be in occupational therapy, that he needed to return to school, and that his mother would have to follow up with intervention strategies. In creating the intervention activities, Sally was able to use *conditional reasoning* by examining the client factors, performance skills, and environmental and personal factors influencing Tim's occupational engagement. She reasoned that adapting and modifying things so Tim could be successful would be a priority, and that as he engaged in those things that were important to him (and with support from the school, friends, and home), Tim would improve his skills, feel good about himself, and continue to make progress.

Sally knows that she can reassess his performance in a few weeks to determine if the interventions have made a significant impact. According to the COPM, a raw score increase of 2 or more indicates clinical significance.

Rehabilitation Team: At the team meeting Sally reports her initial findings to the team. She emailed the neuro-ophthalmologist describing how Tim's vision difficulties impact his function and consequently school performance. During her second session, Sally administered the Beery-Buktenica Developmental Test of Visual-Motor Integration (Beery, 2004) and she shared the findings with the physician. She found Tim needed a break between each of the 3 subtests. During team rounds, the Special Educator asked Sally to provide a brief report she can share with Tim's school about how much assistance he will need when he returns to school and if he will need any adaptive equipment. Sally also created goals for his school Individualized Education Plan (IEP). The physiatrist updated the team on Tim's weight-bearing status and shared that next week given his progress Tim could bear more weight on his foot. Sally and the PT discussed a co-treatment session to complete meal preparation activities in standing to be scheduled next week.

Sally met with Tim's mother. She shared the priorities during treatment to improve his vision and endurance for screen and paper and pencil assignments; help him gain independence getting dressed; and re-engage in social activities with peers. She will share strategies that work in therapy and so they can incorporate these strategies into his routines at home.

BOX 6.6 Principles of the Rehabilitation Approach

- Adapting tasks/methods/substitutes for loss of ROM, strength, use of one side of the body, limited vision, decreased endurance, inadequate stability, or to minimize the effects of spasticity and can simplify work and conserve energy (Rybski, 2012).
- Adapting tasks/objects or using adaptive/assistive devices or orthotics compensates for lack of reach, ROM, grasp, strength, vision, use of one side of the body, and loss of mobility to allow children to engage in proper positioning and overcome barriers (architectural, physical, or social/emotional) for occupational participation (Rybski, 2012).
- Changing the context by modifying the environment will provide access to transportation, home, public and private facilities, work and recreational activities so the child can participate in desired occupations (Rybski, 2012).

TABLE 6.3 Considerations for Telehealth Assessments

What is the safety awareness of the client?
• Do they need supervision by a caregiver?
What is the availability of a caregiver or proxy person to assist with camera positioning, gathering materials and assisting the client?
What telecommunications program will be used?
• What level of security will there be to protect patient information?
Are there copyright laws for the assessments?
What is the validity of assessments delivered over telehealth?
• Check the manual or publisher website for clarification and confirmation that the test is still valid when administered via telehealth rather than in person.
What are licensing laws designated by each state for assessing patients via telehealth?
• Determine if the patient and therapist are in the same state or different states. State licensure may require licensure in their state if you treat a patient who resides in that state.
What are the requirements by the client's insurance when delivering telehealth?
• Will your reimbursement rate be different?
• Clarify insurance requirements and documentation needs prior to scheduling a telehealth visit.
How will a therapist assess daily routines or specific skills?
• Are there readily available household items that may provide a way to assess a variety of skills?
• Contact the patient ahead of the session so they are prepared with materials prior to starting the session to maximize assessment time.
When should you use standardized assessments versus clinical observation?

are validated for tele-visits. For those assessments that are not designed for telehealth, practitioners may decide to administer them but view the results cautiously.

OT practitioners also consider the environment in which they administer an assessment and verify that there is adequate space to complete the items (e.g., gross motor tasks), supportive seating or an appropriate height table, and assure the correct camera angle so the OT practitioner can observe the client's performance.

OT practitioners can complete a client or caregiver interview and observe tasks as part of a telehealth evaluation. For example, the practitioner may observe a cooking activity to assess range of motion, strength, fine motor coordination, bilateral coordination, visual perception and coordination, balance, functional mobility, attention, sequencing, and problem-solving.

■ SUMMARY

OT practitioners use therapeutic reasoning to select and administer assessments that provide information describing performance skills, patterns, client factors, and personal and environmental factors. They use information from the occupational profile, assessments, and clinical observations to inform intervention planning. They synthesize data from the assessment to create hypotheses regarding factors that are influencing a client's occupational performance. They use professional experience and consider theories, models of practice and frames of reference to explain concepts.

OT practitioners synthesize information from multiple sources during the evaluation to hypothesize factors that are interfering with a person's ability to engage in meaningful activities. They use this information to determine the client's strengths and challenges, develop goals, and decide how to best address those goals by using principles of a selected model of practice or frame of reference.

Standardized assessments require specific procedures and directions which some clients may not understand which may affect the findings. The OT practitioner determines if the assessment population is similar to the client and selects the assessment that will provide useful information. Client behaviors, including attention, physical skills, emotions, and the environment may influence the findings. The OT practitioner documents any disruptions in the testing process and uses clinical observations to determine the validity of the assessment in measuring the client's abilities on a given day.

REFERENCES

American Occupational Therapy Association (AOTA). (2020). Occupational therapy practice framework: Domain and process (4th ed.). *American Journal of Occupational Therapy*, 71(Suppl.2), S1–S96.

Asher. I. A. (2014). *Asher's Occupational Therapy Assessment Tools* (4th ed.). Bethesda, MD: AOTA Press.

Ayres. A. J. (2004). *Sensory integration and the child* (2nd ed.). Los Angeles: Western Psychological Services (WPS).

Baron., K., Kielhofner, G., Iyneger, A., Golhammer, V., & Wolenksi, J. (2006). *Occupational Self-Assesemnt (OSA) version 2.2*. Model of Human Occupation Clearinghouse, Department of Occupational Therapy, University of Illinois at Chicago.

Basu, S., Kafkes, A., Schatz, R., Kiraly, A., & Kielhofner, G. (2008). *Pediatric Volitional Questionnaire (PVQ), version 2.1*. Model of Human Occupation Clearinghouse, Department of Occupational Therapy, University of Illinois at Chicago.

Baum, C. M., Bass, J. D., & Christiansen, C. H. (2015). Person-Environment-Occupation-Performance (PEOP) Model. In C. H. Christiansen, C. M. Baum, & J. D. Bass (Eds.), *Occupational Therapy: Performance, Participation, and Well-being* (4th ed., pp. 49–55). Thorofare, NJ: Slack.

Baum, C., & Edwards, D. (1993). Cognitive performance in senile dementia of the Alzheimer's type. The Kitchen Task Assessment. *American Journal of Occupational Therapy*, 47, 431–436.

Baum, C., & Edwards, D. (2008). *Activity Card Sort* (2nd ed.). Bethesda, MD: AOTA Press.

Beery. K. E. (2004). *Beery VMI: The Beery-Buktenica developmental test of visual-motor integration*. Minneapolis, MN: Pearson.

Coster. W. J. (2006). Evaluating the use of assessments in practice and research. In G. Kielhofner (Ed.), *Research in Occupational Therapy: Methods of Inquiry for Enhancing Practice* (pp. 201–212). Philadelphia, PA: FA Davis.

De las Heras, C., Geist, R., Kielhofner, G., & Li, Y. (2007). *The Volitional Questionnaire (VQ), version 4.1*. Model of Human Occupation Clearinghouse, Department of Occupational Therapy, University of Illinois at Chicago.

Granger, C. V., Msall, M. E., Braun, S., Griswald, K., McCabe, M., Heyer, N., & Hamilton, B. B. (1998). *Wee-FIM system clinical guide: Version 5.01*. Buffalo, NY: University of Buffalo.

Haley, S. M., Coster, W. J., Dumas, H. M., Fragala-Pinkham, M. A., & Mood, R. (2012). *Pediatric Evaluation of Disability Inventory-Computer☐aAdaptive Test (PEDI☐CAT)*. Boston: Health and Disability Research Institute, Boston University School of Public Health.

Hinojosa, J., & Kramer, P. (Eds.). (2014). *Evaluation in Occupational Therapy: Obtaining and Interpreting Data* (pp. 322). Bethesda, MD: American Occupational Therapy Association, Incorporated.

Kramer, P., & Grampurohit, N. (2020). *Hinojosa and Kramer's Evaluation in Occupational Therapy: Obtaining and Interpreting Data*. North Bethesda, MD: American Occupational Therapy Association.

Kramer, J., ten Velden, M., Kafkes, A., Basu, S., Federico, J., & Kielhofner, G. (2014). *Child Occupational Self-Assessment (COSA), version 2.2*. Model of Human Occupation Clearinghouse, Department of Occupational Therapy, University of Illinois at Chicago.

Law, M., Baptiste, S., Carswell, A., McColl, M. A., Polatajko, H., & Pollock, N. (2005). *Canadian Occupational Performance Measure* (4th ed.). Ottawa, ON: CAOT Publications ACE.

Mailloux, Z., Parham, L. D., Simth Roley, S., Ruzzano, L., & Schaaf, R. (2018). Introduction to the Evaluation in Ayres Senosry Integrastion® (EASI). *American Journal of Occupational Therapy*, 72(1). https://doi.org/10.5014/ajot.2018.028241.

O'Brien, J., Coker, P., Lynn, R., Pearigen, T., Rabon, S., St. Aubin, M., … Ward, A. (1999). The impact of occupational therapy on a child's playfulness. *Occupational Therapy in Health Care*, 12, 39–51.

O'Brien, J., & Solomon, J. (2021). *Occupational Analysis and Group Process*. Elsevier.

Parkinson, S., Forsyth, K., & Kielhofner, G. (2006). *The Model of Human Occupation Screening Tool (MOHOST), Version 2.0*. Chicago: Model of Human Occupation Clearinghouse.

Skard, G., & Bundy, A. C. (2008). Test of Playfulness. In L. D. Parham & L. S. Fazio (Eds.), *Play in occupational therapy for children* (2nd ed., pp. 71–93). St. Louis, MO: Mosby.

Rocke, K., Hays, P., Edwards, D., & Berg, C. (2008). Developmetna of a performance assessment of executive function: The Children's Kitchen Taskk Assessment. *American Journal of Occupational Therapy*, 62, 528–537.

Rybski. M. (2012). Rehabilitation adaptation and compensation: *Kinesiology for Occupational Therapy* (pp. 355–428). Thorofare, NJ: SLACK Inc.

Taylor. R. R. (2017). *Kielhofner's Research in Occupational Therapy: Methods of Inquiry for Enhancing Practice*. Philadelphia, PA: FA Davis.

Uniform Data System for Medical Rehabilitation. (2004). *WeeFIM II® System*. Buffalo: State University of New York at Buffalo.

Worksheets

WORKSHEET 6.1: OCCUPATIONAL PROFILE

Name:

Background:

Describe where you live:

Members of your household:

Social network:

Interests/hobbies:

Work:

Daily routines:

What brings you joy?

Are you able to participate fully in those things that you want to?

If not, what limits you?

Goals: What would you like to accomplish?

WORKSHEET 6.2: OBSERVATIONS

Document the observations (or example) for each type of therapeutic reasoning.

Brief description of videoclip:

Observations	
Therapeutic reasoning	**Observation from clip**
Scientific	
Narrative	
Pragmatic	
Ethical	
Interactive	
Conditional	

WORKSHEET 6.3: ACTIVITY ANALYSIS

Observe a peer completing an activity and record observations of performance skills, patterns, client factors, context, and activity demands.

Activity Analysis	
Activity description	
Client's goal	
Meaning Describe the meaning and importance of activity to client.	
Sequence of steps List sequence of steps to complete.	
Materials/supplies and their properties Identify materials and their properties (i.e., texture; consistency; size; purpose; shape; color; and sensory properties)	
Space Describe setting in which activity occurs (e.g., outdoors, large space for physical activity).	
Social Describe social and attitudinal requirements.	
Performance pattern Describe when, where, how often, client completes this activity.	
Performance Skills	
• Motor Skills Describe actions related to moving and manipulating objects.	
• Process Skills Describe actions related to selecting, interacting, and using objects (e.g., problem-solving).	
• Social Interaction Skills Describes actions related to communicating and interacting with others (e.g., makes eye contact; acknowledges others).	
Body functions Describe factors required to complete activity.	

Body structures Describe body structures required to complete activity.	
Contexts: Environmental Factors (describe how the environment influences performance)	
Physical (e.g., setting, surroundings)	
Technology	
Social (e.g., supports, attitudes)	
Institution (e.g., services, systems, policies)	
Contexts: Personal Factors (describe how client's experiences influence performance)	
Background Consider age, experiences, education, gender identity and history.	
Culture Describe family culture, identification.	
Social Describe past and current lifestyle choices and interactions.	
Habits and routines Describe past and present habits and routines.	
Professional identity Describe how client views professional roles and expectations.	
Strengths and challenges Describe psychological strengths and challenges.	
Other Describe other health conditions and fitness as they influence performance.	

From: O'Brien, J. & Solomon, J. (2021). *Occupational Analysis and Group Process*. Elsevier.

WORKSHEET 6.4: IDENTIFYING ASSESSMENTS

Identify and describe assessments that measure aspects of each of the models of practice or frames of reference listed.

Identifying Assessments		
Model/Frame of Reference	**Assessment Tool**	**Brief description of aspect that tool measures**
Model of Human Occupation		
Person-Environment-Occupation-Performance (PEOP)		
Biomechanical		
Developmental		
Rehabilitation		
Occupational adaptation		
Motor control/motor learning		
Sensory integration		
Neurodevelopmental		
Cognitive behavioral		

WORKSHEET 6.5: SELECTING AN ASSESSMENT

Select an assessment to administer in 30 minutes on a client (age and diagnosis to be determined by you) and document your considerations by following Worksheet 6.5.

Selecting an Assessment
Brief description of Client:
Brief description of Assessment:
Purpose: What occupations does the client want to address?
Link to theory
• Does the tool address an element or component of the model of practice or frame of reference?
• Will the findings from the assessment help understand concepts related to the model of practice or frame of reference?
Match with client
• Does the assessment provide information that is relevant to the client's identified goals?
• Does the assessment consider the influence of environment, cultural beliefs, or religious practices on the client's performance?
• Does the assessment provide an objective measure of performance that can determine if the client met the goals identified?
Assessment Tool Properties
• Does the assessment provide an objective measure of performance?
• What does the assessment really measure?
• Is there evidence to support the validity of the scores? Does the assessment measure what it says it does? What are the definitions and on what are they based?
• How do we know the information from the measure is reliable? Has it been examined with clients like mine?
• Is the measure responsive to change in the clients and context similar to my clients?
Pragmatics
• What age range and diagnoses does the assessment cover?
• What are the criteria for testing?
• How long does it take to administer the assessment?
• Can the assessment be completed in segments and still be valid?
• What testing materials and space are needed?
• Are there any training requirements for administering and scoring the assessment?

WORKSHEET 6.6: CREATING HYPOTHESES

Use Worksheet 6.6 to identify possible hypotheses regarding occupational performance challenges based on models of practice and frames of reference. Describe data that supports the hypothesis and possible intervention solutions. Refer to Table 6.2 for examples of how to complete the worksheet.

Creating Hypotheses Based on Models of Practice/Frame of Reference			
Model of Practice/Frame of Reference	Hypothesis	Data to support	Possible solutions
Biomechanical			
Model of Human Occupation			
Biomechanical			
Canadian Model of Occupation Participation and Engagement			
Developmental			
Sensory Integration			
Rehabilitation			
Cognitive Behavioral			
Constraint-induced movement therapy			

APPENDIX 6.1 Occupation, Activity, and Task Analysis		
	Explanation	Description of how item is used for specific occupation, activity, or task
Occupation, Activity, or Task	Describe the selected occupation, activity, or task.	
Client's Goal	Client's priorities, interests, and desires to be addressed in therapy.	
Rationale for Selection	Describe who the client is (person, group, or population) and how the occupation, activity, or task address the client's goal.	
Relevance and Importance	Describe the meaning (consider culture, symbolic, subjective)	
Sequence of Steps	List sequence of steps to complete. Describe any timing requirements.	
Preparation	Describe how the client and/or OT practitioner need to prepare.	
Equipment	Identify large objects that remain in setting and are needed for activity, such as table and chairs.	
Technology	List low or high technology needs.	

APPENDIX 6.1   Occupation, Activity, and Task Analysis (Continued)

	Explanation	Description of how item is used for specific occupation, activity, or task
Materials/Supplies and Their Properties	Identify materials and supplies needed and properties (i.e., texture, consistency, size, purpose, shape, color, sensory).	
Space	Describe setting in which activity occurs (e.g., outdoors, large space for physical activity).	
Social	Describe the social and attitudinal requirements.	
Costs	Fees or additional costs.	
Precautions	Include safety, medications effects, supervision needs, dietary requirements, motor, or emotional triggers.	
Performance Skills (observable goal-directed actions that allow client to perform)		
• **Motor**	Describe actions related to moving and interacting with objects (e.g., grips objects; reaches for items)	
• **Process**	Describe actions related to making decisions to select and interact and use objects, carry out steps and problem-solve to engage in and complete activity (e.g., selects correct object for task; seeks help when needed).	
• **Social interaction**	Describes actions related to communicating and interacting with others (e.g., makes eye contact; acknowledges others).	
Client Factors (describe key factors that influence performance).		
Body Function: values, beliefs, spirituality	One's perceptions, motivations, and related meaning that influence occupational performance.	
Body Function: Mental Functions		
• **Specific mental functions**	Includes higher-level cognitive, attention, memory, perception, thought, sequencing, emotional and self-awareness.	
• **Global mental functions**	Includes awareness, orientation, psychosocial, temperament and personality, energy, and sleep.	
• **Sensory functions**	Includes visual, hearing, vestibular, taste, smell, touch, proprioception, pain, interoception, temperature and pressure.	
Body Function: Neuromusculoskeletal and Movement-Related Functions (describe movement required for performance)		
• **Functions of joints and bones**	Describe ROM, integrity of joints for performance.	
• **Muscle functions**	Includes muscle power, and endurance for performance.	
• **Movement functions**	Describe voluntary movement and gait requirements for performance.	
Body Function: cardiovascular, hematological, immunological, respiratory system functions	Describe how systems may influence performance (e.g., is the intensity level appropriate for client with cardiovascular impairment).	
Body Function: voice and speech functions	Describe requirements of voice and speech functions.	
Body Function: skin and related structures	Describe skin and related structures in relationship to occupation, activity, or task.	
Body Structures	Anatomical parts of the body that support body function. Describe what is required when completing occupation, activity or task.	

From: O'Brien, J. & Solomon, J. (2021). *Occupational Analysis and Group Process.* Elsevier.
Reference: American Occupational Therapy Association (AOTA). (2020). Occupational therapy practice framework: Domain and process (4th ed.). *American Journal of Occupational Therapy, 71* (Suppl.2), S1–S96.

Teamwork

Teressa Reidy and Nicole Andrejow

GUIDING QUESTIONS

1. What are the benefits and challenges of working in teams?
2. What are the characteristics of effective teams?
3. What competencies and reasoning strategies promote teamwork?
4. How does practice setting influence therapeutic reasoning?
5. How do group interventions increase the complexity of therapeutic reasoning?

KEY TERMS

Adjourning
Formal communication
Forming
Group therapy
Informal communication
Interdisciplinary
Interprofessional
Multidisciplinary

Norming
Performing
Practice context
Relationship-building
Role overlap
Storming
Team dynamics
Transdisciplinary

INTRODUCTION

Occupational therapy (OT) practitioners work with a variety of team members, including family, health professionals, paraprofessionals, caregivers, and community members to enable clients to participate in valued activities. For example, an OT practitioner working in home health may interact with a nurse, physical therapist, speech therapist, physician, and consult with a social worker, nutritionist, and local builder (e.g., to make home modifications, such as a ramp). An OT practitioner may consult with an audiologist, respiratory therapist, or athletic trainer at a medically oriented gym. Understanding the roles and responsibilities of team members in a variety of practice settings and establishing positive working relationships benefits clients and their families and results in improved continuity of care (Flood et al., 2019; McMurtry, 2013; WHO, 2010).

The authors of this chapter begin by describing the roles of professionals working in teams in a variety of settings. They define the types of teams and examine the competencies and characteristics of effective teams. A description of the benefits and challenges of teamwork leads to a discussion of therapeutic reasoning strategies that support effective collaboration, while advocating for occupational therapy's distinct value. The authors describe the reasoning process and challenges that may present when the OT practitioner is the leader of the team in a group therapy session. They conclude by describing teamwork

in supervisory, administrative, and consultative roles. The authors provide case examples and learning activities to illustrate reasoning strategies for practice.

INTERPROFESSIONAL TEAM MEMBERS

OT practitioners work with many professionals (such as physicians, physical therapists, speech–language pathologists, nurses, social workers, physician assistants, audiologists, dieticians, nutritionists, and mental health workers) in a variety of practice settings. The client is the most important member of the team, but the setting plays a role in the constellation of the team.

For example, teams working in medical settings include other allied health professionals such as physical therapists, speech–language pathologists, physicians, nurses, and rehabilitation aides. Educational teams include teachers, counselors, social workers, and classroom aides. Mental health teams may include psychologists, psychiatrists, and life coaches. Table 7.1 lists examples of the team members and their typical formal communications associated with specific settings. Formal communication may be dictated by institutional policies (e.g., documentation, team meetings, or morning rounds). While each setting has formal meetings or methods for communication between team members, informal communication occurs frequently. Informal communication includes check-ins with team members or short updates. For example, an informal

TABLE 7.1   Team Members and Formal Communication by Setting

Setting	Team Members	Formal Communication
Acute care hospital	• Physicians • Nurses • Physical therapist • Social worker • Case manager • Imaging technicians	Documentation in medical record. Verbal communication regarding client status.
Inpatient hospital	• Orthopedist • Physiatrist • Social worker • Nurse • Neuropsychologist • Radiology	Rounds or team meetings to update the medical team on client progress.
Outpatient hospital	• Physical therapist • Speech–language pathologist • Nutritionist	Documentation and scheduled team meetings.
Community	• Advocacy group members • Planning committees • Department of health/recreation staff • Town supervisors or other personnel	Reports of findings and recommendations. Planning meetings to discuss proposals and findings.
Educational settings	• Special education teacher • Parent • Speech language pathologist • Reading specialist • Counselor • Principal or other school administrator	Documentation and Individualized Educational Meetings (IEP) or 504 plans.
Mental health setting	• Psychologist • Psychiatrist • Aid • Nurse • Counselor • Recreation therapist • Social worker	Team meetings; rounds; family meetings.

check-in with the nurse may provide valuable information to inform an intervention session. As the OT practitioner picks up the child in the classroom, the schoolteacher may indicate the child struggled with an assignment (which the OT may use to address in therapy). Caregivers may provide informal updates on the client's daily status (e.g., "He slept well last night"). Regardless of the setting, to be an effective team member, OT practitioners communicate their reasoning and evidence for decisions as they collaborate with others.

LEARNING ACTIVITY: TEAM MEMBERS

Complete Worksheet 7.1 to identify the roles of team members. Describe the role of the OT practitioner in each setting.
• How does the setting influence the focus of occupational therapy evaluation and intervention?

TYPES OF TEAMS

Teams perform in a variety of ways, which is reflected in terminology to describe the team's style as reflected by Figure 7.1 (Jensenius, 2012).

Multidisciplinary teams refer to members from many disciplines working together, each focusing on their own discipline or professional knowledge. Each team member creates goals and intervention strategies specific to their discipline. They may coordinate intervention schedules and discuss progress together, but they generally work independently from each other.

Transdisciplinary teams work closely together to provide comprehensive care to clients. All team members work on the same goals and consult with each other to reinforce each member's area of expertise. This approach dissolves boundaries allowing professionals to address the client's challenges. For example, the OT practitioner may use knowledge gained from the nutritionist when working on a child's feeding goals. The OT practitioner provides the information to the parent as deemed necessary but does not specifically consult with the nutritionist about the specific client. Transdisciplinary team members may carry out intervention that may be outside of their traditional roles.

Interdisciplinary or **interprofessional** teams work with each other to create intervention plans for clients, while still respecting each profession's practice domains. Team members acknowledge each member's expertise and work to integrate each

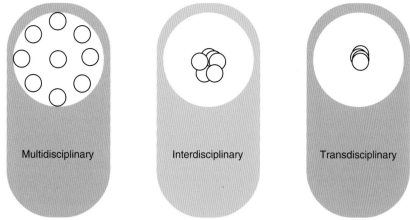

Figure 7.1 Multidisciplinary, Interdisciplinary, and Transdisciplinary Configurations.

profession's knowledge when creating a comprehensive intervention plan that addresses the client's needs. Interprofessional teams collaborate to establish goals and plan, often co-treating and working together to address client issues. They spend time discussing strategies and methods to work towards goals. Together, the interprofessional team creates an intervention plan that all agree upon.

INTERPROFESSIONAL COLLABORATION COMPETENCIES

Lack of teamwork and communication skills among health professionals has been shown to result in adverse health outcomes (Institute of Medicine, 2001). This led the Institute of Medicine (2009) to suggest that health educators and organizations facilitate interprofessional education and interprofessional collaborative practice. The Interprofessional Education Collaborative (IPEC) was formed in 2011, and created core competencies of interprofessional practice which were updated in 2016. The IPEC (2016) identified 4 core competencies for interprofessional collaborative practice as listed in Box 7.1.

BOX 7.1   Core Competencies for Interprofessional Collaborative Practice

1. Work with individuals of other professions to maintain a climate of mutual respect and shared values. (Values/Ethics for Interprofessional Practice)
2. Use the knowledge of one's own role and those of other professions to appropriately assess and address the healthcare needs of patients and to promote and advance the health of populations. (Roles/Responsibilities)
3. Communicate with patients, families, communities, and professionals in health and other fields in a responsive and responsible manner that supports a team approach to the promotion and maintenance of health and the prevention and treatment of disease. (Interprofessional Communication)
4. Apply relationship-building values and the principles of team dynamics to perform effectively in different team roles to plan, deliver, and evaluate patient-/population-centered care and population health programs and policies that are safe, timely, efficient, effective, and equitable. (Teams and Teamwork)

(From IPEC, 2016, p. 10.)

Values/Ethics for Interprofessional Practice

Having mutual respect and shared values opens lines of communication and allows team members to collaborate, communicate, and understand each other. It requires that each member acknowledge the other profession's perspective as important to the success of the intervention plan and the client outcomes. All members of the team, including the client and family, want to be heard and validated. Valuing each member's contribution supports the success of the team. Flood and colleagues (2019) found that effective interprofessional work relied on the team members' attitude towards the process and respect for each other. Working together to achieve outcomes that are valued by all team members (such as client outcomes) includes understanding each profession's roles, practice domain, and philosophy towards client interventions. When teams are forming, they often begin by establishing the vision, values, and purpose of the teamwork which helps members work together towards the same goals. Establishing the team's values makes it possible for each team member to be on the same page, which enhances collaboration and effectiveness (Walton et al., 2019).

Membership in healthcare teams is fluid (as professionals join at different times, and the client changes). Making sure all members are working towards the same outcome is essential and requires effective communication.

LEARNING ACTIVITY: MUTUAL RESPECT AND SHARED VALUES

Use Worksheet 7.2 to reflect upon a team of which you were a member to outline the shared values and feelings of mutual respect. Describe a team situation whereby the members did not share values or did not respect other members.
- How did you observe mutual respect and shared values?
- How did the team function?
- What factors contributed to team performance?

Roles/Responsibilities

It is important for healthcare professionals to understand one's own roles and that of other professions (IPEC, 2016; Walton et al., 2019; Weller, Boyd, & Cumin, 2014). It is helpful to define one's role clearly within a specific practice setting to a variety of people, including clients and family members. Team members seek to understand the full breadth of each profession's services to address client's needs. Weller and colleagues (2014) reported that understanding team members' roles and responsibilities contributed to a collaborative approach for care planning. Understanding each other's roles and responsibilities allows team members to collaborate so they can "be on the same page," "focus on the patient," and "engage in holistic care planning" (Walton et al., 2019).

LEARNING ACTIVITY: ELEVATOR SPEECH

Create a video-clip giving a 1-minute description of the role of occupational therapy services in a specific setting.

Communication

As with any relationship, communication with patients, families, communities, and professionals is key to successful interprofessional team collaboration. Communication may be formal (e.g., team meetings, rounds, Individualized Educational Plan (IEP) meetings, discharge meetings, family meetings) or informal (e.g., check-ins, updates) and may be verbal or written (e.g., reports, documentation, discharge plans, home programs). Communicating clearly and concisely without professional jargon assures that all team members understand the content. All written communication should clearly state the purpose and provide clear accurate information to support the promotion and maintenance of health and the prevention and treatment of disease.

Healthcare professionals attend to non-verbal communication (e.g., body language, facial expressions) to understand the client's or team member's cues. For example, a client may say everything is fine, but give the appearance through facial expressions that they are frustrated, bored, or upset. Reading non-verbal cues is part of interactive reasoning. OT practitioners communicate with clients during all phases of the occupational therapy process. See Chapter 4 for more information on therapeutic use of self as part of one's communication.

Teams and Teamwork

Effective team members use relationship-building practices and the principles of team dynamics to plan, deliver, and evaluate client-centered care and population health programs that are safe, timely, efficient, effective, and equitable (IPEC, 2016). Relationship-building practices include establishing commonalities, listening, responding to each other, and supporting each other to gain trust and collaborate. Team dynamics refers to the interplay and relationships between team members, the power between members, and the roles that members play.

CHARACTERISTICS OF EFFECTIVE TEAMS

Salas and colleagues (2005) identified five key aspects ("Big Five") of teamwork that affect term performance: leadership; mutual performance monitoring; backup behavior; adaptability; and orientation. See Figure 7.2 for descriptions of each component.

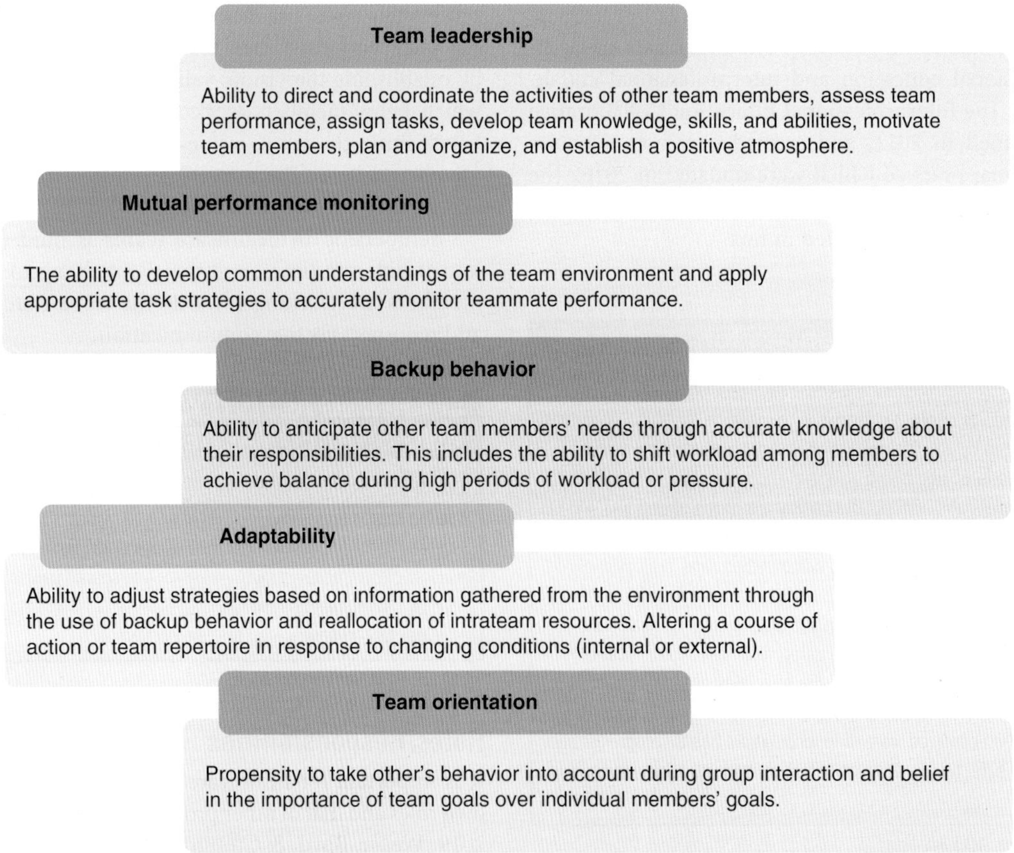

Team leadership

Ability to direct and coordinate the activities of other team members, assess team performance, assign tasks, develop team knowledge, skills, and abilities, motivate team members, plan and organize, and establish a positive atmosphere.

Mutual performance monitoring

The ability to develop common understandings of the team environment and apply appropriate task strategies to accurately monitor teammate performance.

Backup behavior

Ability to anticipate other team members' needs through accurate knowledge about their responsibilities. This includes the ability to shift workload among members to achieve balance during high periods of workload or pressure.

Adaptability

Ability to adjust strategies based on information gathered from the environment through the use of backup behavior and reallocation of intrateam resources. Altering a course of action or team repertoire in response to changing conditions (internal or external).

Team orientation

Propensity to take other's behavior into account during group interaction and belief in the importance of team goals over individual members' goals.

Figure 7.2 The "Big Five" Components of Teamwork. (From Salas et al., 2005, p. 560–561.)

Healthcare teams may have changing leadership, which may interfere with the effectiveness of the team. Effective team leaders show mutual respect for each profession, promote a positive working environment that includes collaboration, and encourage an open communication system (Salas et al., 2005). Teams are more effective when leaders support team members' professional development and engage members in the planning.

Effective teams include team members who follow up and monitor each other's work to catch mistakes, or lapses prior to or shortly after they occur (Salas et al., 2005). The monitoring occurs as part of the team process, especially in stressful situations. This skill requires that team members trust each other and be open and responsive to feedback.

Backup behaviors are used to support a team member who may be experiencing overload and needs assistance. It may include providing feedback and coaching to improve performance, assisting a teammate in performing a task, or completing the task for the teammate (Marks et al. 2000). The flexibility or ability to support teammates as needed contributes to the team's effectiveness. Adaptability refers to the ability to recognize changes and read cues and respond to them which may be accomplished by changing roles, adjusting actions, or changing course. Team adaptability may require creating new plans (Salas et al., 2005).

Team orientation refers to the attitude of team members and refers to one's disposition to work with others (Salas et al., 2005). Flood et al. (2019) found that some professionals expressed a "call to interprofessional practice" and a "spirit of interprofessional practice." Participants focused on the patient in the spirit of interprofessional practice and they sought out team members to benefit the client (Flood et al., 2019).

COMPETENCIES AND REASONING STRATEGIES OF TEAMS

The Interprofessional Education Collaborative (IPEC, 2016) was created to advance interprofessional learning experiences of health professionals to prepare them for enhanced team-based care of clients and improved population health outcomes. Figure 7.3 describes the Core Competencies.

Interprofessional teamwork refers to "the levels of cooperation, coordination, and collaboration characterizing the relationships between professions and delivering patient-centered care" (IPEC, 2016, p. 8). IPEC created a list of sub-competencies for each of the competencies that support interprofessional collaborative practice. The items provide objectives of how professionals can effectively work in teams to provide quality care. Box 7.2 lists the sub-competencies addressing Core Competency 4: Team and Teamwork.

The stages for team development include forming, storming, norming, performing and adjourning (Tuckman & Jenson, 1977). Teams begin in the forming stage by identifying the roles of each member and defining the purpose or practices of the team. Healthcare teams consist of a client and a variety of

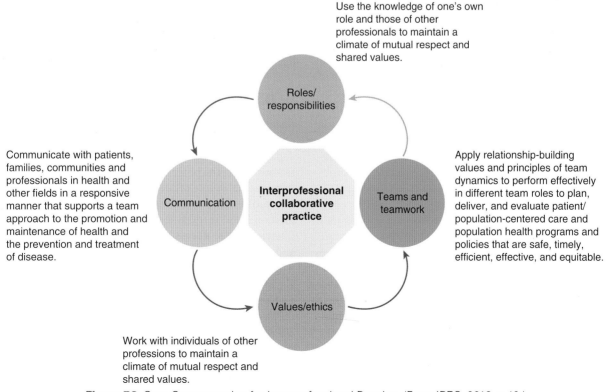

Figure 7.3 Core Competencies for Interprofessional Practice. (From IPEC, 2016, p.10.)

BOX 7.2   Team and Teamwork Sub-competencies

TT1. Describe the process of team development and the roles and practices of effective teams.

TT2. Develop consensus on the ethical principles to guide all aspects of teamwork.

TT3. Engage health and other professionals in shared patient-centered and population-focused problem-solving.

TT4. Integrate the knowledge and experience of health and other professions to inform health and care decisions, while respecting patient and community values and priorities/preferences for care.

TT5. Apply leadership practices that support collaborative practice and team effectiveness.

TT6. Engage self and others to constructively manage disagreements about values, roles, goals, and actions that arise among health and other professionals and with patients, families, and community members.

TT7. Share accountability with other professions, patients, and communities for outcomes relevant to prevention and healthcare.

TT8. Reflect on individual and team performance for individual, as well as team, performance improvement.

TT9. Use process improvement to increase effectiveness of interprofessional teamwork and team-based services, programs, and policies.

TT10. Use available evidence to inform effective teamwork and team-based practices.

TT11. Perform effectively on teams and in different team roles in a variety of settings.

(From IPEC., 2016, p. 14.)

professionals who may enter the team at different stages with different levels of training, experience, and expertise. For example, a new graduate nurse may be assigned to the team with an experienced occupational therapist, physical therapist, and physician assistant. The experience and areas of expertise of the members vary. It is important for team members of healthcare teams to be honest about their level of experience and define their roles to the team. Each professional follows a code of ethics, which guides decision-making and teamwork. For example, the occupational therapy code of ethics include principles of beneficence, nonmaleficence, autonomy, justice, veracity, and fidelity (AOTA, 2020). Effective teams discuss ethical dilemmas as they arise to reach consensus. The ethical decision-making process is much like the therapeutic reasoning process and includes: (1) Gather information; (2) Identify the ethical problem; (3) Use ethical theory or approaches to analyze the problems; (4) Explore alternatives; (5) Complete the action; and (6) Evaluate the process and outcome (Purtillo et al., 2022).

Disagreements about values, roles, goals, and actions may arise during the **storming** stage of the team process. Healthcare professionals work with team members and clients to address disagreements or inevitable events that are part of the therapeutic process. See Chapter 4 for more information on inevitable events. The team's goal is to support clients in reaching their goals. Everyone on the team is responsible for the outcomes. Therefore, team members work through disagreements for the betterment of client outcomes.

During the **norming** stage, teams resolve issues, engage in positive interpersonal communication, and focus on establishing group procedures (Carson, 2022). Group members trust each other and begin to work together. This leads to the **performing** stage, whereby the healthcare team problem-solves and collaborates with each other and the client to create client-centered plans. As part of the process, team members integrate information from their knowledge and experience with the client and community to prioritize intervention goals and strategies. Team members listen to others, ask thoughtful questions, and provide input to support the team in making decisions based on evidence and the individual needs of the client. This is not a linear process and includes communicating changes, results, and outcomes throughout the process. Team members show dedication to the team effectiveness, which is measured as client achievement and satisfaction. Members support each other and exhibit confidence to articulate their findings, question others to find better solutions, and follow through with responsibilities.

The last stage, **adjourning**, signals an end to the team or case. During this stage, teams reflect upon the process, and provide each other feedback to adjust or make changes for the next case. Each member reflects on both their individual and the team's performance to adjust processes as needed for future clients. See Chapter 10 for reflection exercises. The team uses available evidence (such as client satisfaction surveys, client outcomes, and quality discussions) to provide insight into team effectiveness. Examining processes can lead to improved team effectiveness by changing services, programs, and policies. Performing effectively as a team requires members to be invested in the process, willing to do the work necessary, open to communication with others, and clear of their role. Members who work effectively in teams listen to others and value diverse perspectives.

LEARNING ACTIVITY: STRATEGIES DURING STAGES OF TEAM DEVELOPMENT

Complete Worksheet 7.4. Provide personal examples of each stage of the team development. Identify strategies that may be required at each stage.
- How might the stage of development influence one's reasoning?

BENEFITS AND CHALLENGES OF TEAMWORK

The interprofessional approach challenges the traditional model of the physician being in charge as healthcare professionals collaborate with each other (Derrick, 2018). Interprofessional teamwork has the potential to improve patient safety and health outcomes (Institute of Medicine, 2001). Research suggests that interprofessional care decreases inpatient length of stay, readmission rates, medical errors and rates of adverse drug events (Derrick, 2018; Reeves et al., 2012). It improves staff attitudes and satisfaction, interdisciplinary collaboration, and overall patient satisfaction (Derrick, 2018; Walton et al., 2019; Weller et al., 2014). There is an increasing demand for health professionals to work collaboratively and empower the client to be part of the decision-making process (Schot et al., 2020; Walton et al., 2019; Weller et al., 2014).

Sergakis et al., (2016) identified the advantages of engaging in simulated interprofessional experiences as teamwork and collaboration, interprofessional communication, clinical preparation and confidence, and professional identity. Walton and colleagues (2019) examined perceived challenges to interprofessional collaboration during ward rounds and reported time constraints (i.e., takes away from providing care for patients, multiple clinical opinions increases discussion time, case conferences and current process in place are similar), workforce issues (i.e., difficulty in team meeting at an agreed time, team structures not uniform, some patients and discussion irrelevant to different clinicians, power imbalances between disciplines), and care planning (i.e., uncomfortable for patients, too many around bed space, and competing priorities caring for other patients). Team members collaborate to create comprehensive plans, support each other, and identify gaps in the intervention plan.

One of the challenges to interprofessional teamwork includes role overlap. Role overlap refers to two professionals engaging in similar roles with clients (Booth & Hewison, 2002). Understanding one's professional roles, state practice acts, licensure laws, and domain of practice may allow the practitioner to establish different client goals or the focus of the intervention to avoid feeling role overlap. Occupational and physical therapists working in stroke rehabilitation reported that overall, the overlap in care was beneficial to patients, although they felt that it jeopardized their role security (Booth & Hewison, 2002). Healthcare professionals effectively address the overlap in client care and intervention goals by creating an open environment to address these overlaps and collaboratively problem-solve workable solutions (Schot et al., 2020). OT practitioners frequently explain to team members (including clients, families and other professionals) their therapeutic reasoning in relation to occupational therapy's role in client care.

Organizational structures such as the hospital or clinic's policies may minimize role overlap by delineating roles. However, OT practitioners and professionals should make sure the policies do not limit the profession's scope of practice. Each profession establishes goals based on their professional practice domains. For example, the goals of a PT intervention may include strengthening, balance, trunk mobility, and range of motion of the hip, knee, and ankle. The PT focuses on repetitive movement activities and measures the outcome using a biomechanical approach. The focus of the session is to improve the client's underlying abilities for movement.

The OT practitioner may address the same physical factors within a functional activity (such as lifting plates and placing them in a cabinet) with the goal of helping the client effectively and safely maximize independence. The OT practitioner considers the role of vision and cognitive processing as the client performs the activity. The practitioner monitors the client's movement and ability to attend to multiple stimuli and respond while also analyzing the steps of the activity and observing how the physical and social environment influences client performance.

While both professionals address the client's physical performance challenges, they approach intervention differently and support each other by understanding each professional's role in the rehabilitation process. The ability to clearly articulate one's reasoning helps define the professional's role on the team and provides a clearer definition of each profession's unique contribution to client evaluation, intervention, and outcomes.

LEARNING ACTIVITY: ROLE OVERLAP

Complete Worksheet 7.5 to compare roles of OT and speech therapy.

An OT practitioner and speech therapist are developing a summer camp–style life skills group for children with autism at an outpatient pediatric clinic. The camp will run for 1-week sessions for 10 weeks throughout the summer. Children will attend the OT and Speech Therapy sessions once a day. To keep the groups small (6 to 8 children), they will run 3 sessions per day together.

- Create 1 long-term goal to address executive functioning for life skills that both OT and Speech Therapy will target during the summer camp.
  - Create a short-term OT goal and a short-term Speech Therapy goal to address during a group session.
- Describe how each profession will address the goal.
  - Identify specific activities and approaches.
- Compare and contrast each profession's approach to the executive functioning goal.
- Define how OT and ST differ and how they can support each other.

THERAPEUTIC REASONING STRATEGIES WITH TEAMS

Kiesewetter, Fischer, and Fischer (2017) conducted a systematic review to determine the observable factors that make up collaborative therapeutic reasoning. The authors identified the following factors influencing clinical reasoning (although they summarized that there is limited evidence on how the factors influence performance): (1) starting point of reasoning; (2) analysis and hypothesis generation; (3) information generation; (4) information representation; and (5) evaluation and integration.

The team reasoning process begins with the distribution of information among team members. Sharing accurate information is important at this stage and may influence analyses and hypotheses generation. Team members are urged to share information in a clear and concise manner. It is important that the information be shared with all members as this leads to hypothesis generation based upon experience. Information exchange may be influenced negatively by working patterns and increased workloads. Team members who are aware and back each other up may find the process runs more effectively (Salas et al., 2005). Creating an efficient system whereby all team members' information is readily available supports team performance. Finally, evaluating and integrating information for all team members allows all members to work towards the same goals and support each other (Kiesewetter et al. 2017; Salas et al., 2005). These strategies promote collaboration and provide team members with comprehensive information to create plans. They emphasize communication between members.

Strategies for Overcoming Barriers in Communication

Communication is key to successful team performance. Weller and colleagues (2014) provide seven actions to overcome communication barriers:

1. Teach effective communication strategies
2. Train teams together
3. Train teams using simulation
4. Define inclusive teams
5. Create democratic teams
6. Support teamwork with protocols and procedures
7. Develop an organizational culture supporting healthcare teams.

Creating structured methods of communication among team members, such as the "Situation-Background-Assessment-Recommendation" format, may save time and increase transfer of important communication for the client (Weller et al., 2014). Training teams together so that all members develop relationships and understand each other's style as well as the team process benefits all. Using simulation is a safe and low-stakes method for training. Allowing the team to redefine itself as a cohesive whole working towards client outcomes empowers all members of the team. Each member of the team should feel valued and be able to openly communicate with others (Weller et al., 2014). Creating systems by using technology and processes that support communication among team members and recognizing the importance of interprofessional teams supports teamwork.

Healthcare professionals rely on documentation to communicate with team members, including the client and family. Documentation should avoid jargon, be clear and concise, and be written in plain language (6th grade level) so all can understand. The OT practitioner makes sure the client and family understand the documentation by asking the client or family to describe it in their own words or demonstrate the plan or home program. Clients should receive documentation in their first language. All documentation should be written or typed clearly without clutter. Home programs may be more effective if they include pictures.

LEARNING ACTIVITY: COMMUNICATION AND CLIENT EDUCATION

Refer to Worksheet 7.6. Erin is an OTR working in a pediatric outpatient clinic with children who have developmental delay, autism spectrum disorder, and neuromotor disorders. Many of the families are non-English speaking.

- What strategies might Erin use to assure adequate communication between children and their families?
- Provide examples of how pragmatic, narrative, interactive, ethical, scientific, and conditional reasoning influence how she educates family and children.

LEARNING ACTIVITY: COMPREHENSION AND CLIENT EDUCATION

Create a 1-page handout (using 6th grade language, colorful pictures, and illustrations) to describe a movement (e.g., dance step, jump rope, draw a design, fold a paper) of your choice. Once it is completed, ask a peer to follow the handout without asking any questions or having a demonstration.

- Was the peer able to complete the desired motion?
- Describe how you could use this handout in an occupational therapy session.

OCCUPATIONAL THERAPY'S DISTINCT VALUE

OT practitioners focus on helping clients participate in those occupations for which they find meaning and contribute to their sense of identity (Kielhofner, 2008; O'Brien & Kielhofner, 2017). See Chapter 2 for more information on the value of occupation. Performance-based assessments (Fisher, 1998; Gillen, 2013) and occupation-based models of practice (such as the Model of Human Occupation, Person-Environment-Occupation-Performance, Canadian Model of Occupational Performance and Engagement, and Occupational Adaptation) support the use of occupation in practice. Chapter 3 describes the use of models of practice and frames of reference.

While clinical protocols may not emphasize occupation, the OT practitioner integrates occupation into those protocols for best practice. Some practice settings and organizations in which occupational therapists work may not have a culture that values occupation-based interventions. In these settings, the OT practitioner must advocate for occupational therapy service, articulate the value, and demonstrate its usefulness by clearly describing the value of their work. As clients make progress and express satisfaction with occupational therapy services, the culture of the organization may change. Using terminology that all team members understand helps teach others the value of occupational therapy.

LEARNING ACTIVITY: DECODING OT TERMINOLOGY FOR CLIENTS

Pick a treatment setting and client. Make a list of OT terms that might be commonly found in your progress note. Translate this terminology into something understandable for a patient with a sixth grade reading level.

(Hint: use a search engine or word processing program to assess the reading level.)

For example: Bimanual Integration: Using two hands together to get a job done such as cutting with scissors.

The following case example illustrates the contributions of occupational therapy to the team in a rehabilitation setting and provides examples of how the OT practitioner worked as a valued member of the team contributing to client success.

Case Example: Occupation-Focused Intervention

Mark is an OT working in an outpatient clinic. He conducts a 90-minute group twice a week for clients recovering from total knee replacement. The other three days a week, a physical therapist (PT) runs the group. Mark designs client-centered occupational therapy group activities to address each client's goal during the group. He includes intervention activities that are meaningful to each client and activities that are part of their daily routines. He adjusts the activities so that each member is challenged to promote self-efficacy and confidence upon discharge.

Mark understands that protocols for total knee replacement rehabilitation exist. He decides that individualizing sessions and using the motivation from feeling a part of a group will help members of the group engage in their rehabilitation to its fullest for better recovery. Mark uses knowledge of each client's story and their interpersonal styles to personalize the activities (while following guidelines from the protocol) to ensure each client feels valued and heard while engaging in occupational therapy.

He focuses each session on instrumental activities of daily living (IADL) tasks (e.g., meal preparation, care of pets, household chores) that become progressively more challenging over time and have meaning and purpose to the group participants. He collaborates with members to create activities that address their concerns. Mark measures each client's physical gains and improvements in daily activities (occupations). He evaluates the outcome of the group sessions by recording attendance and client satisfaction. He documents changes in each client's ability to perform IADL, attendance, follow up with home exercise program, and satisfaction. By staying true to occupational therapy philosophy, Mark created an innovative group session resulting in improved patient outcomes, illustrating the value of his work.

THE ROLE OF SETTING (CONTEXT) IN THERAPEUTIC REASONING

Practice setting influences the dominant type of reasoning a therapist uses to evaluate and intervene with clients (Alnervik & Svidén, 1996; Carrier, Levasseur, Bedard, & Desrosiers, 2012; Munroe, 1996; Ward, 2003). Research suggests that working within a client's home or personal space influences all steps, stages, and facets of the therapeutic reasoning process (Carrier et al., 2012; Munroe, 1996). Munroe (1996) reported that in home health settings, the practitioner is a guest, invited into a client's personal home to empower them with independence, and subsequently practitioners made decisions based on interactive reasoning most often. In a qualitative study examining the practice of an expert clinician in a mental health setting, Ward (2003) found that practitioners used interactive reasoning and consistently appraised the role of the practice setting on the intervention. The occupational therapist was "tuned in" not only to their clients, but also to the center staff and the interpersonal interactions occurring between all of them (Ward, 2003). Additionally, OT practitioners use pragmatic reasoning as they consider organizational and administrative policies, such as safety procedures, billing, and documentation rules and regulations when making practice decisions in each setting. Context plays a role in therapeutic decisions, which requires that OT practitioners understand the practice setting in which they provide intervention.

> ### LEARNING ACTIVITY: CONTEXT-DEPENDENT PRACTICE
>
> Using Worksheet 7.7 as a guide, contact two OT practitioners who work in different practice settings. Ask them to share one case (no names or identifying information) to determine the similarities and differences in their reasoning.

GROUP THERAPY

Group therapy refers to intervention where there is more than one client and at least one practitioner. The type and makeup of the group depends upon many factors including payer reimbursement, treatment setting, and client profiles. Group therapy provides services to more clients at the same time, which can increase overall access to treatment when there are limited available therapists. Group therapy sessions facilitate social interactions and connections between people experiencing the same disability or life event. Clients often feel additional support from their peers in a group therapy setting which motivates them to work towards goals (Komar et al., 2016). Yang et al. (2017) found that clients with Parkinson's disease participating in group-based Tai Chi were more compliant in their home program than those participating in the individual-based intervention. The authors suggest that the increased social interaction and competitive dynamics of the group sessions increased clients' motivation to complete more independent practice to improve their performance (Yang et al, 2017).

OT practitioners consider the advantages of group therapy to the client and ensure that quality occupational therapy intervention is delivered during the group therapy session. Through ethical reasoning, they determine if the client is benefiting from the group therapy session. They use pragmatic reasoning to plan an activity that can be safely executed and monitored in a setting with multiple patients. During the group session, the practitioner uses interactive reasoning to make decisions to manage group dynamics and social responses between clients.

Challenges in Group Therapy

Group therapy also comes with challenges that may be difficult for a novice practitioner. Group interventions require monitoring multiple clients' status and their responses to the intervention, adjusting activities, and changing plans as needed. The OT practitioner uses conditional reasoning to simultaneously understand the needs of clients who are at varying cognitive, physical, and social–emotional abilities while engaging them in group activities. The OT practitioner plans the group session with specific activities in mind, but grades tasks as needed based on each group member's social emotional, physical, or cognitive abilities. Groups may include clients with similar characteristics (i.e., homogenous) or groups with clients who have diverse abilities (i.e., heterogenous).

Group sessions look different in each treatment environment. For example, in a rehabilitation setting, members of a group session to address upper extremity strengthening may engage in preparatory exercises followed by activities to develop strength. Alternatively, in a mental health setting an OT practitioner may work with several clients using arts and crafts to facilitate problem-solving, seeing a project through to completion, and dealing with unexpected challenges.

OT practitioners frequently co-treat with other professionals in group sessions. For example, an OT practitioner may work with a nutritionist on a meal preparation group for community dwelling adults at risk for diabetes or with a speech therapist in a school-based group for teens with executive functioning challenges. The following case describes the therapeutic reasoning process used to plan and implement a group occupational therapy session for teens recovering from concussion.

Case Example: Group for Teens with Concussion

Ingrid is an occupational therapist who runs a weekly community living skills group for teens recovering from concussion in a sports medicine clinic. The teens commonly complain of persistent headaches, fatigue, visual disturbances, and loss of roles as student and student athletes. Clients can attend one to 10 sessions depending on their needs and severity of injury.

Figure 7.4 provides examples of how each type of reasoning informs practice decisions within this group.

As Ingrid begins to design the community living skills group for teens with concussions, she reviews the signs, symptoms, and characteristics of concussions. She relies on *scientific reasoning* to understand the severity of concussions and the factors that may influence prognosis (such as multiple concussions, time post injury). She examines current research evidence on assessment and intervention for mild concussion. Ingrid further explores assessments and interventions to address client factors that interfere with community living skills. She uses scientific reasoning to structure occupational therapy sessions to address memory loss and executive functioning while being mindful that the clients may have headaches, dizziness, and visual disturbances requiring frequent breaks.

As Ingrid plans the first session, she integrates *pragmatic reasoning* relating to the students' activity tolerance and scheduling demands. For example, since the group members attend school from 9 am to 12 pm and then attend the group sessions from 1 pm to 3 pm, she hypothesizes that the academic demands of school may cause them to be tired during the group sessions. In addition, since the group meets in the sports medicine clinic which requires transportation from school, and may require members to rush from school, possibly missing lunch, they may feel stressed and unable to participate adequately in the group. Ingrid is not sure this time will work for the teens and she is concerned that they will not be invested in the group.

To better understand the needs of each teen, Ingrid uses *narrative reasoning*, which allows her to understand their stories. Ingrid decides that the first session will be dedicated to getting to know the stories of each member and will include creative and fun games. Narrative information such as the teen's background, past experiences (e.g., academic, social, family), perspective on their identity (i.e., past, and present), and description of experiences dealing with change (i.e., resilience) inform intervention activities. As Ingrid gathers this information, she may decide to consult with other team members for advice. For example, she may decide that the social worker can help the teens with transportation, housing, financial assistance, and emotional counseling. She may invite the physical therapist to identify strategies to provide support to the teens regarding returning to sports.

While creating ideas for the group sessions, Ingrid uses *ethical reasoning* by contemplating how she can attend to each member's individual needs, while providing high quality, skilled occupational therapy. She maintains confidentiality of each client's medical and social history during group sessions. As the teens are vulnerable, she acknowledges that she must be truthful to them and maintain professional boundaries. Ingrid feels protective of the teens and will consult with other professionals (e.g., psychologist, social worker) as needed.

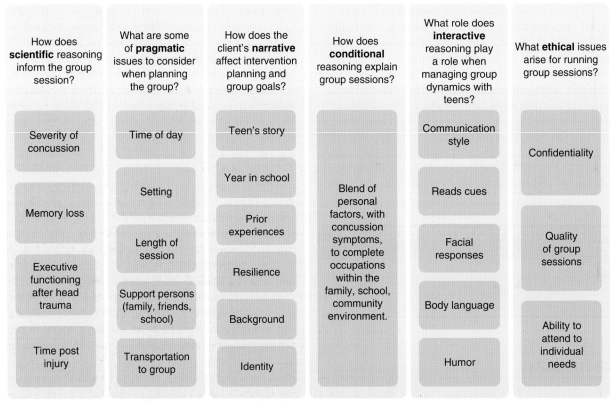

Figure 7.4 Examples of Types of Therapeutic Reasoning for Group for Teens.

As the group sessions begin, Ingrid uses *interactive reasoning* to understand the members' communication style, personalities, and interactions with others. She pays attention to their use of humor, attitudes, facial responses, and body language. Ingrid observes how each member gives and responds to cues from others. She also observes their attention to details, awareness levels, and behaviors that may be viewed as impulsive. By observing the teens' interactions, Ingrid identifies group dynamics that support or hinder group processes. She may use this reasoning to facilitate group dynamics. This may include adjusting seating, seeking assistance from group members, clarifying instructions, or allowing group members to lead activities.

As the group sessions develop, Ingrid uses *conditional reasoning* to create and carry out the sessions. For example, Ingrid integrates knowledge of each teen's severity of concussion (scientific), personal stories (narrative), and personality style (interactive), to determine group activities that are possible at the center in the afternoon from 1 pm to 3 pm with 8 teens at varying levels of recovery (pragmatic) and that effectively address each member's occupational therapy goals (ethical).

In this group setting, the team consists of the OT and the teens. The therapist is the leader of the team but seeks to collaborate with the teens, so they are invested in the group and learn from each other. The OT is mindful of the team dynamics and uses therapeutic use of self to promote collaboration and empower the teens to take on leadership roles within the group.

TEAMWORK IN SUPERVISORY ROLES

The novice occupational therapy practitioner benefits from mentorship and guidance from a supervisor to facilitate reasoning. Coates and Crist (2004) report that in the fieldwork setting students' initial reasoning is primarily procedural but as the clinical experience progresses reasoning becomes more client centered and shifts to interactive and conditional modes. Working as a team provides a novice clinician or fieldwork student the benefit of experiencing and hearing various perspectives on the client's occupational performance.

Guided reflection and feedback from supervisors is integral to advancing one's reasoning skills. Providing constructive feedback to fieldwork students on specific therapeutic reasoning skills while assisting them to find avenues to improve may be more effective than just affirming students that they are using the right type of reasoning (De Beer & Mårtensson, 2015). Reflecting on the things that went well and things that did not with one's supervisor allows the opportunity to improve and advance a student's knowledge. See Chapter 10 on reflection in practice.

Certified occupational therapy assistants (COTA) use their reasoning skills to monitor the client's response to intervention and adjust activities accordingly. Expert COTA use procedural reasoning to customize intervention to each client (Lyons & Creapeau, 2001). They also use pragmatic and conditional reasoning as they monitor changes in client performance and inform their supervising occupational therapist of the client's progress towards goals. As members of the interprofessional team, they engage in reflection and discussion of outcomes.

The following case example describes how a rehabilitation team uses the strengths and skills of each of its team members to improve the client-centered care.

Case Example: Collaborative Intervention

Mary is a COTA who is treating a teenage girl who recently had a concussion on an inpatient rehabilitation unit. The client's primary concerns are decreased endurance, headaches, dizziness upon standing resulting in difficulty completing her schoolwork, and baking (a hobby she enjoyed prior to her injury). The Rehabilitation Unit Manager, an OT, assigned a physical therapist (PT) who has advanced training in vestibular rehabilitation therapy to the case. The client was also evaluated by a speech–language pathologist (SLP) and a neuropsychologist to determine the impact of her injury on cognitive and language performance. All patients on the unit are followed by a hospitalist (physician) and receive nursing as needed.

In team meetings Mary reports that the client's ability to complete meal preparation activities is severely impacted by her dizziness when standing. The SLP reports the patient is having significant difficulties with comprehension and recall when reading longer passages of text. The PT examined the client and attributes the dizziness to vestibular dysfunction.

The team (COTA, OT manager, SLP, and PT) discuss strategies to maximize the client's functional abilities. The team decides that the client may do better in occupational therapy if it is scheduled after physical therapy sessions which address vestibular processing. The COTA decides to use recipes that have simple 1-step directions to reinforce reading comprehension during a baking task, which also requires physical skills of standing, bending, and reaching. The SLP provides a list of reading comprehension strategies that team members can use for written materials. The SLP decides to treat the client weekly in the morning when the client is rested to work on memory and comprehension. The OT will inform the SLP of the activities they engaged in so the SLP may ask questions about those (reinforcing the sequence of steps).

The COTA focused occupational therapy sessions on meal management since the client expressed interest in returning to baking. The interprofessional team collaborated to provide comprehensive care that reinforced all members' goals and supported the client. They reinforced strategies from each profession's intervention. They communicated often with each other to make sure that the client was making progress.

They used scientific reasoning when they identified the need to address vestibular impairments before completing functional standing activities. The team used pragmatic reasoning to schedule sessions in a logical manner to benefit the client. Team members used interactive reasoning while working in sessions with the client to read her cues and respond. They used narrative reasoning to understand the client's interests (e.g., baking), the importance of returning to school, and the frustrations she felt about how her physical limitations were interfering with her abilities to engage in daily activities. They used ethical reasoning by providing quality services within their practice domains recognizing each professional's expertise. The team was able to collaborate to use conditional reasoning to create a comprehensive intervention plan.

TEAMWORK IN ADMINISTRATIVE AND CONSULTATIVE ROLES

Occupational therapists may also supervise allied health professionals in other disciplines. For example, a rehabilitation manager may supervise physical therapists, occupational therapists, rehabilitation technicians and speech–language pathologists. It is the manager's job to ensure all therapists are providing appropriate, evidence-based care within the appropriate scope of their practice while adhering to regulatory agencies' guidelines. For example, the OT manager ensures that therapists' licenses are up to date, and documentation reflects the interventions that they are performing.

OT practitioners may also lead community projects or use their OT skills as consultants. Pairing one's passion and curiosity with occupational therapy's skill set may lead an entrepreneurial OT to fill a need in a niche market. Possibilities are limitless but may include consulting on playground design, specializing in travel services for the aging population, or becoming a telehealth expert.

◼ SUMMARY

OT practitioners work with interprofessional teams to benefit clients and their families. Teams are made up of a variety of people and most importantly include the client and their family. Understanding the practice setting informs the team's goals and communication styles. Communication (e.g., written, verbal, non-verbal) is key to team dynamics and can sometimes be challenging in busy work settings. Understanding team members' roles and responsibilities, clearly outlining one's goals, and articulating in clear language without jargon are all strategies to ensure positive team experiences. Entering teams with a collaborative and curious attitude and willingness to provide and receive feedback promote team dynamics. These same strategies may be used in group sessions to facilitate group dynamics. The OT practitioner is responsible for monitoring all members' progress, facilitating communication, adapting activities, and helping each member work towards their goals. OT practitioners use therapeutic reasoning to work in interprofessional teams to promote client-centered intervention in a variety of practice settings.

REFERENCES

Alnervik, A., & Svidén, G. (1996). On clinical reasoning: patterns of reflection on practice. *The Occupational Therapy Journal of Research, 16*(2), 98–110.

American Occupational Therapy Association. (2020). AOTA 2020 occupational therapy code of ethics. *American Journal of Occupational Therapy, 74* 7413410005.

Booth, J., & Hewison, A. (2002). Role overlap between occupational therapy and physiotherapy during in-patient stroke rehabilitation: an exploratory study. *Journal of Interprofessional Care, 16*(1), 31–40.

Carrier, A., Levasseur, M., Bedard, D., & Desrosiers, J. (2012). Clinical reasoning process underlying choice of teaching strategies: A framework to improve occupational therapists' transfer skill interventions. *Australian Occupational Therapy Journal, 59,* 355–366.

Carson, N. (2022). Interpersonal relationships and communication. In J. OBrien & J. Solomon (Eds.), *Occupational Analysis and Group Process* (2nd ed., pp. 23–32). Elsevier.

Coates, G. L. F., & Crist, P. A. (2004). Brief or new: Professional development of fieldwork students: Occupational adaptation, clinical reasoning, and client-centeredness. *Occupational Therapy in Health Care, 18*(1–2), 39–47.

De Beer, M., & Mårtensson, L. (2015). Feedback on students' clinical reasoning skills during fieldwork education. *Australian Occupational Therapy Journal, 62*(4), 255–264.

Derrick, H. (2018). Interdisciplinary healthcare teams. *SPNHA Review, 14*(1), 93–109.

Fisher, A. G. (1998). Uniting practice and theory in an occupational framework. *American Journal of Occupational Therapy, 52*(7), 509–521.

Flood, B., Hocking, C., Smythe, L., & Jones, M. (2019). Working in a spirit of interprofessional teamwork: a hermeneutic phenomenological study. *Journal of Interprofessional Care, 33*(6), 744–752.

Gillen, G. (2013). 2013 Eleanor Clarke Slagle lecture: A fork in the road: An occupational hazard? *American Journal of Occupational Therapy, 6*(67), 643–652.

Grajo, L. C., & Rushanan, S. G. (2022). Ethical decision-making in occupational therapy practice. In J. O'Brien & J. Solomon (Eds.), *Occupational Analysis and Group Process* (2nd ed., pp. 174–184). Elsevier.

Institute of Medicine. Committee on Quality of Health Care in America (2001). *Crossing the quality chasm. A new health system for the 21st century.* National Academy of Press.

Institute of Medicine. (2009). *The future of nursing: Acute care.* Institute of Medicine.

Interprofessional Education Collaborative (IPEC). (2016). *Core competencies for interprofessional collaborative practice: 2016 update.* Interprofessional Education Collaborative.

Jensenius, A. R. (2012). Disciplinarities: intra, cross, multi, inter, trans. Available at: https://www.arj.no/2012/03/12/disciplinarities-2/

Kielhofner, G. (2008). *A Model of Human Occupation: Theory and Application* (4th ed.). Baltimore, MD: Lippincott, Williams & Wilkins.

Kiesewetter, J., Fischer, F., & Fischer, M. R. (2017). Collaborative clinical reasoning - a systematic review of empirical studies. *Journal of Continuing Education in the Health Professions, 37*(2), 123–128.

Komar, A., Ashley, K., Hanna, K., Lavallee, J., Woodhouse, J., Bernstein, J., & Reed, N. (2016). Retrospective analysis of an ongoing group-based modified constraint-induced movement therapy program for children with acquired brain injury. *Physical & Occupational Therapy in Pediatrics, 36*(2), 186–203.

Lyons, K. D., & Crepeau, E. B. (2001). Case Report—The clinical reasoning of an occupational therapy assistant. *American Journal of Occupational Therapy, 55,* 577–581.

Marks, M. A., Matthieu, J. E., & Zaccaro, S. J. (2000). A temporarily based framework and taxonomy of team processes. *Academy of Management Review, 26,* 356–376.

McMurtry, A. (2013). Reframing interdisciplinary and interprofessional collaboration through the lens of collective and sociomaterial theory of learning. *Issues in Interdisciplinary Studies, 31,* 75–98.

Munroe, H. (1996). Clinical reasoning in community occupational therapy. *British Journal of Occupational Therapy, 59*(5), 196–202.

O'Brien, J., & Kielhofner, G. (2017). The interaction between the person and the environment. In R. Taylor (Ed.), *Kielhofner's model of human occupation* (5th ed., pp. 24–37). Philadelphia, PA: Wolters Kluwer.

Purtillo, R. (2005). *Ethical Dimensions in the Health Professions* (4th ed.). American Occupational Therapy Association.

Reeves, S., Tassone, M., Parker, K., Wagenr, S. J., & Simmons, B. (2012). An overview of key developments in the past three decades. *Work, 41,* 233–245.

Salas, E., Sims, D., & Burke, C. S. (2005). Is there a "big five" in teamwork? *Small Group Research, 36*(5), 555–599.

Sergakis, G., Clutter, J., Hothaus, V., et al. (2016). The impact of interprofessional clinical simulation on attitudes, confidence, and professional identity: The added value of integrating respiratory therapy. *Respiratory Care Education Annual, 25,* 11–16.

Schot, E., Tummers, L., & Noordegraaf, M. (2020). Working on working together. A systematic review on how healthcare professionals contribute to interprofessional collaboration. *Journal of Interprofessional Care, 34*(3), 332–342.

Tuckman, B. & Jensen, M. (1977). Stages of small group development revisited. *Group & Organizational Studies, 2*(4), 419–127.

Ward, J. D. (2003). The nature of clinical reasoning with groups: A phenomenological study of an occupational therapist in community mental health. *American Journal of Occupational Therapy, 57,* 625–634.

Walton, V., Hogden, A., Long, J. C., Johnson, J. K., & Greenfield, D. (2019). How do interprofessional healthcare teams perceive the benefits and challenges of interdisciplinary ward rounds. *Journal of Multidisciplinary Healthcare, 12,* 1023–1032.

Weller, J., Boyd, M., & Cumin, D. (2014). Teams, tribes, and patient safety: overcoming barriers to effective teamwork in healthcare. *Postgrad Medicine Journal, 90,* 145–154.

World Health Organization (WHO). (2010). *Framework for Action on Interprofessional Education and Collaborative Practice.* Geneva: WHO. Available at. http://apps.who.int/iris/bitstream/handle/10665/70185/WHO_HRH_HPN_10.3_eng.pdf;jsessionid=E83BDF5E42C1BE6BAA1186A22930AB31?sequence=1.

Yang, J. H., Wang, Y. Q., Ye, S. Q., Cheng, Y. G., Chen, Y., & Feng, X. Z. (2017). The effects of group-based versus individual-based tai chi training on nonmotor symptoms in patients with mild to moderate Parkinson's disease: A randomized controlled pilot trial. *Parkinson's Disease,* 1–9.

WORKSHEET 7.1: TEAM MEMBERS

Complete Worksheet 7.1 to identify the roles of team members. Describe the role of the OT practitioner in each setting.

• How does the setting influence the focus of occupational therapy evaluation and intervention?

Team Members		
Setting	**Members – Describe the role of each member**	**Role of OT (setting specific)**
Acute care hospital	• Physicians • Nurses • Physical therapist • Social worker • Case manager • Imaging technicians	
Inpatient hospital	• Orthopedist • Physiatrist • Social worker • Nurse • Neuropsychologist • Radiology	
Outpatient hospital	• Physical therapist • Speech–language pathologist • Nutritionist	
Community	• Advocacy group members • Planning committees • Department of health/recreation staff • Town supervisors or other personnel	
Educational settings	• Special education teacher • Parent • Speech language pathologist • Reading specialist • Counselor • Principal or other school administrator	
Mental health setting	• Psychologist • Psychiatrist • Aid • Nurse • Counselor • Recreation therapist • Social worker	

WORKSHEET 7.2: MUTUAL RESPECT AND SHARED VALUES

Use Worksheet 7.2 to reflect upon a team of which you were a member to outline the shared values and feelings of mutual respect. Describe a team situation whereby the members did not share values or did not respect other members.

Mutual Respect and Shared Values
Name:
Description of a team situation:
How did you observe mutual respect and shared values?
How did the team function?
What factors contributed to team performance?

WORKSHEET 7.3: TEAM EFFECTIVENESS

Complete Worksheet 7.3 to learn more about team effectiveness. Describe a team or group project for which you participated and analyze the team components by providing examples.

Team Effectiveness	
Name:	
Brief description of team or group project:	
Your role:	
Team members:	
Describe the effectiveness of the team:	
Components of Teamwork	Examples (from your team)
Team leadership	
Mutual performance monitoring	
Backup behavior	
Adaptability	
Orientation	
What factors contributed to the effectiveness of the team?	
Upon reflection, how might you do things differently?	

WORKSHEET 7.4: STRATEGIES DURING STAGES OF TEAM DEVELOPMENT

Complete Worksheet 7.4. Provide personal examples of each stage of the team development. Identify strategies that may be required at each stage.

Strategies during Stages of Team Development		
Stage of Team Development	**Example**	**Strategies**
Forming		
Storming		
Norming		
Performing		
Adjourning		
How might the stage of development influence one's reasoning?		

WORKSHEET 7.5: ROLE OVERLAP

Complete Worksheet 7.5 to compare roles of OT and speech therapy.

An OT practitioner and speech therapist are developing a summer camp–style life skills group for children with autism at an outpatient pediatric clinic. The camp will run for 1-week sessions for 10 weeks throughout the summer. Children will attend the OT and Speech Therapy sessions once a day. To keep the groups small (6 to 8 children), they will run 3 sessions per day together.
- Create 1 long-term goal to address executive functioning for life skills that both OT and Speech Therapy will target during the summer camp/
  - Create a short-term OT goal and a short-term Speech Therapy goals to address during a group session.
- Describe how each profession will address the goal.
  - Identify specific activities and approaches.
- Compare and contrast each profession's approach to the executive functioning goal.
- Define how OT and ST differ and how they can support each other.

Role Overlap		
	Occupational Therapy	**Speech Therapy**
Long-term goal to address executive functioning for life skills		
Short-term goal		
How will each profession address goal?		
Identify specific activities and approaches.		
Compare and contrast each profession's approach to the executive functioning goal.		
Define how OT and ST differ and how they can support each other.		

WORKSHEET 7.6: COMMUNICATION AND CLIENT EDUCATION

Refer to Worksheet 7.6. *Erin is an OTR working in a pediatric outpatient clinic with children who have developmental delay, autism spectrum disorder, and neuromotor disorders. Many of the families are non-English speaking.*

- What strategies might Erin use to assure adequate communication between children and their families?
- Provide examples of how pragmatic, narrative, interactive, ethical, scientific, and conditional reasoning influence how she educates family and children.

Communication and Client Education	
Name:	
List strategies to assure adequate communication with children and their families.	
Type of Reasoning	Provide examples of how reasoning influences communication and client education
Scientific	
Narrative	
Pragmatic	
Interactive	
Conditional	

WORKSHEET 7.7: CONTEXT-DEPENDENT PRACTICE

Using Worksheet 7.7 as a guide, contact two OT practitioners who work in different practice settings. Ask them to share one case (no names or identifying information) to determine the similarities and differences in their reasoning.

Context-dependent Practice		
Name:		
	Practitioner 1 (Name):	Practitioner 2 (Name):
Setting:		
Patient population:		
Team members:		
Brief description of case:		
What influenced their decision-making?		
How did they decide upon the specific activities for the intervention?		
Describe the similarities and differences between the two settings.		

Applying Knowledge to Develop Therapeutic Reasoning

Mary Elizabeth Patnaude, Teressa Garcia Reidy and Jane O'Brien

GUIDING QUESTIONS

1. What are the characteristics of critical thinkers?
2. How do OT students and practitioners use cognitive processes and strategies to engage in therapeutic reasoning?
3. What practices and strategies facilitate therapeutic reasoning skills?
4. What are the critical thinking and evidence-informed practice behaviors operationalized in therapeutic reasoning assessments?
5. How can fieldwork educators and supervisors facilitate therapeutic reasoning?

KEY TERMS

Abstract thought
Cognitive strategy
Critical thinking
Deductive reasoning
Evidence-informed practice
Inductive reasoning

Formal operations stage
Guided discovery
Metacognition
Socratic questioning
Threshold concepts

INTRODUCTION

Therapeutic reasoning is a complex process that challenges OT students and practitioners (both novice and experienced) as highlighted in the following classroom encounter.

A faculty member provides students information on a case of a 48-year-old woman with multiple sclerosis, and questions them about how they would approach the assessment and intervention to stimulate therapeutic reasoning. A student, frustrated with the process, asks, "What would you do?" The faculty member responds, "There are many correct answers to this case. The goal is to learn to think it through considering the multiple factors that influence decisions along the way, assess the outcomes, and be flexible in your approaches." The entire class sighs.

Therapeutic reasoning requires OT students and practitioners to consider many factors when creating intervention plans, using evidence, and applying knowledge of the client's motivations, interests, culture, and abilities. There are many different correct answers for each client's situation.

For example, when thinking about the best way to treat the woman mentioned above with multiple sclerosis, OT practitioners consider the client's condition, stage, and symptoms. They assess the practice setting (e.g., acute care setting focuses on medical status; home health setting focuses on her ability to function at home), client's environment, and community resources. The practitioner also reflects on their own interactive style and professional strengths and challenges to create client-centered intervention plans. They integrate knowledge of

all these areas in combination with the client's lived experience, performance skills, performance patterns, and client factors to make decisions throughout the process.

Healthcare educators strive to educate students and practitioners who will engage in effective therapeutic reasoning by synthesizing information from multiple sources to make decisions and create effective intervention plans. They may use a variety of strategies (such as guided discovery, Socratic questioning, and video analysis) to promote analysis, application of knowledge in practice, problem-solving, and reflection. OT students and practitioners develop therapeutic reasoning skills by engaging in discussions regarding authentic cases, such as those included in problem-based learning (PBL), case-based learning, experiential learning (such as simulation, service learning, and fieldwork experiences), and team-based learning (Baird et al., 2015; Knecht-Sabres, 2010; Keiller & Hanekom, 2013; Murphy & Radloff, 2019; Murphy & Stav, 2018; O'Brien & McNeil, 2013).

Critical thinkers engage in a process of prioritizing goals, making decisions, perceiving responses, anticipating outcomes, examining evidence, and applying knowledge to practice. Habits of mind that support therapeutic reasoning include curiosity, self-awareness, flexible thinking, and evidence-informed practice. **Evidence-informed practice** refers to the use of intellectual habits and beneficial professional activities that provide practitioners the skills and knowledge to practice effectively (Benfield & Johnston, 2020). These include engaging in lifelong learning, critiquing evidence, using reflection to assess one's effectiveness, and collaborating with peers to develop intervention plans to achieve the most desirable client outcomes (Benfield & Johnston, 2020). These characteristics and habits of mind are operationalized in assessments measuring therapeutic reasoning (Benfield & Johnston, 2020; deCarvalho et al., 2017; Jenkins, 1985; Lasater, 2007; Murphy & Stav, 2018).

The authors of this chapter examine the characteristics of critical thinkers and outline cognitive processes and strategies used during therapeutic reasoning. A description of assessments used to measure therapeutic reasoning provides readers with skills and abilities that support therapeutic reasoning. They describe strategies and techniques to enhance the development of therapeutic reasoning. Learning activities and case examples reinforce content and can be used by educators to help the student synthesize and apply concepts in practice.

CHARACTERISTICS OF CRITICAL THINKERS

Critical thinking refers to the ability to analyze, examine, and evaluate information to make decisions, synthesize information, and prioritize (Sahamid, 2014). Critical thinking is part of the therapeutic reasoning process and is included in each step as the OT practitioner generates questions, gathers information, identifies occupational challenges, creates an occupational

therapy plan, implements the intervention plan, and assesses the outcomes. Figure 8.1 lists characteristics of critical thinkers as compiled from the literature on therapeutic reasoning.

Critical thinkers show a curiosity for information and figuring things out. They ask questions. For example, OT practitioners ask questions about human behaviors, the client's goals, lived experience, and the physical, social, and attitudinal environment. They inquire about the client's culture to make intervention decisions. They also search for answers and examine the quality of the evidence. See Chapter 6 on evidence-based practice. They use their curiosity for learning to link concepts together and make sense of the situation which leads to creative solutions. Critical thinkers are open-minded, while also being critical of the information. They use their knowledge of occupational therapy to judge the source of information and its suitability to the specific client. Given that they value the underlying philosophy of the profession, OT practitioners who critically think about the process, follow occupational therapy theory. By showing a curiosity for learning, asking questions, and finding evidence, critical thinkers can cite reasons for choices, justify approaches and decisions at each step. and provide support for their decisions.

For example, an OT practitioner evaluating a young child for the first time creates questions based on the Model of Human Occupation (as it has evidence to support its use in practice) and

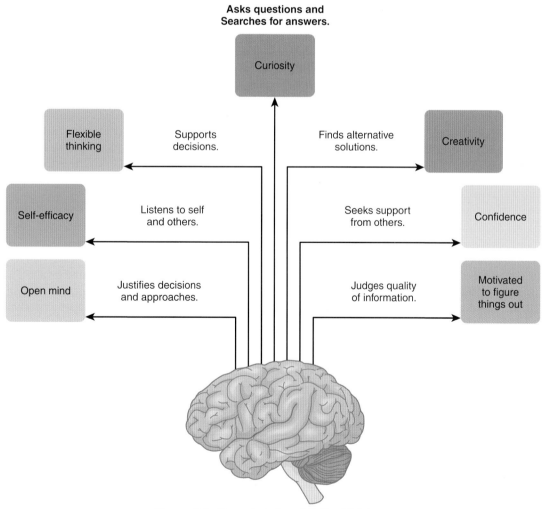

Figure 8.1 Characteristics of Critical Thinkers.

uses knowledge of therapeutic communication (use of modes) to interview the parent. The practitioner observes that the parent is concerned and worried about the child. After learning about the parent's concerns and observing the child, the practitioner decides which assessments to administer. She selects an assessment that is suitable for the child's age, diagnosis, and temperament and one that will provide objective measures of which she can make further decisions. The practitioner informs the parent of the choices. For example, she says "this short assessment will help us know if your child is having difficulty with touch." The practitioner collaborates with the parent throughout the process, checking in to make sure the parent understands what is happening at each step, and showing interest in the child and the family dynamics. The practitioner uses critical thinking to justify each decision, and to calmly explain the reasoning to the parent. This therapeutic use of self helps to ease the parent's anxiety. As a collaborative team, they problem-solve the next steps. By keeping the parent informed of the reason for the choices made during the assessment, the parent (and child) are part of the process, and feel at ease throughout the occupational therapy process.

LEARNING ACTIVITY: CURIOSITY

Use Worksheet 8.1. Select a topic related to therapeutic reasoning. List 10 questions you would like answered on this topic.
* How does curiosity enhance learning?

Benfield and Johnston (2020) identified the habits and practice skills of effective therapists as behaviors related to both critical reasoning and evidence informed practice (i.e., integrating research into practice). Hours spent reading, reflection on level of knowledge, consideration of new interventions, and demonstration of confidence through the willingness to trial new interventions correlated with evidence-informed practice. Using data from peer-reviewed sources to assess the accuracy of clinical decisions, evaluate the effectiveness of intervention outcomes, and formulate alternate theories of the situation all correlated with evidence-informed practice (Benfield & Johnston, 2020).

Behaviors that were associated with critical reasoning included examining decisions related to knowledge (conditions, client populations, evidence), accuracy of perceptions and beliefs, and formulation of client problems. The ability to seek information, advice, or feedback from colleagues and examine outcomes were associated with critical reasoning (Benfield & Johnston, 2020). These behaviors imply that questioning, searching for answers, and seeking support and advice from others are characteristics of critical thinkers.

Behaviors that support critical thinking include self-efficacy, which is one's belief in their skills and abilities (Audétat, et al., 2012; Kielhofner & Forsyth, 2008). As OT practitioners gain skills in therapeutic reasoning resulting in client successes, they are reinforced to engage in those behaviors, and they gain confidence. Self-efficacy and confidence support flexible thinking leading to creativity and the ability to find more options for intervention plans. Attitudes of open-mindedness, belief in change, and the power of engaging in occupations also support a practitioner's ability to engage in the therapeutic reasoning process.

LEARNING ACTIVITY: CHARACTERISTICS OF CRITICAL THINKERS

Using the list provided in Worksheet 8.2, indicate behaviors you possess that are characteristic of critical thinkers. Provide personal examples.
* How could you develop abilities in the other behaviors?

THE PROCESS OF APPLYING KNOWLEDGE

Metacognition refers to thinking about one's thinking. As OT practitioners provide their rationale for decisions, justify choices, and reflect upon their problem-solving regarding occupational therapy, they engage in metacognition. OT students and practitioners engage in metacognition throughout the reasoning process as they select strategies from frames of reference; analyze theory, principles, and research findings; and judge the quality of the evidence. Metacognition involves thinking about one's decisions, line of inquiry, and conceptualization of the client's occupational challenges and intervention choices.

OT practitioners use both inductive and deductive reasoning to interpret client situations.

Inductive reasoning is the process by which individuals make sense of the world by creating rules about the situations they encounter, remembering the instances to which the rule applies, and developing new hypotheses related to the rules (Babcock & Vallesi, 2015). For example, OT practitioners who structure intervention based on protocols or follow established guidelines are using inductive reasoning. They combine knowledge of the rules of the protocol to the new information they learn about the client to develop new hypotheses related to the rules. Inductive reasoning suggests that if the premises are correct (and the new information supports it), the conclusions are probable.

Deductive reasoning involves determining if logical conclusions follow a given set of premises that are based on prior beliefs, observations, and/or suppositions that are not explicit in the initial premise (Stephens et al., 2018). The individual determines how to respond to the situation by making inferences based on previous knowledge. For example, OT practitioners may begin with understanding the client's condition and during the assessment determine how the client matches previous known knowledge and experiences of that condition. If all the premises are true, the conclusions reached are true.

Figure 8.2 illustrates the reasoning involved as an OT practitioner completes the steps (i.e., generate questions based on theory, gather data, identify occupational challenges, create intervention plan, implement plan, and assess outcomes) of the process. The OT practitioner begins by using metacognition to prepare for the client interview by reviewing occupation-based models of practice (such as Model of Human Occupation, Person-Environment-Occupation-Participation, Canadian Model of Occupational Performance and Engagement) and frames of reference that may be suitable to the setting (such as biomechanical, cognitive behavioral, or rehabilitation). The practitioner generates questions based on the theory from the model. Next, the OT practitioner prepares to gather information by getting all the materials needed and making decisions on the types of assessments, time requirements, training, and set up.

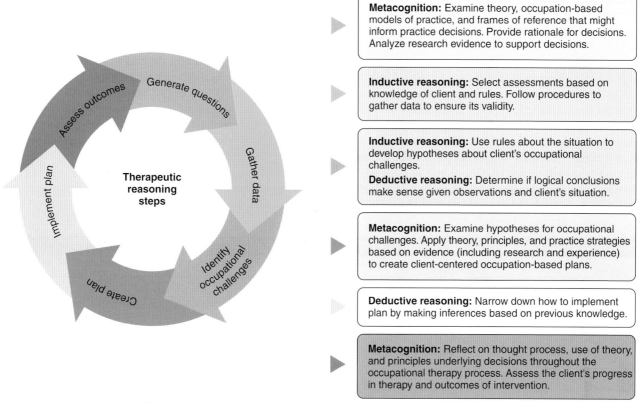

Metacognition: Examine theory, occupation-based models of practice, and frames of reference that might inform practice decisions. Provide rationale for decisions. Analyze research evidence to support decisions.

Inductive reasoning: Select assessments based on knowledge of client and rules. Follow procedures to gather data to ensure its validity.

Inductive reasoning: Use rules about the situation to develop hypotheses about client's occupational challenges.
Deductive reasoning: Determine if logical conclusions make sense given observations and client's situation.

Metacognition: Examine hypotheses for occupational challenges. Apply theory, principles, and practice strategies based on evidence (including research and experience) to create client-centered occupation-based plans.

Deductive reasoning: Narrow down how to implement plan by making inferences based on previous knowledge.

Metacognition: Reflect on thought process, use of theory, and principles underlying decisions throughout the occupational therapy process. Assess the client's progress in therapy and outcomes of intervention.

Figure 8.2 Applying Knowledge at Each Therapeutic Reasoning Step.

The OT practitioner uses scientific and pragmatic reasoning in these initial steps. As the OT practitioner enters the client's room to gather data they incorporate therapeutic use of self (interactive reasoning) by attending to their communication style, body language and the client's cues and reactions to both verbal and non-verbal communication. The OT practitioner uses inductive reasoning to select assessments based on the client's age, setting, and diagnoses. Specifically, the OT practitioner surmises that if the assessment is suitable for the client's age, addresses factors for which clients with this diagnosis typically present, and can be administered in this setting, then the assessment results will probably be accurate and inform the occupational therapy evaluation.

The practitioner synthesizes information about the client from the interview, observations, and assessments to identify occupational challenges. At this stage, the practitioner uses inductive reasoning to use rules about the situation to create hypotheses to focus intervention. The OT practitioner also uses deductive reasoning to determine if conclusions based on theory make sense given the client's situation. This conceptualization is based on conditional reasoning which integrates information from narrative, interactive, scientific, pragmatic and ethical reasoning.

The OT practitioner creates a client-centered intervention plan using metacognition. The practitioner examines all the available information to create a logical and client-centered plan based on theory and the best available evidence. As the OT practitioner engages the client in the plan, they make decisions, judge information, analyze information, and anticipate responses. The practitioner uses deductive reasoning to narrow down how to implement the plan by making inferences based on previous knowledge.

OT practitioners assess the client's progress towards their goals and reflect using metacognition throughout the process as they justify decisions, provide rationales for decisions, and adjust intervention or processes based on new knowledge. Throughout each step of the therapeutic reasoning process, OT practitioners use cognitive strategies to process information.

Cognitive Strategies

The ability to critically think and apply reason to situations begins in early adolescence in Piaget's formal operations stage as adolescents imagine different possibilities, make judgments, analyze problems, and determine solutions to a variety of situations (deCarvalho et al., 2017; Sahamid, 2014). During this stage, adolescents engage in abstract thought as they contemplate solutions for situations that may present. Abstract thought is the ability to think about things that are not actually present (Merriam-Webster, 2021). Healthcare professionals use abstract thinking for therapeutic reasoning as they anticipate the client's needs, future possibilities, and imagine how the client may respond to intervention.

As OT practitioners engage in therapeutic reasoning, they use a variety of cognitive strategies to gather, sort through, prioritize, and analyze information regarding the client, environment, and occupations. "A cognitive strategy is a mental plan of action that helps a person to learn, problem solve, and perform. The use of cognitive strategies can improve an individual's learning, problem solving, and task performance in terms of efficiency, speed, accuracy, and consistency" (Toglia et al., 2012, p. 227).

Everyone uses cognitive strategies to manage performance. For example, cognitive strategies include such things as organizing one's space before studying, creating lists of assignments, rehearsing before giving a presentation, and verbalizing what one is thinking. These strategies support the person's performance and allow the person to look at information more deeply to apply knowledge. Table 8.1 provides a list of cognitive strategies.

Toglia and colleagues (2012) present a framework (Table 8.2) to guide practitioners' reasoning regarding the use of cognitive strategies with clients. This framework may also be used to explain the practitioner's therapeutic reasoning process.

This framework can be applied to a practitioner's use of strategies to promote reasoning. Figure 8.3 provides an example of using the framework to describe the cognitive strategies used by the OT practitioner involved in conducting an OT evaluation. For example (as depicted in Figure 8.3), the OT prepares for the OT evaluation using strategy knowledge which includes knowledge of models of practice and frames of reference. As the OT conducts the evaluation, they translate the information into more manageable chunks for the client. The therapist switched cognitive strategies during the evaluation and was aware when the strategies were not working as they engaged in the post-session review. The therapist reflected on the effectiveness of their use of strategies and made decisions about how they might modify strategies for the next session. Cognitive strategies can and should be taught to clients to promote occupational performance. The framework provided by Toglia et al. (2012) provides a tool to organize one's thoughts, analyze the use of cognitive strategies, and reason using strategies to enhance occupational performance.

TABLE 8.1   A Descriptive Typography of Cognitive Strategies

Strategies	Description
Modality-specific Strategies	Visual, tactile, auditory, or kinesthetic cues.
Mental or Self-verbalization Strategies	A broad category of techniques that involve mental operations, inner speech, or imagery, or thinking and talking aloud.
• Rehearsal	Repeating information mentally or verbally such as key words, rules, procedures, action steps, or facts to enhance retention of information or procedures.
• Mnemonic techniques	Forming associations between words, sets of words, pictures, or images to cue actions or recall.
• Rote scripts	Repeating information that has been coded or abbreviated to guide a sequence of actions or enhance recall of information.
• Association	Linking similar information together based on previous experiences, knowledge of categories, or physical similarities.
• Elaboration (mental, verbal)	Expands or adds to new information (adding new words, sentences, images, symbols or actions) and relates it to previous information.
• Imagery	Mental images involve transforming physical objects, events, actions, or experiences into images, symbols, or representations. Mental imagery is not just visual as it can involve imagining smells, textures, sounds, or the feel of movements.
• Reconstruction (mental verbal)	Thinking back involves replaying, imagining, or verbalizing a previous activity, experience, or context to assist in guiding performance in a new situation.
• Anticipation (mental verbal)	Imagining or verbalizing potential challenges or obstacles, possible scenarios, or outcomes to assist in preparing for a task.
• Translation	Translation of information such as written instructions, procedures, or actions into images, phrases, or more manageable chunks of information.
• Self-guidance	Provide oneself instructions, self-cues, or reminders to prepare or guide oneself through a task (self-instruction, self-talk, talk aloud).
• Self-coaching	Positive self-talk, thinking, and encouragement to increase persistence or to help regulate and control emotions (e.g., you can do this, stay calm).
• Self-questioning	Imagining or asking oneself key questions related to the task or performance.
• Knowledge	Identifying, verbalizing, or thinking about what one knows about a task before beginning.
Task Specification/ Modification	
• Stimuli reduction	Decreasing the amount of information or number of items presented at any one time, covering, or removing part of task stimuli.
• Organization	Reorganizing task materials or steps so that similar items or steps are together (association, categorization).
• Task simplification	Breaking apart steps or reducing steps or activity into more manageable parts.
• Lists	Creating or using a written, pictorial, or audiotaped list of steps to guide performance or cue actions.
• Pacing strategies	Actions that assist with the timing of activities, e.g., taking breaks, spreading activities throughout the day, completing partial tasks.
• Task specifications	Identify specific relevant features or components of a task prior to an activity that requires careful consideration, planning or attention.
• Attention to doing	Identifying key cues or features to pay attention to during performance.
• Finger pointing	Pointing to relevant task stimuli to enhance attention to details to pace timing within a task.

From Toglia, J. P., Rodger, S. A., & Polatajko, H. J. (2012). Anatomy of cognitive strategies: A therapist's primer for enabling occupational performance. *Canadian Journal of Occupational Therapy, 79*(4), 225–236.

TABLE 8.2 Framework for Analysis of Cognitive Strategy Use: A Clinical Reasoning Tool

	Therapist Observations and Comments
A. Prerequisites to Effective Strategy Use	
1. Strategy knowledge *Does the client know what a strategy is, how a strategy operates, and when and why it should be applied?* 2. Strategy repertoire *Is the client's range or repertoire of strategies adequate?* 3. Strategy beliefs *What are the client's beliefs about strategies (e.g., strategies will influence outcome or strategies will not help performance)?* 4. Anticipation and recognition of need *Does the client anticipate and recognize task challenges? Does the client identify the need to use a strategy within an activity context?* 5. Strategy generation and selection *Does the client self-generate, state, or self-select strategies for activities or are strategies selected and provided by others?*	
B. Strategy Execution	
1. Initiation *Is strategy spontaneously initiated by the client?* 2. Implementation *Are strategies carried out completely and accurately?* 3. Number of strategies *Can the client use and coordinate multiple strategies simultaneously? Single strategies only?*	
C. Quality of Strategy Use	
1. Degree of effort *What is the degree of effort or resources needed to use strategies (e.g., does degree of effort negatively affect performance or speed)?* 2. Temporal pattern *What are the timing and frequency of strategy use (e.g., are strategies used too late, over-used, finding too soon, or fluctuating?* 3. Flexibility of strategy use *Does the client adjust or switch strategies when needed?* 4. Monitoring and evaluating strategy use *Does the client know when strategies have not been efficient or effective? Are performance errors recognized?*	
D. Effectiveness of Strategy Use	
Are positive changes in learning, problem-solving, or performance outcomes associated with strategy use?	

From Toglia, J. P., Rodger, S. A., & Polatajko, H. J. (2012). Anatomy of cognitive strategies: A therapist's primer for enabling occupational performance. *Canadian Journal of Occupational Therapy, 79*(4), 225–236.

LEARNING ACTIVITY: ANALYSIS OF COGNITIVE STRATEGIES

Use Worksheet 8.3 to apply the Framework for Analysis of Cognitive Strategy Use (Toglia et al., 2012) to a challenging occupation for which you engage. Describe the activity and the cognitive strategies you use.
- How would this framework be used to inform decisions in practice?

EDUCATIONAL METHODOLOGIES TO PROMOTE THERAPEUTIC REASONING

Faculty teaching in healthcare professions prepare students to become practitioners in a variety of practice settings (e.g., acute care, rehabilitation, community, schools, and home) and work with clients of all ages and from diverse backgrounds. While students want to know "what to do," faculty want to teach them "how to think" to educate lifelong learners. Faculty seek to inspire students to be lifelong learners who can problem-solve, anticipate, prioritize, synthesize, and integrate information from multiple sources to create sound practice decisions in a variety of settings with people of all ages. The educational goal is to create practitioners who blend the art and science of occupational therapy.

The scholarship of teaching and learning in occupational therapy supports a variety of educational methods to prepare students and practitioners to engage in therapeutic reasoning for practice. Educational methods that require students to apply theory-driven knowledge to complex clinical problems promote therapeutic reasoning (Benson et al., 2013; Bowyer et al., 2019; Giles et al., 2014; Murphy & Radloff, 2019; O'Brien & McNeil, 2013; Reichl et al., 2019). These experiences can be provided through formalized learning opportunities, such as coursework and continuing education and by applying reasoning to real life situations, such as provided in problem-based learning,

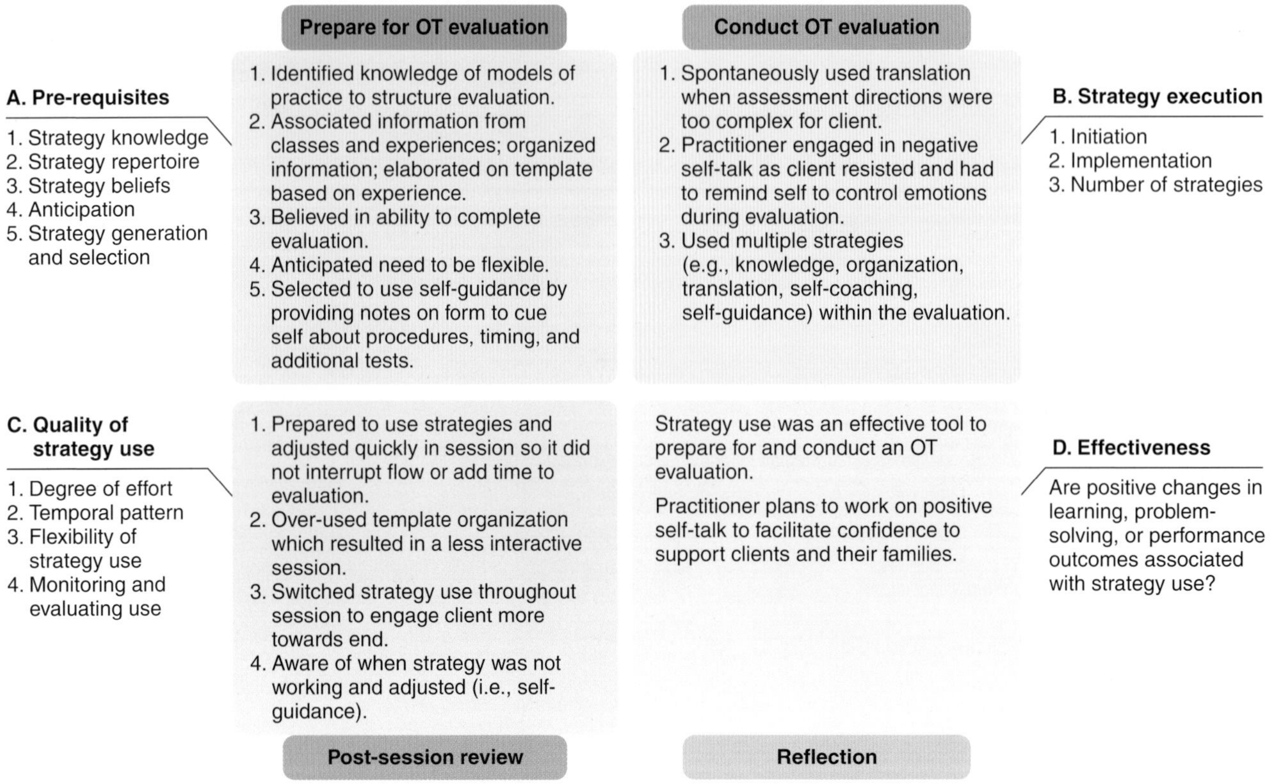

Figure 8.3 Framework for Analysis of Cognitive Strategy.

case-based learning, and experiential learning (Bowyer et al., 2019; Keiller & Hanekom, 2013; Knecht-Sabres, 2010, O'Brien & McNeil, 2013; Murphy & Stav, 2018).

OT students and practitioners continue to advance their therapeutic reasoning skills as they engage in practice experiences with clients, discuss concepts with colleagues, seek feedback on practice, and participate in continuing education.

TECHNIQUES TO FACILIATE THERAPEUTIC REASONING

Therapeutic reasoning requires active learning experiences where OT students and practitioners practice engaging in the process that they use in practice and delve deeply into concepts, which will be used to further understand practice. The process involves exploration, discovery, reflection, feedback, and metacognition. A variety of techniques, such as Socratic questioning, guided discovery, and video analysis facilitate therapeutic reasoning in educational and practice settings.

Socratic Questioning

Socratic questioning uses questions to prompt students and OT practitioners to think deeply about concepts (Sahamid, 2016). It is an educational technique that engages students in the thinking process by asking questions in a prescribed manner using the same set of procedures to guide that thinking. By repeating the thinking process, students and practitioners raise their standard of thinking and learn to provide a rationale for their decisions (Dinkins & Cangelosi, 2019; Paul & Elder, 2007; Sahamid, 2014; Sahamid, 2016).

For Socratic questioning to be effective, educators and supervisors must provide a supportive and open environment that will stimulate thought, in which students and practitioners feel safe in taking risks (Sahamid,2014). Questions give direction and help the practitioner focus. Figure 8.4 lists the Socratic elements of questions that stimulate thought and identifies sample questions from occupational therapy. Asking the right questions stimulates the OT practitioner's thinking and promotes a deeper understanding of concepts that promote professional growth and benefit clients and their families.

Torabizadeh et al., (2018) conducted a study whereby one group received instruction using Socratic questioning techniques and another group received a four-hour lecture-based workshop. The students in the Socratic questioning group performed significantly better than the workshop group on their ability to respond to ethical dilemmas (Torabizadeh et al, 2018).

LEARNING ACTIVITY: SOCRATIC QUESTIONING

Complete Worksheet 8.4. Imagine you are the fieldwork educator about to meet with a student who just completed their first intervention session. You observed the session. The client, who has mental health issues, showed difficulty paying attention, initiating actions, and completing simple verbal steps to a project. The student made good attempts to adjust the activity, but at times appeared disappointed in the client's performance (and it showed on his/her/their face).

- Using the elements of thought (Figure 8.4), create questions to allow the student to describe his reasoning and facilitate self-awareness to promote change.
- What is the advantage of using Socratic questioning techniques?

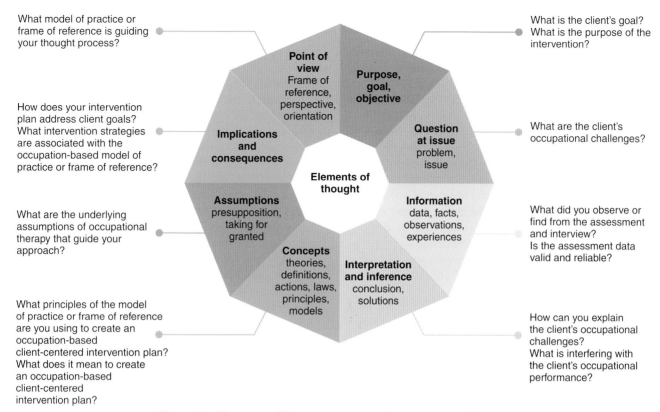

What model of practice or frame of reference is guiding your thought process?

What is the client's goal? What is the purpose of the intervention?

How does your intervention plan address client goals? What intervention strategies are associated with the occupation-based model of practice or frame of reference?

What are the client's occupational challenges?

What are the underlying assumptions of occupational therapy that guide your approach?

What did you observe or find from the assessment and interview? Is the assessment data valid and reliable?

What principles of the model of practice or frame of reference are you using to create an occupation-based client-centered intervention plan? What does it mean to create an occupation-based client-centered intervention plan?

How can you explain the client's occupational challenges? What is interfering with the client's occupational performance?

Figure 8.4 Elements of Thought. (Adapted from Elder & Paul, 2001.)

Guided Discovery

Guided discovery and reflection can be used to promote communication between students and fieldwork educators (Tanner, 2011). It is a collaborative approach whereby the supervisor encourages the practitioner to find their own solutions (Overholser, 2018). Using guided discovery may help students and practitioners identify challenges they experience in practice so that fieldwork educators and faculty can better prepare them for practice. Key struggles can also be identified as threshold concepts (termed by Meyer & Land, 2003). Threshold concepts refer to knowledge that begins as troublesome or difficult but grasping the concept leads to learner transformation of thinking and professional growth (Meyer & Land, 2005; Nicola-Richmond et al., 2016). Nicola-Richmond et al. (2016) identified therapeutic reasoning threshold concepts in occupational therapy that help transform individuals from student to practitioner as thinking critically, reasoning, reflecting, and utilizing evidence-based practice. Tanner (2011) explored the threshold concepts related to occupational therapy fieldwork education through focus groups and identified three skills that need to be mastered for students to transform into competent practitioners: client-centered practice and use of self; development of a professional self-identity; and practicing in the real world (Tanner, 2011).

The supervisor guides the student or practitioner in a collaborative manner using Socratic questioning techniques, highlighting useful ideas, focusing on major themes, and redirecting as needed. The practitioner may complete assignments and self-monitoring activities on their own (Overholser, 2018). This learning process uses inductive reasoning to help clients (or students) search for new information to find effective solutions (Overholser, 2018).

LEARNING ACTIVITY: GUIDED DISCOVERY

Complete Worksheet 8.5. You are working with patients who are all status post total knee replacements. Using guided discovery, reflect on what you know and need to know.

- What OT models of practice and frames of reference will guide your session?
- Why did you select these?
- What are the protocols for total knee replacements?
- How comfortable are you working with orthopedic conditions?
- What else would you like to know?
- What do you anticipate the client will feel like doing?
- How will you use scientific (procedural), narrative, and conditional reasoning in practice?
- What would you like to review for the session?

Video Analysis

Video analysis may be used during an evaluation, administration of a standardized assessment tool, or when facilitating individual or group interventions. Giles et al. (2014) examined the effectiveness of using reflective video analysis to prepare students for level II fieldwork. Students were videotaped during a comprehensive practical exam. They analyzed their performance related to the clinical skills they demonstrated, such as their ability to safely execute an evaluation and intervention (Giles et al., 2014). After completing a self-assessment, students reviewed their reflection with a faculty member and received feedback on their performance. More than 75% of the students reported that they valued the use of video for self-reflection and to improve performance (Giles et al., 2014).

In another study, looking at the use of video as a teaching tool, students who engaged in video case studies and video to clarify points in class in a clinical reasoning course scored higher on the Health Science Reasoning Test (HSRT) than students who engaged in the course with written case studies and text-based learning tools (Murphy & Stav, 2018). Students who received the additional instruction with video clips demonstrated improved performance in all areas of reasoning (Murphy & Stav, 2018).

Video analysis may be used in practice settings to provide OT practitioners with the opportunity to view their work with clients with a supervisor or peer. The reflection and analysis may allow the practitioner to see things more clearly and understand practice decisions for the future. Debriefing by discussing specific questions (see Worksheet 8.6) provides structure to the analysis and may result in a deeper conversations.

LEARNING ACTIVITY: DEBRIEFING TO IMPROVE THERAPEUTIC REASONING

Record a 5-minute intervention or evaluation session with a client. Complete Worksheet 8.6 and then meet with a peer and discuss the session.
• How does this information inform your next session?

THERAPEUTIC REASONING ASSESSMENT TOOLS

Researchers create assessments by operationalizing concepts into observable behaviors which can be addressed to promote professional development. A closer look at the items measured in these assessments provides insight into how OT practitioners demonstrate reasoning skills. The assessments highlighted in this chapter explore reasoning. Additional assessments promoting self-reflection of one's reasoning are reviewed in Chapter 10.

Macauley and colleagues (2017) conducted a systematic review of assessments that evaluate clinical decision-making, clinical reasoning, and critical thinking for measuring changes after participation in simulation experiences. Table 8.3 lists some of the items from each assessment to provide readers with an indication of behaviors associated with reasoning.

A review of the assessment tools may help OT students and practitioners understand the behaviors that make up therapeutic reasoning in practice. Many of the items overlap, reinforcing the key concepts of making decisions based on current evidence, reflecting on practice, and looking for options. Additional behaviors, such as anticipating possibilities, exhibiting curiosity for learning, and seeking support are part of therapeutic reasoning. The following case example, Brinlee, shows how information gained from an assessment of the student or practitioner may enhance therapeutic reasoning for practice.

Case Example: Brinlee

Brinlee is a level II fieldwork student working at a community reintegration program at a shelter for women experiencing homelessness as well as those who are newly housed. There is

one occupational therapist onsite. Brinlee's university provides support to the program through service-learning activities. Brinlee is the first level II student at this site, so she is also working closely with her OT faculty mentor to create a good learning experience.

The faculty mentor suggests that it might be helpful for Brinlee to reflect upon and assess her current skills in relation to therapeutic reasoning within the community mental health practice setting. The faculty mentor, clinical supervisor, and Brinlee all complete the Lasater Clinical Judgement Rubric (Lasater, 2007) during the first week of fieldwork to determine a baseline level of reasoning.

All three rated Brinlee's skills in interpreting at the "Beginning" level and skills in noticing at the "Developing" level. They saw her skills on some items as approaching "Accomplished": commitment to improvement (reflecting); and calm confident manner (responding). See Figure 8.5 for a description of the categories of clinical judgment based on the Lasater rubric.

Brinlee found the rubric helpful when creating weekly goals to discuss with her supervisor during their scheduled meetings. The measure provided her with information on the next logical steps to work towards to enhance her reasoning. Her clinical supervisor used the rubric to provide learning activities to address Brinlee's strengths and challenges. Overall, the team found the rubric helpful in facilitating communication regarding therapeutic reasoning strengths and challenges.

FOSTERING THERAPEUTIC REASONING IN FIELDWORK

Occupational therapy fieldwork educators play an important role in the development of therapeutic reasoning skills in OT students and practitioners. Qualities of fieldwork educators that promote students' reasoning include: supportive supervisory attitudes, effective instructional strategies, cultural competency, and they provide structure to the experience and grade the fieldwork activities to increase expectations gradually (Coviello et al., 2019; Raphael-Greenfield et al., 2017).

Emotional intelligence has been linked to intuition and therapeutic reasoning (Chaffey et al., 2012). Students who have emotional intelligence demonstrate resilience, competency, and self-initiative when challenging situations arise and they perform better on fieldwork (Raphael-Greenfield, et al., 2017). They use their knowledge, experiences, and resiliency to flexibly reason and consider alternatives. They read cues more quickly than those students with low emotional intelligence.

Peer supervision supports long-term learning and professional development as practitioners develop collaborative relationships to allow them to problem-solve safely (Raphael-Greenfield et al., 2017). Coviello and colleagues (2019) examined the fieldwork experiences that supported development of therapeutic reasoning skills in ten occupational therapy assistant (OTA) students (completing a level II fieldwork) using journals, focus groups, and questionnaires. The eight themes that emerged when examining the students' perspectives on

TABLE 8.3 **Behaviors Measured in Clinical Decision-Making, Clinical Reasoning, and Critical Thinking Assessments**

Assessment	Description	Subscales/Categories and Sample Behaviors of Critical Thinkers
California Critical Thinking Disposition Inventory (Facione, Facione, & Sanchez, 1994; Insight Assessment, 2013a)	75 Likert scale items that measure attributes contributing to the inherent qualities (i.e., disposition) to engage in problems and make decisions using critical thinking.	**Truth Seeking or bias**: Truth-seekers ask hard questions; do not ignore relevant details; they strive not to let bias or preconception color their search for knowledge and truth. **Open mindedness vs. intolerance:** Open-minded people act with tolerance toward others, knowing that we hold beliefs from our own perspective. **Analytical vs. heedless of consequences:** Analyticity is the tendency to be alert to what happens next (or anticipate). **Systematic or disorganized**: Habit of approaching problems in an orderly way. **Confident in reasoning or hostile toward reasoning:** Trust reflective thinking to solve problems and make decisions. **Inquisitive or indifferent:** Intellectual curiosity to want to know things. **Judicious or imprudence:** Seeing the complexity of issues and yet striving to make timely decisions.
California Critical Thinking Skills Test (Insight Assessment, 2016; Pike, 1997).	Multiple choice test that examines one's critical thinking abilities in complex situations.	**Overall Reasoning Skills:** Overall strength of using reasoning to form judgments about what to do. **Analysis:** Identify assumptions, reasons, claims and elements of a situation. **Evaluation:** Assess credibility of sources of information and the claims they make. **Inference:** Draw conclusion from reasons and evidence. **Deduction:** Decision-making in precisely defined context where rule, operating conditions, core beliefs, values, policies, principles, procedures and terminology determine the outcome. **Induction:** Draw inferences about what we think must probably be true based on case studies, prior experience, simulations, and familiar circumstances. **Interpretation:** Make sense of information provided. **Numeracy:** Figure out and interpret data, charts, figures.
Clinical Decision-Making Nursing Scale (Jenkins, 1985)	The 40-item Likert scale measures perceived decision-making abilities in 4 processes.	Sample items from scale: 1. **Search for alternatives or options:** I mentally list options before making a decision. 2. **Canvassing of objectives and values:** When I have a clinical decision to make, I consider the institutional priorities and standards. 3. **Evaluation and reevaluation of consequences:** I consider even the remotest consequences before making a choice. 4. **Search for information and unbiased assimilation of new information**: I go out of my way to get as much information as possible to make decisions.
Health Sciences Reasoning Test (Facione & Facione, 2007; Insight Assessments, 2013b).	33-item multiple choice test to assess clinical thinking in health professions education.	**Analysis:** Identify intended meaning of actions. **Induction:** Determining what is most likely true or not true with information provided. **Inference:** Draw conclusions based on reasons and evidence. **Evaluation:** Address the credibility of claims and the strength and weakness of arguments. **Deduction:** Understand the content of the premise requires the conclusion to be true and use this awareness to make judgments. (Adapted from Huhn, Black, Jensen, & Deutsch, 2011.)
Lasater Clinical Judgment Rubric (Lasater, 2007)	Rubric completed by observer during nursing simulation. 11 items, rated on 4-point Likert scale of expertise: beginning, developing, accomplished, and exemplary.	**Noticing** (i.e., focused observation, recognizing deviations from expected patterns, information seeking): Regularly observes and monitors the client and environment. **Interpreting** (i.e., prioritizing data, making sense of data): Focuses on most important and relevant data for explaining the situation. **Responding** (i.e., calm confident manner, clear communication, well-planned intervention, being skillful): Communicates effectively and clearly; explains interventions reassures patient and family. **Reflecting** (evaluation/self-analysis, commitment to improvement): Reflects on and evaluates experience accurately identifying strengths and challenges.
Yoon's Critical Thinking Disposition Tool (Yoon, 2008)	Self-assessment 27-item Likert scale to measure qualities of thinking.	*Sample statements from the tool representing each category (Shin et al., 2015).* **Objectivity:** I have reasonable proof. **Prudence:** I don't rush to judgment. **Systematicity:** I have a reputation for being a rational person. **Intellectual eagerness & curiosity:** When I have a question, I try to get the answer. **Intellectual fairness:** I willingly accept criticism of my opinion. **Healthy skepticism:** I continually evaluate whether my thought is right or not. **Critical thinking confidence:** I think I can get through any complicated problem.

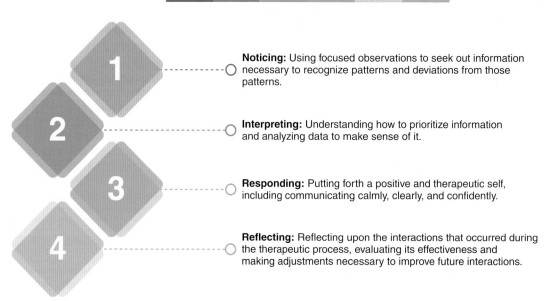

Figure 8.5 Lasater Clinical Judgment Rubric: 4 Categories.

promoting reasoning are listed in Box 8.1. The themes reveal the need for structure, communication, consistency, clear expectations, feedback, and the importance of collaboration.

Strategies for the Fieldwork Educator and Supervisor

Novice practitioners preferred checklists and used standardized tools to organize their therapeutic reasoning and the flow of their sessions, whereas expert clinicians drew on previous experiences to create practice strategies (Mitchell & Unsworth, 2005). Expert clinicians used more conversational descriptions and had greater fluidity in reporting how they used various types of reasoning in practice, whereas novice clinicians identified aspects of clinical reasoning they aspired to but did not readily use it in client sessions (Mitchell & Unsworth, 2005). Novice clinicians valued client-centered practice and realized the influence of the client's context, but they were not able to effectively use conditional reasoning to deliver client-centered care consistently (Mitchell & Unsworth, 2005).

Setting clear expectations and communicating clearly with students and OT practitioners, including providing constructive feedback, facilitates learning. Asking thoughtful questions encourages the student or practitioner to examine and reflect on their progress and challenges made during each week of fieldwork. Modeling habits of reflection after each session promotes reasoning.

LEARNING ACTIVITY: GUIDED REFLECTION

Worksheet 8.7 includes a student fieldwork experience and an excerpt from the fieldwork site student manual. Complete the worksheet from Lana's point of view.
- How can you approach a supervisor for constructive feedback to set appropriate goals related to therapeutic reasoning during this stage of fieldwork?

BOX 8.1 OTA Students' Perspectives on Promoting Therapeutic Reasoning

Theme	Example
Onboarding	• Introduction to site staff • Provision of site-specific orientation • Checklist of learning objectives • Observations of client population
Knowing expectations	• Understanding supervisor's feedback on progress towards goals and objectives
Experience of fieldwork experience	• Supervisor's level of expertise • Supervisory skills • Training in fieldwork education • Prompt and receptive responses to student concerns
Importance of feedback	• Written • Verbal • Regularly scheduled meetings • Debriefing • Use of probing questions
Value of collaboration	• Intraprofessional • Interprofessional • Provided opportunities to work in partnerships • Allowed students to learn from and ask questions of other professionals to create suitable intervention plans
Hands-on learning	Improved the students' ability to... • Recognize the needs of their clients in various environments • Create intervention plans • Adapt or grade interventions • Accurately document services provided
Consistency of caseload	• Homogeneity of the client population's clinical presentation • Treating the same clients over the course of the fieldwork • Treating a smaller caseload and gradually ramping up caseload responsibility
Self-reflection	• Critical examination • Statements about progress • Statements about areas to improve

(From Coviello et al., 2019.)

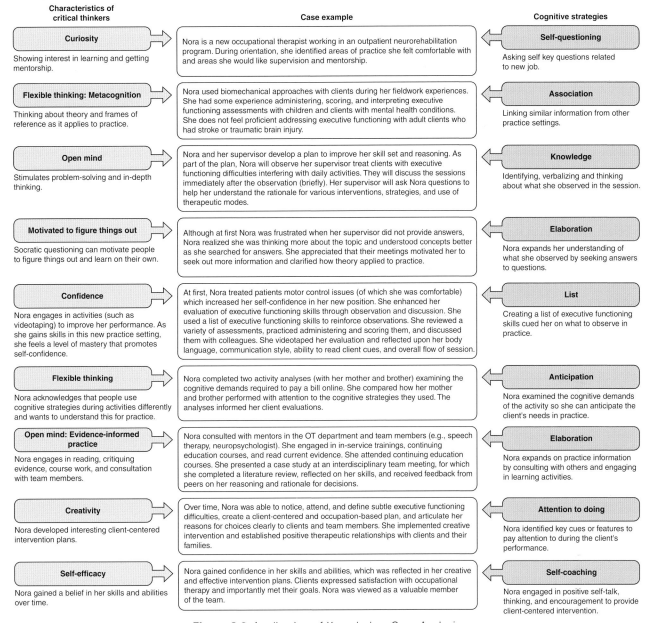

Figure 8.6 Application of Knowledge: Case Analysis.

APPLICATION OF THERAPEUTIC REASONING CONCEPTS IN PRACTICE: A CASE ANALYSIS

OT students and practitioners learn by taking part in the thinking process and making explicit what they observe or do. The case provided in Figure 8.6 explicitly names characteristics involved in critical thinking (from Fig. 8.1) and the cognitive strategies (listed in Table 8.1) used while engaging in the OT process.

Nora's story shows the intention, thought process, and engagement required to become a proficient practitioner. She is an active participant in the supervisory process and uses the meetings with her supervisor to identify challenges in practice so that she is able to address them for the benefit of her clients.

As you read through the case analysis provided in Figure 8.6, identify additional ways that Nora's actions could illustrate these concepts. How would you approach the challenges of being a new OT practitioner?

LEARNING ACTIVITY: APPLICATION OF CONCEPTS

Complete Worksheet 8.8. Describe a short case scenario from the Evolve learning site, or from a practice experience. Provide examples of characteristics of critical thinkers and cognitive strategies used in practice.

SUMMARY

Critical thinking forms the basis of therapeutic reasoning. Critical thinkers exhibit a curiosity for learning, flexible thinking, creativity, confidence, self-efficacy, open-mindedness, and motivation to figure things out. They ask questions and search for answers. Their inquisitiveness allows them to find creative solutions to address occupational performance challenges for a variety of clients. OT students and practitioners use metacognition along with deductive and inductive reasoning as they engage in the steps of therapeutic reasoning. They engage in a variety of types of reasoning (i.e., scientific, narrative, conditional, pragmatic, ethical, and interactive) and cognitive strategies to analyze, anticipate, prioritize, judge, evaluate, synthesize, and problem-solve at each step. This complex process requires practice, reflection, self-awareness, and support from faculty, supervisors, and/or peers. Critical thinking behaviors and evidence-informed practice behaviors form therapeutic reasoning. Using assessment tools to identify one's strengths and challenges is useful when addressing reasoning in practice.

Active authentic learning experiences, such as those created for problem-based learning, case-based learning, and experiential learning methodologies, promote therapeutic reasoning. Techniques such as Socratic questioning, simulation, guided discovery, and video analysis reinforce learning. These same strategies and techniques can be reinforced in practice settings during supervision, team meetings, and through informal/formal discussions with colleagues. Practitioners who show curiosity for learning continue to develop therapeutic reasoning skills.

REFERENCES

Audétat, M. C., Dory, V., Nendaz, M., Vanpee, D., Pestiaux, D., Junod Perron, N., & Charlin, B. (2012). What is so difficult about managing clinical reasoning difficulties? *Medical Education, 46*(2), 216–227.

Babcock, L., & Vallesi, A. (2015). The interaction of process and domain in prefrontal cortex during inductive reasoning. *Neuropsychologia, 67*, 91–99.

Baird, J. M., Raina, K. D., Rogers, J. C., O'Donnell, J. O., & Holm, M. B. (2015). Wheelchair transfer simulations to enhance procedural skills and clinical reasoning. *American Journal of Occupational Therapy, 69*(S2), 1–7.

Benfield, A., & Johnston, M. (2020). Initial development of a measure of evidence-informed professional thinking. *Australian Journal of Occupational Therapy, 67*, 309–319.

Benson, J. D., Provident, I., & Szucs, K. A. (2013). An experiential learning lab embedded in a didactic course: Outcomes from a pediatric intervention course. *Occupational Therapy in Healthcare, 27*(1), 46–57.

Bowyer, P., Munoz, L., Tkach, M. M., Moore, C. C., & Tiongco, C. G. (2019). Long-term impact of model of human occupation training on therapeutic reasoning. *Journal of Allied Health, 48*(3), 188–193.

Chaffey, L., Unsworth, C. A., & Fossey, E. (2012). Relationship between intuition and emotional intelligence in occupational therapists in mental health practice. *American Journal of Occupational Therapy, 66*, 88–96.

Coviello, J. M., Potvin, M. C., & Lockhart-Keene, L. (2019). Occupational therapy assistant students' perspectives about the development of clinical reasoning. *The Open Journal of Occupational Therapy, 7*(2), 1–14.

deCarvalho, E. C., Oliveira-Kumamura, A. R. D. S., & Morais, S. C. R. V. (2017). Clinical reasoning in nursing: Teaching strategies and assessment tools. *Revista Brasileira de Enfermagem REBEn, 70*(3), 662–668.

Dinkins, C. S., & Cangelosi, P. R. (2019). Putting Socrates back in Socratic method: Theory-based debriefing in the nursing classroom. *Nursing Philosophy, 20*(2), e12240.

Elder, L., & Paul, R. (2001). Critical thinking: Thinking to some purpose. *Journal of Developmental Education, 25*(1), 40.

Facione, N., & Facione, P. (2007). *The Health Science Reasoning Test Manual.* Insight Assessment.

Facione, N. C., Facione, P. A., & Sanchez, C. A. (1994). Critical thinking disposition as a measure of competent clinical judgment: the development of the California Critical Thinking Disposition Invention. *Journal of Nursing Education, 33*(8), 345–350.

Giles, A. K., Carson, N. E., Breland, H. L., Coker-Bolt, P., & Bowman, P. J. (2014). Use of simulated patients and reflective video analysis to assess occupational therapy students' preparedness for fieldwork. *American Journal of Occupational Therapy, 68*, S57–S66.

Huhn, K., Black, L., Jensen, G. M., & Deutsch, J. E. (2011). Construct validity of the Health Science Reasoning Test. *Journal of Allied Health, 40*(4), 181–186.

Insight Assessments (2016). California Critical Thinking Skills Test.

Insight Assessments (2013a). California Critical Thinking Disposition Inventory.

Insight Assessments (2013b). Health Sciences Reasoning Test.

Jenkins. H. M. (1985). A research tool for measuring perceptions of clinical decision making. *Journal of Professional Nursing, 1*, 221–229.

Keiller, L., & Hanekom, S. D. (2013). Strategies to increase clinical reasoning and critical thinking in physiotherapy education. *South African Journal of Physiotherapy, 70*(1), 8–12.

Kielhofner, G., & Forsyth, K. (2008). Therapeutic reasoning: Planning, implementing, and evaluating the outcomes of therapy. In G. Kielhofner (Ed.), *Model of human occupation: Theory and Application* (4th ed.). Baltimore, MD: Lippincott Williams & Wilkins.

Knecht-Sabres. L. J. (2010). The use of experiential learning in an occupational therapy program: Can it foster skills for clinical practice? *Occupational Therapy in Health Care, 24*(4), 320–334.

Lasater. K. (2007). Clinical judgment development: Using simulation to create an assessment rubric. *Journal of Nursing Education, 46*(11), 496–503.

Macauley, K., Brudvig, T. J., Kadakia, M., & Bonneville, M. (2017). Systematic review of assessments that evaluate clinical decision making, clinical reasoning, and critical thinking changes after simulation participation. *Journal of Physical Therapy Education, 31*(4), 64–75.

Merriam Webster (2021). Abstract thought. In Merriam-Webster.com dictionary. Retrieved from https://www.merriam-webster.com/dictionary/abstractthought.

Meyer, J., & Land, R. (2003). *Threshold concepts and troublesome knowledge: Linkages to ways of thinking and practising within the disciplines* (pp. 412–424). Edinburgh: University of Edinburgh.

Meyer, J. H. F., & Land, R. (2005). Threshold concepts and troublesome knowledge (2): Epistemological considerations and a conceptual framework for teaching and learning. *Higher Education, 49* 673–388.

Mitchell, R., & Unsworth, C. A. (2005). Clinical reasoning during community health home visits: Expert and novice differences. *British Journal of Occupational Therapy, 68*(5), 215–223.

Murphy, L., & Radloff, J. (2019). Facilitation of clinical reasoning through case-based learning in OT education. *American Journal of Occupational Therapy, 4*(1), S1.

Murphy, L. F., & Stav, W. B. (2018). The impact of video cases on clinical reasoning in occupational therapy education: A quantitative analysis. *The Open Journal of Occupational Therapy, 6*(3), 1–10.

Nicola-Richmond, K. M., Pepin, G., & Larkin, H. (2016). Transformation from student to occupational therapist: Using the Delphi technique to identify the threshold concepts of occupational therapy. *Australian Journal of Occupational Therapy, 63,* 95–104.

O'Brien, J. C., & McNeil, S. D. (2013). Teaching effectiveness: Preparing occupational therapy students for clinical practice. *Open Journal of Occupational Therapy, 1*(3), 1–11.

Overholser. J. C. (2018). Guided discovery: a clinical strategy derived from the Socratic method. *Journal of Cognitive Therapy, 11,* 124–139.

Paul, R., & Elder, L. (2007). Critical thinking: The art of Socratic questioning. *Journal of Developmental Education, 31*(1), 36.

Pike, G. R. (1997). The California critical thinking skills test. *Assessment Update, 9*(2), 10–11.

Raphael-Greenfield, E., Miranda-Capella, I., & Branch, M. (2017). Adapting to a challenging fieldwork: understanding the ingredients. *The Open Journal of Occupational Therapy, 5*(1), 1–14.

Reichl, K., Baird, J. M., Chisholm, D., & Terhorst, L. (2019). Measuring and describing occupational therapists' perceptions of the impact of high-fidelity, high-technology simulation experiences on performance. *American Journal of Occupational Therapy, 73* 7306205090.

Sahamid, H. (2014). Fostering critical thinking in the classroom. *Advances in Language and Literary Studies, 5*(6), 166–172.

Sahamid, (2016). Developing critical thinking through Socratic questioning: An action research study. *International Journal of Education & Literacy Studies, 4*(3), 62–72.

Stephens, R. G., Dunn, J. C., & Hayes, B. K. (2018). Are there two processes in reasoning? The dimensionality of inductive and deductive inferences. *Psychological Review, 125*(2), 218–244.

Tanner, B. (2011). Threshold concepts in practice education: Perceptions of practice educators. *British Journal of Occupational Therapy, 74*(9), 427–434.

Toglia, J. P., Rodger, S. A., & Polatajko, H. J. (2012). Anatomy of cognitive strategies: A therapist's primer for enabling occupational performance. *Canadian Journal of Occupational Therapy, 79*(4), 225–236.

Torabizadeh, C., Homayune, L., & Moattari, M. (2018). Impacts of Socratic questioning on moral reasoning of nursing students. *Nursing Ethics, 25*(2), 174–185.

Wang, L., Zhang, M., Zou, F., Wu, X., & Wang, Y. (2020). Deductive reasoning brain networks: A coordinate-based meta-analysis of the neural signatures in deductive reasoning. *Brain and Behavior, 10,* e01853.

Yoon, J. (2008). A study on the critical thinking disposition of nursing students-Focusing on a school applying integrated nursing curriculum. *Journal of Korean Academy of Nursing Administration, 14*(2), 159–166.

Worksheets

WORKSHEET 8.1: CURIOSITY

Use Worksheet 8.1. Select a topic related to therapeutic reasoning. List 10 questions you would like answered on this topic.

- How does curiosity enhance learning?

Curiosity
Name:
Describe a topic related to therapeutic reasoning:
List 10 questions you would like to answer related to this topic. 1. 2. 3. 4. 5. 6. 7. 8. 9. 10.
How does curiosity enhance learning?

WORKSHEET 8.2: CHARACTERISTICS OF CRITICAL THINKERS

Using the list provided in Worksheet 8.2, indicate behaviors you possess that are characteristic of critical thinkers. Provide personal examples.

- How could you develop abilities in the other behaviors?

Characteristics of Critical Thinkers	
Name:	
Characteristics of Critical Thinkers	**Personal Example**
Curiosity	
Creativity	
Confidence	
Flexible thinking	
Motivated to figure things out	
Open-minded	
Possessing self-efficacy	
Asks questions	
Searches for answers	
Finds alternative solutions	
Seeks support from others	
Judges quality of information	
Justifies decisions and approaches	
Listens to self and others	
Support decisions	
How could you develop abilities in the other behaviors?	

WORKSHEET 8.3: ANALYSIS OF COGNITIVE STRATEGIES

Use Worksheet 8.3 to apply the Framework for Analysis of Cognitive Strategy Use (Toglia et al., 2012) to a challenging occupation for which you engage. Describe the activity and the cognitive strategies you use.

- How would this framework be used to inform decisions in practice?

Framework for Analysis of Cognitive Strategy Use: A Clinical Reasoning Tool (from Toglia et al., 2012)	
A. Prerequisites to Effective Strategy Use	**Therapist Observations and Comments**
1. Strategy knowledge *Does the client know what a strategy is, how a strategy operates, and when and why it should be applied?* 2. Strategy repertoire *Is the client's range or repertoire of strategies adequate?* 3. Strategy beliefs *What are the client's beliefs about strategies (e.g., strategies will influence outcome or strategies will not help performance)?* 4. Anticipation and recognition of need *Does the client anticipate and recognize task challenges? Does the client identify the need to use a strategy within an activity context?* 5. Strategy generation and selection *Does the client self-generate, state, or self-select strategies for activities or are strategies selected and provided by others?*	
B. Strategy Execution	
1. Initiation *Is strategy spontaneously initiated by the client?* 2. Implementation *Are strategies carried out completely and accurately?* 3. Number of strategies *Can the client use and coordinate multiple strategies simultaneously? Single strategies only?*	
C. Quality of Strategy Use	
1. Degree of effort *What is the degree of effort or resources needed to use strategies (e.g., does degree of effort negatively affect performance or speed)?* 2. Temporal pattern *What are the timing and frequency of strategy use (e.g., are strategies used too late, over-used, found too soon, or fluctuating?* 3. Flexibility of strategy use *Does the client adjust or switch strategies when needed?* 4. Monitoring and evaluating strategy use *Does the client know when strategies have not been efficient or effective? Are performance errors recognized?*	
D. Effectiveness of Strategy Use	
Are positive changes in learning, problem-solving, or performance outcomes associated with strategy use?	

WORKSHEET 8.4: SOCRATIC QUESTIONING

Complete Worksheet 8.4. Imagine you are the fieldwork educator about to meet with a student who just completed their first intervention session. You observed the session. The client, who has mental health issues, showed difficulty paying attention, initiating actions, and completing simple verbal steps to a project. The student made good attempts to adjust the activity, but at times appeared disappointed in the client's performance (and it showed on their face).

- Using the elements of thought (Figure 8.4), create questions to encourage the student to describe his reasoning and facilitate self-awareness to promote change.
- What is the advantage of using Socratic questioning techniques?

Socratic Questioning	
Name:	
Describe the student's strengths and challenges:	
Elements of Thought	**Questions**
Purpose, goal, objective	
Question at issue (problem, issue)	
Information	
Interpretation and inference	
Concepts	
Assumptions	
Implications and consequences	
Point of view	
What are the advantages of using Socratic questioning technique?	

WORKSHEET 8.5: GUIDED DISCOVERY

Complete Worksheet 8.5. You are working with patients who are all status post total knee replacements. Using guided discovery, reflect on what you know and need to know.

Guided Discovery
Name:
What OT models of practice and frames of reference will guide your session? Why did you select these?
What are the protocols for total knee replacements?
How comfortable are you working with orthopedic conditions?
What else would you like to know?
What do you anticipate the client will feel like doing?
How will you use scientific (procedural), narrative, and conditional reasoning in practice?
What would you like to review for the session?

WORKSHEET 8.6: DEBRIEFING TO IMPROVE THERAPEUTIC REASONING SKILLS

Record a 5-minute intervention or evaluation session with a client. Complete Worksheet 8.6 and then meet with a peer and discuss the session.

- How does this information inform your next session?

Debriefing to Improve Therapeutic Reasoning Skills
Name:
Briefly describe the session.
1. Describe your reasoning skills immediately after the session (and without feedback): • What went well? • Were you prepared? • What would you do differently next time? • Did you change your interactions or style at any point? Why? • What methods did you use to get the information? Why did you choose them? • What theories (models or frames of reference) did you use to select your questions? Why did you select those?
2. Meet with the peer and discuss the session. • What did you learn from listening to your peer? • Were your perspectives similar or different? • What is the advantage of getting feedback from peers, clients, supervisors?
3. Based on your reflection and your peer's input, what would you like to learn about for next time? • What questions do you have?
4. How does this information inform your next session?

WORKSHEET 8.7: GUIDED REFLECTION

Worksheet 8.7 includes a student fieldwork experience and an excerpt from the fieldwork site student manual. Complete the worksheet from Lana's point of view.

Lana is a student in a Master of Occupational Therapy program completing her second level II fieldwork in an inpatient neurorehabilitation unit. She is in her third week of fieldwork and is gradually taking on more responsibilities and clients on her caseload. As agreed upon during her orientation with her FWE, Lana has reflected on her past week of clinical interactions prior to her supervision meeting and has come prepared to discuss the designated topics on the meeting template. At her orientation she was provided with a week-by-week competency checklist of clinical skills to master (excerpt from manual below). She and her supervisor have 30 minutes once a week blocked out of their clinical schedules to meet formally for the first 6 weeks of her fieldwork.

Guided Reflection

Name:

Inpatient Rehabilitation Fieldwork Student Weekly Competency Checklist (Week 3)

1. *Caseload Expectation:* 1–2 clients, similar diagnoses, or profiles if available
2. *Assessments and Evaluations:* Student completes chart review and identifies appropriate performance areas to address in assessment. Student administers the whole or part of a standardized measure pre-approved by the supervisor. Student observes the client in a group session and documents observations. The student observes and documents observations of all evaluations completed by the supervisor. The student completes electronic health record documentation of at least one section of the evaluation template with minimal revisions. Supervisor writes most of the report with input from the student as appropriate. The student observes assessments of the designated client by other disciplines as appropriate.
3. *Group Treatment Planning:* The student uses the group session planning template to plan and co-lead at least one group this week. The student meets with interdisciplinary staff as appropriate to plan and execute group treatment.
4. *Individual Intervention Session Plans:* The student uses the individual session planning template to plan and carry out 2 treatment sessions with moderate to maximal assistance of supervisor. Written treatment plans are required to be submitted to the supervisor at least one day in advance of the session. The student observes all individual sessions this week and provides observations to the supervisor. Supervisor completes most documentation/progress notes.
5. *Progress Notes:* The student completes a progress note for one session. May require significant revisions to content.
6. *Team Meetings/Interdisciplinary Encounters:* The student generates at least one comment about the designated client to present at weekly team rounds. The student rehearses a presentation of comment with the supervisor at least one day prior to rounds meeting.
7. *Client/Caregiver Education:* Student observes education of client and caregivers as available. The student generates at least one strategy to provide education to clients.

Sample Supervisory Meeting Template

Student Name: Lana Rodriquez_____

Supervisor's Name:_Mariana Campbell_____

Week number:_____3

Topics Discussed:
1. Behavioral strategies and modifications for patients experiencing fatigue
2. Evidence for electrical stimulation for the UE

Student Self-Identified Strengths This Week:
1. Better on my feet thinking to observe response to intervention and grade tasks to make them more challenging during dynamic balance/LB ADL

Supervisor Identified Strengths/Progress Noted this Week:
1. Becoming more assertive with interdisciplinary staff and rehabilitation techs

Student Self-Identified Areas for Improvement:
1. Use more narrative reasoning when planning meaningful activities for clients
2. Observe meal prep group and meet with SLP to learn about their role on the unit

Supervisor Identified Areas for Improvement:
1. Provide more feedback during sessions to student instead of only post session debriefings.

This Week's Goals for Student (refer to weekly orientation checklist):
1. Lana will independently identify at least one instance where she used both scientific reasoning and narrative reasoning to modify activities based on patient response to treatment by providing a verbal report to the supervisor during debrief.

This Week's Goals for Supervisor:
1. Marianna will assure the student schedule has at least initial and one discharge evaluation observation on it for next week.

The above items have been discussed and agreed upon by the student and supervisor.

Student's Signature:_____Lana Rodriquez OTS_____

Date:_____5/26/21_____

Supervisor's Signature:_____Marianna Campbell MS, OTR/L_

Date:_____5/26/21_____

WORKSHEET 8.8: APPLICATION OF CONCEPTS

Complete Worksheet 8.8. Describe a short case scenario from the Evolve learning site, or from a practice experience. Provide examples of characteristics of critical thinkers and cognitive strategies used in practice (see Figure. 8.6 for an example).

Application of Concepts		
Name:		
Brief description of case scenario:		
Characteristics of Critical Thinkers (with brief explanation)	**Example (from case)**	**Cognitive Strategies (with brief explanation)**
Describe 3 therapeutic reasoning types you used and provide an example.		
Describe where you used: • Metacognition • Inductive reasoning • Deductive reasoning		
Identify steps of the therapeutic reasoning process you used in this case scenario.		

Creative Intervention Planning

Jane O'Brien

GUIDING QUESTIONS

1. What are the steps, types of therapeutic reasoning, and cognitive processes used to plan and implement occupational therapy?
2. How do OT practitioners use principles and strategies of frames of reference/models of practice to develop creative intervention plans?
3. How can OT practitioners develop creative intervention plans?
4. How does creativity enhance occupational therapy intervention?

KEY TERMS

Brainstorming
Cognitive processes
Conceptualization
Creativity
Environmental factors

Personal factors
Playfulness
Principles
Schematic processes
Search processing

INTRODUCTION

Therapeutic reasoning is a complex skill that involves more than just applying knowledge. Therapeutic reasoning involves synthesizing information from many sources and making decisions, attending to responses, and adjusting decisions. It is a dynamic process that is influenced by the practice setting, the client's **personal factors** (i.e., client's background and life experiences that are not part of health condition [American Occupational Therapy Association AOTA, 2020]) and **environmental factors** (i.e., physical, social, and attitudinal surroundings of client [AOTA, 2020]), and the OT practitioner's experience (professional and personal). One way to understand a process more clearly is to describe the components that are involved in the process. Research on therapeutic reasoning often examines parts of each step or the types of reasoning practitioners use when making decisions in practice (Bonsall, 2012; Bowyer et al., 2019; Mahaffey, 2009; Mitchell & Unsworth, 2004; O'Brien et al., 2010). Examining the steps, types of reasoning, and cognitive processes provide insight into the skills and strategies that enhance therapeutic reasoning.

The author examines the therapeutic reasoning processes involved in creating an intervention plan. The author describes the types of reasoning, process, and guidelines to create intervention plans considering multiple factors with an emphasis on the dynamic interactions that contribute to intervention planning. Strategies to develop one's creativeness are presented. Case examples and learning activities are interspersed throughout the chapter to reinforce concepts.

HOW DO OT PRACTITIONERS DEMONSTRATE THERAPEUTIC REASONING IN PRACTICE?

Figure 9.1 illustrates the interconnectivity of the components of the therapeutic reasoning process. As OT practitioners work through the steps of therapeutic reasoning to create intervention plans, they use multiple types of reasoning, thought processes, skills, and strategies which are influenced by factors, such as practice setting, environment, beliefs, and experiences of both the client and the OT practitioner. The process is dynamic and the OT practitioner returns to steps, and adjusts reasoning, thoughts, skills, strategies throughout the process as they gain more information.

Researchers discuss therapeutic reasoning by outlining the steps of reasoning (Kielhofner & Forsyth, 2008; Mahaffey, 2009; O'Brien et al., 2010), while others examine the types of reasoning used during practice (Bonsall, 2012; During et al., 2011; Ward, 2003). The types of reasoning used as OT practitioners proceed through the steps include scientific (sometimes referred to as procedural), narrative, conditional, ethical, pragmatic, and interactive. Each type of reasoning relies on making sense of information. For example, OT practitioners use narrative reasoning to understand a client's story, lived experiences,

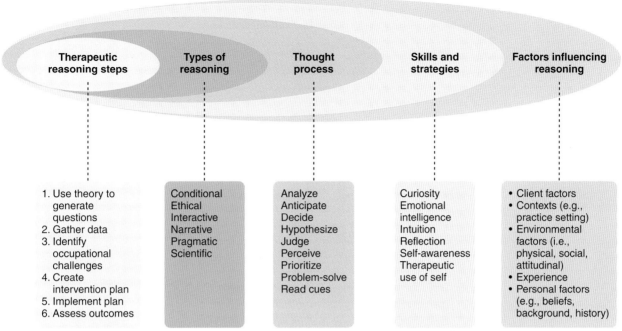

Figure 9.1 Therapeutic Reasoning Process Connectivity Between Components.

and history to plan client-centered intervention (Bonsall, 2012; Mattingly, 1994; Skarpaas et al., 2016).

Procedural or scientific reasoning has been examined in terms of diagnostic decisions (Baird et al., 2015; Rogers & Holm, 1991; Schaaf, 2015; Schell & Cervero, 1993). For example, decision trees indicate the pathway to follow when making diagnostic decisions (Bissessur et al., 2009: Montgomery et al., 2001). OT practitioners use this approach when following protocols based upon evidence (Rogers & Holm, 1991; Schaaf, 2015). However, many of the protocols or decision trees do not consider the multitude of factors influencing occupational therapy intervention. Deciding upon occupational therapy intervention activities is not a linear process. There is not one activity or intervention plan for specific conditions, rather activities are created based on client factors, goals, and contexts. OT practitioners follow the guidelines of the protocol while creating client-centered intervention activities. Therefore, understanding the principles of intervention using an occupation-based model of practice and frame of reference provides structure and guidance as OT practitioners use cognitive processes to sort out material and create a client-centered intervention plan.

Thought Process

Cognitive processing refers to making sense of information through one's thoughts, experiences, and senses (Cherry, 2020). It involves paying attention to stimuli, acquisition, storage (short- and long-term memory), interpretation, manipulations, transformation and use of knowledge (American Psychological Association APA, 2018). Cognitive processing involves attention, perception, learning, and problem-solving (APA, 2018). Thought is a type of cognitive processing that allows people to engage in decision-making, problem-solving, and higher reasoning (such as analyze, anticipate, hypothesize, judge, perceive, prioritize, and read cues) (Cherry, 2020).

As OT practitioners reason, they use thought processes to analyze data to make decisions (such as when engaged in procedural or diagnostic reasoning). After practitioners gather data, they synthesize the information by relating it to past experiences. They anticipate future performance, prioritize the information, and create hypotheses that consider the client's occupational strengths and challenges. Throughout the OT process, practitioners judge the client's performance and responses by problem-solving and reading cues. They make decisions while analyzing responses and adjusting activities to challenge the client to meet their goals.

Skills and Strategies

OT practitioners make clinical decisions based on their perceptions of the client's behavior changes (Cheung et al., 2018). They use therapeutic use of self skills and strategies to listen to the client to understand the client's goals and motivations, and to adjust the way they give information (such as providing visual or tactile cues). OT practitioners reflect on the effectiveness of their approaches in practice. They use self-awareness as they consider how their actions influence clients' responses. OT practitioners react to clients therapeutically by anticipating responses based on experience and using their intuition for how a client may interpret activities. They rely on emotional intelligence to read cues, respond to clients' feelings, and maintain boundaries. OT practitioners remain curious about the client and their life experiences. These skills and strategies are used during the therapeutic reasoning process.

Factors influencing reasoning

OT practitioners consider client factors, contexts (such as practice setting), environment (e.g., physical, social, and attitudinal), personal (e.g., client's beliefs, background and history) and one's experience when engaging in therapeutic reasoning. Therapeutic

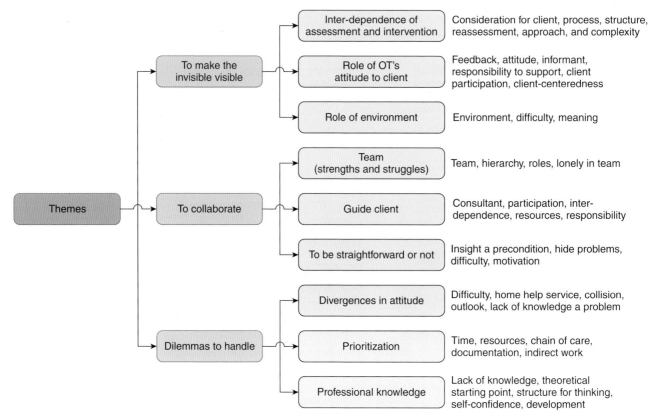

Figure 9.2 Summary of Themes (From Holmqvist, Kamwendo, & Ivarsson, 2009.)

reasoning involves considering the complex nature of the person within their environment and anticipating and facilitating change. Therapeutic reasoning is complex and requires experience, self-awareness, reflection, and curiosity to learn.

For example, Holmqvist and colleagues (2009) asked 12 occupational therapists to describe their work in a community setting. Figure 9.2 summarizes the themes found in the study. The themes included: (1) making the invisible visible (which referred to identifying factors that interfere with occupational performance, defining the role of the OT, and therapeutic use of self); (2) collaborating for success included comments regarding team dynamics and supporting clients; and (3) handling dilemmas referred to communication (e.g., difficult conversations), self-awareness, and prioritizing. The themes from this study are consistent with concepts illustrated in Figure 9.1.

NOVICE VERSUS EXPERIENCED REASONING

Therapeutic reasoning requires OT practitioners to synthesize information from multiple sources and continually examine, adapt, and adjust decisions and procedures as they gain new information. OT practitioners may develop advanced (or expert) reasoning skills in specific areas or with specific populations and be challenged (or at the novice level) when presented with a new area or population. Therapeutic reasoning may be challenged when a practitioner begins a new service or introduces a new intervention approach. The process is dynamic and requires that practitioners continue to engage in lifelong learning and reflection on their therapeutic reasoning.

Many researchers have examined reasoning between novice and experienced occupational therapists to better understand the reasoning process (Gibson et al., 2000; Glaser & Chi, 1988; Hagedorn, 1996; Mitchell & Unsworth, 2004; Rassafiani et al., 2009). Rassafiani et al. (2009) identified decision-making characteristics of occupational therapy experts. Instead of using years of experience as the criteria for expertise, the authors examined responses based on case vignettes. Therapists with high ability to discriminate (and recognize differences among cases) and greater consistency were considered high performers, whereas those who showed less ability to discriminate, and less consistency were considered low performers. Both groups had similar experience with children or adolescents with cerebral palsy. High performers used more information to facilitate their decision-making than low performers (Rassafiani et al., 2009).

The findings of Rassafiani et al. (2009) suggest that novices use a search processing model in which they look for relevant information, whereas experts use a schematic processing of which they match decisions against stored patterns of information. Schematic processing is rapid and automatic, and the expert is often not conscious of using it (Hagedorn, 1996). Experts have also been found to have superior short- and long-term memory and see problems at a deeper level (Glaser & Chi, 1988).

Mitchell and Unsworth (2004) examined the perceptions of therapeutic reasoning among occupational therapists working in community health and conducting home visits. Participants' responses to four case scenarios indicated that they used procedural, interactive, and conditional reasoning to identify the most important factors to consider, the action they would take, and whether they would see the client again.

Gibson et al. (2000) examined the reasoning of a novice (1 year or less of experience) and an experienced occupational therapist (5 years or more in the same setting) using a qualitative focus. They observed therapists in clinic settings and conducted semi-structured interviews after each therapist reviewed a sample case study to elicit the clinical reasoning process. Both experienced and novice therapists used multiple sources of information and past professional experience; factored the patient's discharge destination, changes in health care (i.e., insurance), time restraints, and setting (or specific place of employment); and reported a way of doing things for the setting (Gibson et al., 2000). They both mentioned personal style and education as influencing their reasoning.

Experienced therapists reported using additional factors, such as the patient's culture, secondary diagnosis, and motivation, to guide goal selection. They emphasized the ability to establish priority areas during treatment planning and identified experience, personal characteristics, and good clinical reasoning as main factors in the ability to establish priorities. The novice therapists alluded to the concepts of prioritizing but did not mention deviating from standard protocols (Gibson et al., 2000).

Both novice and experienced therapists expressed the importance of looking at each patient as an individual and identified that patients have a role in the intervention process. While the novice practitioner stated the importance of the client making the decision, when asked to describe her clinical reasoning she used "I" statements, indicating she was making the decisions (Gibson, et al., 2000).

APPLICATION OF THEORY IN PRACTICE

The thought process that practitioners apply when creating an intervention plan involves working through the steps of therapeutic reasoning, and engaging in different types of reasoning (i.e., scientific, pragmatic, conditional, ethical, narrative, and interactive). They use a variety of thought processes to sort through, prioritize, make decisions, respond, adapt, and analyze. OT practitioners rely on experience and personal factors (including therapist's and client's beliefs, attitudes, and culture), environmental factors (including practice setting, physical, social, and attitudinal), and knowledge of client factors and activity analysis to design intervention.

They create intervention plans based on theory and principles (from models of practice and frames of reference) which are specific to the client's situation and life history. OT practitioners who engage in therapeutic reasoning can articulate their rationale for their decisions and adjust and modify as needed. They understand the rationale for practice decisions.

Mahaffey (2009) and O'Brien et al., (2010) used the 6 steps of the therapeutic reasoning process to demonstrate how the Model of Human Occupation (MOHO; Taylor, 2017) can be applied in practice. Table 9.1 provides a summary of one case example from each of the studies.

The OT practitioners used information gained throughout the process to form hypotheses about what was interfering with the clients' occupational performance. They created client-centered intervention plans which were occupation-centered. Using MOHO helped them focus on occupation, by better understanding the client's needs and occupational identity. Using theory to guide one's practice allowed OT practitioners to clarify concepts and create intervention plans based on evidence. They described their decisions and reflected upon the

TABLE 9.1   Application of MOHO in Practice

Steps of Therapeutic Reasoning	Examples of process with older adults with mental illness (Mahaffey, 2009)	Examples of process with children (O'Brien et al., 2010)
Setting	Short-term acute care	Community outpatient center
Case	Marion	Emma
Generate clinical questions based on theory	Occupational identity: How does the client describe herself? Occupational competence: Does she feel she can accomplish the tasks she needs and wants to do? Volition: Does she feel she has control of her day? Habituation: What is her daily routine? Performance capacity: Are there factors that interfere with her ability to participate in self-care? Environment: Does she have the transportation and monetary support to stay active and meet her role expectations?	Volition: What does she like to do? What would she like to do more? How does she feel about her abilities? Habituation: What is her school day like? What does she do after school? What does she do for fun? Performance capacity: What helps her control her movement? What interferes with her motor skills? Environment: Where does she play? Where does she live?
Gather information	Occupational Performance History Interview (OPHI) (Kielhofner et al., 2004) Occupational Self-Assessment (Baron, Kielhofner, Iyenger, Goldhammer, & Wolenski, 2008) Role checklist (Oakley, Kielhofner, Barris, & Reichler, 1986) Model of Human Occupation Screening Tool (Parkinson, Forsyth, & Kielhofner, 2008) Performance test (cognition, motor)	Peabody Picture Vocabulary Test (Dunn & Dunn, 1998) Clinical observation Family and child interview (based on MOHO concepts)

Continued

TABLE 9.1	**Application of MOHO in Practice—cont'd**	
Steps of Therapeutic Reasoning	**Examples of process with older adults with mental illness (Mahaffey, 2009)**	**Examples of process with children (O'Brien et al., 2010)**
Conceptualize	Client is currently not engaging in roles that she identifies as important to her since her husband died. She is proud of her life, but currently is not engaged and is worried about her future. Habituation: She is currently sleeping a lot and having trouble focusing. She was happiest when she owned a gift shop. Performance: Good communication and social interactions in the past. Currently, minor difficulty with task management, frustration, memory. Was diagnosed with Alzheimer's type dementia. Volition: Most important to her is reconnecting with her social supports and finding things to do that give her a sense of purpose. Environment: Will return home, able to drive, gift shop nearby and several volunteer options. Family will assist with home maintenance.	Volition: Emma is a social child who enjoys being around other children, likes to be active, tell jokes, and be silly. She values her family and friends as evidenced by her approaching friends quickly and with smiles. Habituation: Emma has a consistent routine and can assist in many areas of occupation although she remains dependent upon others. She is on a strict dietary intake program and participates in leisure, academics, and free play. Performance capacity: Emma's athetoid muscle tone and extraneous movement interfere with her ability to perform gross- and fine-motor skills. Emma's poor oral motor skill interferes with her speech and communication. Environment: Emma has more difficulty moving around in unfamiliar and crowded environments. She becomes easily distracted in new environments and exhibits extraneous movements.
Generate the intervention plan (goals)	Arrange to return to the gift shop and to volunteer to regain a sense of control and to explore and understand the changes in her cognitive states, which will require modification for future occupations.	Emma will show improved fine-motor control to access her communication device. Emma will use her communication device consistently. • Given proximal stability, Emma will use her index finger to directly point to pictures or objects within 30 seconds of verbal request. • Emma will tell a joke to her friends by pressing the correct buttons on her communication device once during a 10-min play session.
Implement the plan	Provide her with resources she needs to explore her community, setting up opportunities for her to discuss her goals with her family and friends, and keeping her discharge plans achievable. She also appreciates the frank discussion about her Alzheimer's diagnosis and the need to have a plan for her future.	Play using the communication device and with her peers. Opportunities to be "silly" and joke. Address proximal stability to assist children with communication and timing.
Evaluate outcomes	Focus on a person's function within the hospital. Marion expressed a greater sense of self-control and comfort now that she has direction and some things to look forward to. She feels more hopeful, and her fear is under control. Her family states that they also have a better idea of how to help her.	Emma enjoyed the sessions, followed directions, and interacted with peers. She met her short-term objective related to using her communication device and especially enjoyed using it to tell jokes. Her motor skills continue to interfere with her gross- and fine-motor abilities required for dressing, bathing, academics, and play. The OT will continue to work with her on these skills while allowing her to be social and choose fun activities.
Key reasoning concepts	• Promotion of mental and physical health through engagement in occupation • Occupation-centered theory • Client-centered goals • Collaboration to empower client and family • "I have the structure and language to explain to teammates the benefits of helping someone engage in meaningful occupations, thus creating a unique and valued place for occupational therapy on the treatment team." (Mahaffey, 2009, p. 7)	• Promotion of social participation through fun activities • Promotion of physical skills during play • Increasing her use of communication device by understanding her volition to engage with peers • Collaboration to empower child and family • Occupation-centered theory

client's and their performance. This format may be used with other models.

The authors suggest that using the case analysis process distinguishes characteristics of models and helps students and practitioners enhance their therapeutic reasoning by considering multiple factors influencing occupational performance. O'Brien and Patnaude (2022) found that students' scores on the Self-Assessment of Clinical Reflection and Reasoning measure (SACRR; Royeen et al., 2001) improved after a course on therapeutic reasoning using a case-based approach.

LEARNING ACTIVITY: CASE ANALYSIS

Use Worksheet 9.1 to complete an analysis of another case from Mahaffey (2009) and O'Brien et al. (2010).

TYPES OF REASONING

As OT practitioners engage in the steps of therapeutic reasoning, they rely on types of reasoning approaches to problem-solve and make decisions. The thought process that practitioners use

TABLE 9.2   Example of Types and Processes Used During Steps

Steps	Tasks	Type of reasoning	Thought processes
Generate questions	Use theory to develop questions and structure thought processes.	Scientific Conditional	• Decide on model of practice or frame of reference. • Anticipate occupational performance challenges based on diagnostic conditions. • Problem-solve how to create questions based on the client's condition, culture, age, and within practice setting.
Gather data	Collect information about the client's occupational performance (e.g., physical, cognitive, psychosocial). Use assessment tools to gather objective data.	Narrative Pragmatic Scientific	• Anticipate challenges to select assessments. • Problem-solve variety of assessments to administer. • Decide on appropriate assessments. • Analyze evidence.
Identify occupational challenges	Synthesize information to hypothesize what supports and interferes with a client's occupational performance.	Conditional	• Judge findings from multiple sources (person, occupation, environment) to create conceptualization. • Hypothesize factors that are interfering with client's occupational performance.
Create an intervention plan	Create goals, objectives, activities, and strategies (based on principles of frame of reference) to intervene.	Conditional Ethical	• Prioritize goals. • Analyze evidence related to frames of reference. • Decide on a frame of reference and strategies to use during intervention. • Document accurately and in a timely manner.
Implement intervention plan	Implement plan, adjusting and modifying during the session to create the just right challenge.	Interactive Pragmatic Conditional Ethical	• Anticipate the client's needs to be ready to adapt and modify activities in session. • Perceive the client's reactions to activities during the session. • Read cues from the client. • Problem-solve to create activities that challenge the client and address goals of session. • Decide how to provide fair and equitable high-quality services to all clients within the practice setting. • Judge one's level of expertise to determine if consultation is needed to provide best care to the client.
Assess outcomes	Measure progress towards goals, patient satisfaction. Revise or adapt plan as needed based upon outcome data.	Scientific Conditional	• Analyze outcomes of intervention based on outcome measurements. • Adjust or modify intervention.

while reasoning includes abilities to analyze, anticipate, decide, hypothesize, judge, perceive, prioritize, problem-solve, and read cues. Table 9.2 provides some examples of the types of reasoning and thought processes that may be involved during each step of the process. It is not meant to describe all possibilities but rather to give readers an idea of how reasoning types and thought processes may be used to inform practice decisions. For example, ethical reasoning is used during all stages of the reasoning process as the OT practitioner considers the quality of services, equitable provision of services, fairness, and truthfulness.

LEARNING ACTIVITY: TASKS, TYPES AND THOUGHT PROCESSES

Complete Worksheet 9.2. Provide examples to illustrate the types of reasoning and thought processes that may occur at each stage of therapeutic reasoning.

IDENTIFY OCCUPATIONAL CHALLENGES

Once OT practitioners gather data from interviews, assessments, and observation, they analyze, prioritize, problem-solve, and judge the quality of observations or information to identify occupational challenges. This is an important step in the therapeutic reasoning process. OT practitioners synthesize information from a variety of sources and hypothesize what is interfering with the client's occupational performance. They

identify the client's strengths and challenges. Using knowledge from the client's condition along with evidence from models of practice and frames of reference, they make decisions about how occupational therapy may influence occupational performance specific to the client. At this stage of the therapeutic reasoning process, experienced OT practitioners use conditional reasoning to pull information from multiple sources to create a hypothesis about what is interfering in the client's occupational performance. The conceptualization refers to formation of an idea of something (Merriam-Webster, n.d.), which may be the formation of hypotheses regarding what is influencing behaviors. Conceptualization is based upon theory and evidence from one's model of practice and frames of reference and identifies occupational strengths and challenges.

Box 9.1 provides a conceptualization of occupational challenges for a client named Ali (see description of case in O'Brien

BOX 9.1   Identify Occupational Challenges

Conceptualization

Ali is a 9-year-old girl who likes being social, doing things with peers, and going to school. Ali seeks out social opportunities (e.g., girl scouts, community center) which provide her with positive role models and friends. Her behaviors (i.e., poor attention, anger, aggression, mood swings, demanding nature) and inconsistent family routines and limited family support, interfere with her school performance.

et al., 2010). The conceptualization incorporates information on her volition (i.e., social participation in the community); habituation (i.e., attendance at school, inconsistent family routines); performance capacity (i.e., behaviors, such as poor attention, anger, aggression, and mood swings); and environment (i.e., community activities, lack of family support). The therapist relies on her experience volunteering in the community setting (where she first met Ali, who walked to the community center on her own) and information that Ali's family struggles with consistency in her care (e.g., mother has mental health issues, brother was recently incarcerated). The OT practitioner also knows Ali struggles in school and is being followed by a case manager at home. The therapist believes Ali is a resilient child (e.g., she found girl scouts and a community center on her own) who would benefit from positive role models (such as OT student volunteers). The OT practitioner hypothesizes that Ali will benefit from learning behavioral strategies and being involved in positive community activities where she may forge friendships with adults and peers. This conceptualization becomes the basis for the intervention plan. The OT practitioner revisits their hypotheses and conceptualization as they gather new information and learn more about the client and their situation, performance abilities, and environment. As the OT practitioner interacts with and learns about the client during the intervention process, they may change, modify, or refine hypotheses, adjust priorities, and evaluate progress towards goals. Therapeutic reasoning is ongoing.

CREATING AN INTERVENTION PLAN

Once the OT practitioner has identified the client's strengths and challenges and created hypotheses on those things interfering with the client's occupational performance, they collaborate with the client to create long- and short-term goals. Goals require the OT practitioner to understand the client's circumstances, environment, client factors, habits, routines, and personal factors (such as beliefs and values, background, history). The OT practitioner anticipates how the intervention will address the goals and considers past experiences with clients who have similar diagnoses, knowledge of the science of the condition, along with the client's current level of functioning to design achievable goals. Developing goals requires the OT practitioner to understand the components that make up the occupation. OT practitioners examine hypotheses to determine the strategies they will use during intervention and this information informs activity selection. See Table 9.3 for sample goals and strategies for intervention associated with hypotheses based on selected frames of reference.

> **LEARNING ACTIVITY: IDENTIFY OCCUPATIONAL CHALLENGES**
>
> Use Worksheet 9.3 to identify hypotheses describing occupational challenges for selected case examples (see Evolve learning site).

> **LEARNING ACTIVITY: STRATEGIES AND PRINCIPLES OF FRAMES OF REFERENCE**
>
> Use Worksheet 9.4 to provide descriptions of the principles and strategies of each frame of reference. Use Tables 3.1 and 3.2 for a list of principles of frames of reference.
> - How does this information inform intervention planning?

TABLE 9.3 Sample Goals

Frame of Reference	Hypotheses	Goal	Strategies for Intervention
Biomechanical	Client's limited R upper extremity strength interferes with his ability to complete daily activities.	Client will lift 2 pounds × 5 times with her R UE within 30 seconds. Client will carry a full laundry basket (3 pounds) from the bedroom to the laundry room (10 feet) × 1/week.	Gradually increase the weight of objects used in therapy to strengthen R UE. Engage client in meaningful activities that require her to lift objects with R UE repeatedly to strengthen extremity.
Cognitive behavioral therapy	Client's negative thinking interferes with her confidence, limiting her social participation.	Client will participate in 1 new social event with a friend × 60 minutes within 1 week. Client will record 3 positive things she did to plan the social event with a friend.	Engage client in role play and exercises to support positive self-talk. Begin with activities that are achievable to promote success and confidence. Encourage client to articulate and record her achievements (self-assessment).
Model of Human Occupation	Client displays lack of motivation adapting to physical limitations, resulting in poor performance at work and with self-care.	Client will demonstrate 2 methods to complete his morning routine within 30 minutes × 3 consecutive days. Client will demonstrate 5 possible strategies to adapt his work environment so he can return to work.	Validate client's concerns. Physically support client as they engage in demonstrations. Collaborate and problem-solve with client to identify adaptations. Engage client in meaningful occupations, daily routines within his/her environment.
Motor control/motor learning	Client has difficulty with bilateral coordination interfering with daily activities and play.	Client will use B UEs and B LEs to pump a swing × 10 times consecutively. Client will use B UEs to dress herself for school within 30 minutes.	Use motor learning strategies (such as demonstration, feedback, knowledge of result/performance, verbal directions, mental rehearsal) to teach the client to complete bilateral coordination activities, such as pumping swing, hopping, jump rope. Engage the client in whole, meaningful activities within their environment using objects that are familiar to them.

Intervention activities are designed to address the goals and follow the frame of reference strategies (based on the conceptualization of the client's situation). The OT practitioner uses the principles of the frame of reference or model of practice to design activities specific to the client.

Principles are the underlying assumptions regarding how factors interact to result in the outcome being examined. Understanding the principles of the model of practice or frame of reference provides the foundation for the intervention plan. The principles provide the direction of the intervention. See Tables 3.1 and 3.2 in Chapter 3 for a description of principles associated with models of practice and frames of reference. Principles and the strategies associated with them are based upon research evidence.

LEARNING ACTIVITY: RESEARCH NOTE: EVIDENCE

Complete Worksheet 9.5. Summarize the findings from a research article that examines a principle of a selected frame of reference.
- Based on this article, how would you apply the principle in practice?
- Describe some strategies and activities that follow this principle.

After creating long-term and short-term goals, the OT practitioner plans activities to address those goals. The OT practitioner considers multiple factors when deciding on the specific activities for the intervention.

CREATIVE INTERVENTION PLANS

Creativity is defined as "the skill and imagination to create new things" (Merriam-Webster, n.d.). Figure 9.3 presents a word cloud of synonyms for creativity. OT practitioners use their sense of creativity and therapeutic reasoning to develop client-centered intervention plans. Creativity in occupational therapy practice may be inspired by examining the client's interests, background, history, and integrating this information with the client's skills, abilities, client factors, and the practical aspects of the practice setting, time, and resources.

Creativity includes inventing new ways of doing things, creating adaptations, and incorporating the client's interests, background, and culture into the activities. For example, an OT practitioner finds out the client's family celebrates birthdays by making lemon squares (like their mother always did) and incorporates this into the intervention session, as she learns the client's birthday is coming up. The OT practitioner incorporates a dance from the client's culture by bringing in music to facilitate movement in the session. Other clients observe the dancing and ask to learn the movements. The OT practitioner skillfully adapts the steps so that clients at all levels can learn. Together, they decide to have a "dance show" at the end of the week. Creativity involves expanding ideas, adapting them, and being flexible and playful in one's approach to activities. Playfulness is one's approach or attitude towards activities or play (Bundy, 1993). It may involve using objects in unconventional ways, approaching a situation flexibly, reading and giving cues (Bundy, 2010). Adding creativity to one's intervention sessions may help clients adapt and flexibly approach activities.

Brainstorming is a technique that may facilitate creativity. The goal of brainstorming is to expand one's thinking to create new ideas. For example, asking clients to come up with activities for intervention engages them in their intervention and encourages them to problem-solve and collaborate with the practitioner. To promote ideas, clients must feel safe to express thoughts during a brainstorming session. The OT practitioner does not judge their ideas, but rather encourages the client to express ideas. Once the ideas are generated, the OT practitioner and client make decisions on which activities best address goals. Allowing clients to brainstorm may provide insights into future goals and activities that were not addressed earlier. For example, a client in a brainstorming session, became excited about the possibility of learning to make a ceramic mug for her sister. The OT practitioner learned during the brainstorming session that the client previously did ceramics and was artistic ("when she was younger").

OT practitioners may need to be resourceful to create intervention activities. For example, the OT practitioner may use household items during a telehealth intervention session. Incorporating music, making the activity a "game," or including other people may encourage clients to engage more actively. For example, during one telehealth session, the OT learned of the client's favorite actor. The OT practitioner included a short clip of the actor as part of the next session and also changed her picture on the computer to be the actor's. Although it was a small part of the session, the client enjoyed the session and appreciated the personal touch.

Box 9.2 provides a list of tips to incorporate creativity into an intervention plan. The purpose of being creative is to engage

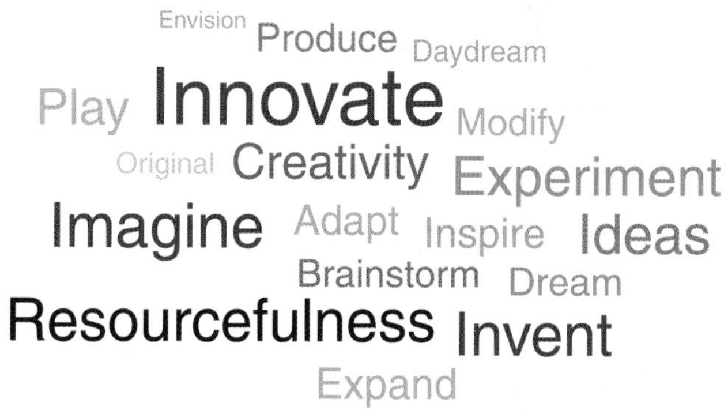

Figure 9.3 Creativity: Word Cloud.

BOX 9.2   Tips to Promote Creativity

- Know the client: implement interests, family, routines into sessions.
- Collaborate with client: engage client in creating activities for session.
- Use principles of frames of reference.
- Curiosity: try new things yourself.
- Incorporate therapeutic use of self.
- Add humor to the session.
- Ask others for ideas.
- Make simple changes to known activities.
- Read and search for new ideas.

clients in the occupational therapy process. Research shows that clients perform better and complete more repetitions when the activities are whole, completed in the natural environment, and use authentic objects as opposed to simulated activities (Persson et al., 2001; Sorman et al., 2019; Stav et al., 2012; Weinstock-Zlotnick & Mehta, 2018). For example, pretending to swing a golf club is not as effective as asking a client to swing his/her actual golf club.

Clients enjoy novel, interesting, and meaningful activities (Fisher, 1998; Gillen, 2013). For example, cooking with actual food is preferred to "pretending" to cook with food. Selecting a novel dish may elicit more engagement. Cooking requires many skills and abilities. OT practitioners analyze the directions, movements, timing and sequencing, and activity demands to determine if the client will be able to successfully complete the specific recipe. Since there is variation in simple to complex recipes, cooking or meal preparation is often a preferred activity. For example, an OT practitioner may design a cooking activity to address a client's memory, sequencing, and timing strategies. Cooking activities (such as repetitive stirring or kneading dough) may be used to improve hand strength or engage the client in standing activities. Clients should clearly see the benefits of the activity.

Integrating family or support persons into intervention may encourage clients to engage. For example, a client who was working on initiating a weight shift and reaching with his right arm across midline for objects engaged in the intervention session with minimal interest, engagement, or effort. His spouse entered the session holding their toddler daughter. The OT practitioner positioned the spouse to the left of the client and adjusted the activity by asking the client to touch his toddler's arm. As the client did this, the toddler giggled and smiled at her father. The father continued the activity with great interest and motivation. He initiated the weight shift and reached to his daughter repeatedly. The OT practitioner watched as the father and daughter interacted. The client showed improved effort, interest, and motivation to engage in this social activity with a valued member of his family. The client stated he felt like "dad" again.

As OT practitioners develop intervention activities, they consider the principles and strategies of the frame of reference as they adjust or modify tasks. OT practitioners engage clients in different activities based on the hypotheses they make. For example, Table 9.3 describes biomechanical goals, hypotheses, and intervention strategies for a client who is unable to complete household chores of doing laundry. After hypothesizing that the client's limited right upper extremity (R UE) strength interferes with his ability to complete daily activities, the practitioner creates a goal that he will lift 2 pounds to complete daily activities. The OT practitioner selected the goal after observing the client and considering factors such as his living situation (e.g., he lives alone, and his laundry room is 10 feet from his bedroom) and learning that he prides himself that he lived independently, even doing his own laundry. The client is an elderly man who will be satisfied with doing his own laundry and light household tasks, so 2 pounds is a reasonable weight goal. The OT practitioner chooses activities to strengthen the client's R

UE functioning using meaningful activities, progressing from lightweight to heavier weight, with the goal of having the client lift 2 pounds.

The OT practitioner may create different intervention activities for the same goal for a 10-year-old client who has difficulty with play, school, and dressing due to R UE strength problems. The goal may focus on laundry (as with the older client) if the child assumes family chores such as taking the laundry from his room to the laundry room. However, the activities for the young child may include play activities, such as tennis, ball games, writing or crafting on an easel/vertical surface or swinging. The OT may decide to include activities required for school, such as carrying his books or backpack or using both hands to hold his lunch tray. Intervention activities are designed to progress from lighter weight to heavier as the child gains strength.

Using therapeutic reasoning to understand the purpose of the intervention, principles guiding the activities and the client's background, lived experience, history, and culture informs creative intervention planning. The OT practitioner integrates all the information to design client-centered activities that address the client's goals. As OT practitioners engage in the intervention process, they use interactive reasoning to respond to cues and to provide support as needed. Therapeutic use of self (see Chapter 4) includes understanding the client and their culture and being self-aware of one's own interacting style and the situation (and environment). It requires creativity and flexibility along with self-awareness.

LEARNING ACTIVITY: CREATIVITY

Complete Worksheet 9.6. Design an interesting activity that could be used in occupational therapy intervention.
- Identify the materials, steps, and sequence for completing the activity.
- Describe the performance skills required.
- Identify contextual (personal and environmental) factors related to the activity.
- How would you change the activity?

LEARNING ACTIVITY: CREATIVITY AND FLEXIBILITY IN PRACTICE

Since intervention sessions do not always go as planned, OT practitioners often have "back pocket" activities readily available, such as a balloon, deck of cards, beach ball, pen, or paperclips. Use Worksheet 9.7 to list the items you might use as back-up intervention ideas. Identify 10 activities that you could use from one of the items that address different performance skills. (For example, given a beach ball, you can throw it for UE strength, pick it up for dynamic standing, blow it up for pacing/energy conservation, hold with 2 hands for bimanual coordination).
- Gather the item and demonstrate the activities to peers.

SELECTING INTERVENTION ACTIVITIES

Understanding the client's interests, background and lived experiences allows the practitioner to develop creative activities. Furthermore, asking the client specifically what they would like to accomplish in therapy and what type of activities they enjoy involves them in their process, which promotes learning. For example, the Cognitive Orientation to daily Occupational Performance (CO-OP) model involves children in creating their own goals, identifying strategies, and evaluating their performance (Missiuna et al., 2001). The "goal-can-do-check" format teaches children to problem solve and gives them a sense of accomplishment and self-efficacy that they may use after therapy.

The following case study by Dr. Brittany Conners illustrates the use of therapeutic reasoning to design meaningful activities for a client with anxiety preventing her from engaging in her previously held roles of entrepreneur, money management, community mobility, and community management. Dr. Conner collaborates with the client throughout the process. See the Evolve learning site for a video (Video 9.1) reflection regarding this case.

Case Application: Breonna by Dr. Brittany Conners
Occupational Therapy Case Study Template
Client's Name (Change to protect PHI): Breonna
Date of report: 11/18/20
DOB: June 5th, 1993
Chronological age: 27 years, 5 months and 5 days
Setting: Co-Working Space (called Light Work in downtown St. Louis)
Primary Diagnosis: Anxiety
Reason for referral to OT: Breonna self-referred to OT for evaluation and intervention for coping skills for role as entrepreneur, budgeting, routines, and instrumental activities of daily living. Breonna is a frequent member of preventative wellness groups in a co-working space called Light Work.
Client History
Family: Breonna lives with her boyfriend in a quiet neighborhood near her sneaker shop. They just recently moved to St. Louis from Louisville. They relocated for the opening of her new store as the brand (Just Us Shoes) expanded into a budding market in St. Louis' bustling downtown district from launching a successful online store.

Educational: Breonna is currently attending hybrid classes part time due to Covid-19. She is studying to obtain a Bachelor of Science in Entrepreneurial Studies from Howard University. Breonna chose a historically black college to further her studies and achieve her dream of becoming a first-generation college student.

Housing: Breonna has been unhoused in the past while building her sneaker business. She moved to Los Angeles to be closer to a business partner who backed out at the last minute. The experience was traumatic as she had never lived in shelters before and did not know how to tell her family what happened. Breonna was unhoused for 8 months before landing a job that paid enough money to allow her to save up for rent and a security deposit. She lived in a small apartment in LA for 5 months until she met her boyfriend. The couple decided to move to St. Louis as the market was great for business and he could return home to be closer to family. Currently, she

and her boyfriend are stably housed in a loft in St. Louis overlooking the city near The Arch. There is a tent city not too far from her loft and she finds herself becoming anxious when seeing people finding refuge on the streets. Breonna has vivid dreams about her time living outdoors.

Financial: Breonna has had a hard time managing finances due to new responsibilities of managing business funds and trauma with losing all her money in Los Angeles. Breonna's boyfriend has managed the couple's finances to reduce her anxiety and panic attacks. Breonna would like to eventually hire a financial advisor as the recent encounters with money management have not been positive. She finds herself collecting business and personal mail to organize yet she is unable to open due to fear of receiving bills, eviction notices, court dues, etc. The business is doing well in its first physical brick and mortar, yet she delays many financial processes because she will not open correspondence from key stakeholders, customers, and buyers.

Background Information from Other Professionals
- Information from other disciplines involved in case: None
- Other disciplines involved in care: None
Volition
Client's concerns/goals: Breonna is concerned that anxiety, past trauma, and lack of coping skills will negatively impact performance in her role as an entrepreneur. She wants to feel confident in her ability to manage both personal and business finances without fear of the past repeating itself. One major goal Breonna would like to achieve is opening physical mail and invoices online. She reports tremendous anxiety when attempting to engage in these critical activities. Her boyfriend is concerned that poor money management skills may deter personal and professional growth.

Client//family interests: Breonna enjoys spending time with her boyfriend, family, and friends. She enjoys reading fashion blogs, writing articles for stylish brands, and listening to podcasts about sneaker trends. Breonna wants to visit local attractions in St. Louis to engage in leisure exploration to feel more connected to the city. She has a huge love for volunteering and helping others in need. She would like to find an organization that serves Black women through the hardships of entrepreneurship.

Habituation
Typical day: Breonna wakes up at 4:00am to read and write in her journal. She sages her apartment and office to bring in good energy before the workday begins. She works from 9am–5pm at a full-time job with a local tech startup as a Community Engagement Specialist. After work, she drives straight to her sneaker shop to network, manage social media accounts, ship orders, research consignment opportunities, and monitor the store until the shop closes at 9pm. Breonna attempts to FaceTime with family and friends back home for an hour. Then, she and her boyfriend enjoy a late dinner and quality time together until she goes to bed around 11:30pm.

Work and leisure activities: As an entrepreneur, Breonna is constantly working towards the business in some way or another. From networking, attending virtual conferences, and developing partnerships, Breonna is both the power behind the brand and the face towards the public. Her leisure activities are closely tied to sneaker culture, but she also enjoys cooking, hiking, and collecting crystals.

Roles and responsibilities: Breonna's roles include entrepreneur, daughter, girlfriend, sister, mentor, mentee, transplant, and volunteer. She is responsible for growing her company, bookkeeping, accounting, scouting new looks, analyzing data from social media, and managing operations of the Just Us Shoes physical store and e-commerce website.

Environment (include cultural, physical): As a Black woman, Breonna reports experiencing microaggressions in the workplace since she started working at age 16. She wants to build opportunities for diverse and inclusive workforces due to this experience. She experienced her first panic attack while working when she was 24 years old. Ongoing microaggressions throughout her career soon negatively impacted her mental health. She stayed at home for days at a time before going to see her family doctor in Louisville. There, she was diagnosed with generalized anxiety disorder. During the time off, Breonna sketched up the ideas for what would become her sneaker business.

Description of Assessments:

AOTA Occupational Profile Template: The occupational profile is a summary of a client's occupational history and experiences, patterns of daily living, interests, values, and needs. The information is obtained from the client's perspective through both formal interview techniques and casual conversation and leads to an individualized, client-centered approach to intervention.

The Canadian Occupational Performance Measure (COPM): The COPM (Law et al., 2015) is a personalized, client-centered instrument designed to identify the occupational performance problems experienced by the client. Using a semi-structured interview, the therapist initiates the COPM process by engaging the client in identifying daily occupations of importance that they want to do, need to do, or are expected to do but are unable to accomplish. Areas of everyday living explored during the interview include self-care, productivity, and leisure.

Clinical observations and informal interview comprised the remainder of this evaluation.

Behavioral Observations. Breonna was her bubbly self during engagement in the Occupational Profile via our virtual session. As we ventured through the COPM, Breonna became unsure of which problems to work on and needed more cueing to answer questions directly. She became tearful as she reflected on her performance in productivity. Therapist employed a quick 4-7-8 breathing technique to help her find a sense of calm and relief. After 5 minutes of guided breathing, Breonna identified 5 out of 5 problems to address with OT.

Findings (Include Scoring and Findings with Interpretation, Use Table Format)

Canadian Occupational Performance Measure – Web App (COPM via smartphone): Clients rate the importance of daily activities and identify their top occupational performance problems and rate their performance and satisfaction. Scores range from 1 (lowest) to 10 (highest).

	Daily Activity Categories	Step 2: Rating Importance
Step 1A: Self-Care	**Personal Care:**	
	Mani/Pedi	7
	Moisturizing	9
	Cooking	10
	Functional Mobility:	
	Drive car	7
	Ride share app	4
	Walking	3
	Community Management:	
	Shopping at local businesses	7
	Going to the credit union	1
	Building new support system	6
Step 1B: Productivity	**Paid/Unpaid Work:**	
	Volunteer	2
	Managing finances	1
	Running own business	3
	Household Management:	
	Cleaning house and office	4
	Grocery shopping	8
	Decorating house and office	9
	Play/School:	
	Trying sex toys	9
	Part time student	8
	Board games with bae	10
Step 1C: Leisure	**Quiet Recreation:**	
	Reading	5
	Meditation	9
	Eating edibles	7
	Active Recreation:	
	Hiking	10
	Biking	8
	Pole dancing classes	9
	Socialization:	
	Networking	10
	Zoom calls w/friends & fam	9
	Virtual fashion shows	6

Initial Assessment	Occupational Performance Problem	Performance	Satisfaction
	Opening mail and invoices	2	1
	Past trauma affecting current life	6	7
	Anxiety while managing finances	4	1
	Wants to volunteer in new city	5	6
	Going to the credit union	1	1

Performance Capacity

- *Subjective experience:* Breonna enjoyed the individual session and stated the time "felt like a great way to reclaim life." She chose to video chat her boyfriend near the end to let him know she was feeling more confident already.
- *Occupation:* Breonna was able to open mail with verbal and visual cues from the therapist after one envelope was opened as an example. Using visualization and breathing techniques, she opened mail that had been sitting in her kitchen for over six months.
- *Performance skills:* Breonna followed simple 1-step directions and used her right pointer finger to identify current mental health pain level on a colorful scale. Whenever she became nervous, she fidgeted a keychain in the shape of her hometown in her left hand. She took breaks spontaneously and asked for feedback often throughout the session.
- *Client factors:* Breonna's acute experience with bouts of anxiety arise sharply when presented with a challenging situation. When she is alone, she tends to cease or avoid the activity. With verbal support and/or physical supervision, she can complete about 75% of the task at hand. Sights, smells, and even songs from LA artists evoke emotions from her.

Assessment

Breonna exhibits anxiety which interferes with her ability to engage in her role as entrepreneur, money management, community mobility, and community management.

Strengths: Regular attendee of wellness groups in coworking space, supportive boyfriend, supportive family, motivated to learn new techniques to assist in completion of critical IADLs

Areas of Improvement: Asking for help, opening mail in a timely fashion, managing "flashbacks," becoming upset with friends and family who are trying to help her, wants to make weekly trips and/or phone calls to local credit union to manage finances.

Plan

Long term goal: Breonna will consistently complete all financial business tasks independently using 3-5 effective coping techniques as needed from OT sessions by the end of 2021.

Frame of Reference: Psychodynamic approach. This approach is based on Freud's work and focusing on bringing the individual's unconscious thoughts and beliefs into the conscious providing insight into personal behavior (Carson, 2020).

Short-term Goals (2)	FOR Principle used to address goals	Intervention Approach/Methods (Be specific on how you will use this FOR principle in your session)
Breonna will independently collect and open mail 4 out of 7 days every week for 3 months	Meaningful occupation that will assist in reducing financial stress in personal and professional life.	Breonna will examine emotions, environment, and context of mail delivery to incorporate opening envelopes in her daily routine. The therapist will grade tasks and ask for self-report from Breonna to monitor progress. Once Breonna can show bills being paid on time and bring in opened mail spontaneously, she can uncover the benefits on accomplishing this task in other areas of life.
Breonna will utilize at least 1 new coping strategy per week via modeling from an evidence-based mental health app.	Using existing forms of repetitive learning through technology will allow Breonna to monitor progress and readjust accordingly.	Using an app will require Breonna to practice coping techniques in real time. She can role play with boyfriend and get feedback from the app on ways to improve current satisfaction and performance.

Creative Intervention Session

Short term goal: Breonna will independently collect and open mail 4/7 days every week for 3 months.

Describe activities	Rationale (why did you select these activities)	Role of the therapist	Grading: How would you make it easier for the client?	Grading: How would you make it more challenging for the client?
Warm-up	Choose fun exercises to encourage positive body movements and squeeze in physical activity for a busy individual	Leading Breonna through an exercise routine that encourages movement in all major muscle groups and relieves tension, nervousness	Seated exercises, shorten the time, decrease number of reps	Add weights, have Breonna lead therapist in exercise routine, increase reps, perform exercise on uneven terrain
Application	Review and teach Breonna new breathing and calming techniques	Educate about neuro system through app, impact of stress on the body, how anxiety manifests, how anxiety impacts occupation, give relevant examples, talk about Mental Health First Aid	One topic at a time, start with worksheets, show videos	Ask her to complete a task without cues, fun quiz, teach bf or family over video chat, incorporate stress-inducing activity for Breonna to employ techniques in the moment

Continued

Describe activities	Rationale (why did you select these activities)	Role of the therapist	Grading: How would you make it easier for the client?	Grading: How would you make it more challenging for the client?
Activity	She needed to achieve simple tasks and techniques to prepare to attempt the more difficult activity of opening mail with decreased assistance	Emotional support, coaching, modeling how to set the mood to complete a hard task	Therapist opens one envelope, ask Breonna to come to session with envelopes partially opened, make phone calls to senders instead, have bf collect and rubber band mail together	Open more than one envelope at a time, Breonna must collect all unopened mail to bring to session, open one invoice, open credit union online portal.
Cool down	Reflect and share calming activities, like her favorite songs, to safely and therapeutically end session	Listener, motivational interviewing, ask questions, recap, give personal experiences, offer praise	Save reflections for next session, keep calming period brief, have her write in journal in lieu of speaking	Leading a cool down activity, tell family the scope of experience using written or verbal reflection, reflect on tough LA memory

Infection Control Measures/Issues

- Temperature checks before entering building. Complete symptom checklist upon arrival to building.
- Decrease in number of clients seen per day with a 30-minute free block between visits.
- Breonna could cancel the session if she or boyfriend experienced any symptoms in the last 24 hrs.

Precautions/Safety Considerations

- Session held in open, ventilated area.
- Decreased traffic overall in the space.
- Therapist booked session for quieter time in the day.
- Disinfectant wipes, hand sanitizer, and face shields used throughout the session.
- Assessment for harm and suicide employed during each session for each person.
- Therapist shares and asks for pronouns of all guests in groups and 1:1.

Discharge Plan and Plan for Follow Up Care

- Breonna will continue to attend weekly virtual groups for community support.
- Breonna will begin to meet with OT once a week virtually or in person for the next 6 months.
- Once Breonna has chosen primary care team in St. Louis, will attempt to collaborate to increase quality of care.

LEARNING ACTIVITY: APPLY THEORY IN PRACTICE

Use Template 9.1 A to complete a case analysis on a sample case (see Evolve learning materials), showing your reasoning throughout the process. A description of each section is provided.

SUMMARY

OT practitioners use a variety of types of therapeutic reasoning as they work through the steps of the therapeutic reasoning process to design creative intervention plans. This requires they use cognitive processes and skills and strategies in a dynamic and flexible manner and consider influences of experience (the practitioner's and client's), contexts, and client factors. OT practitioners use curiosity, imagination, originality, and innovativeness as they collaborate with clients and problem-solve to design creative intervention plans. They may engage in brainstorming or be inspired by reading or engaging with a client to adapt and change intervention activities for the client. Creative intervention planning is an ongoing process that requires OT practitioners to apply knowledge gained about the client to select a frame of reference that adequately addresses the client's occupational strengths and challenges and match activities specifically for that client in a specific environment.

REFERENCES

American Occupational Therapy Association (AOTA) (2020). Occupational therapy practice framework: Domain and process (4th ed.). *American Journal of Occupational Therapy*, 74(2), 1–87.

American Psychological Association (APA). (2018). *Cognition. APA Dictionary of Psychology*. Washington, DC: American Psychological Association.

Baird, J. M., Raina, K. D., Rogers, J. C., O'Donnell, J., & Holm, M. B. (2015). Wheelchair transfer simulations to enhance procedural skills and clinical reasoning. *American Journal of Occupational Therapy*, 69(Suppl. 2), 6912185020.

Baron, K., Kielhofner, G., Iyenger, A., Goldhammer, V., & Wolenski, J. (2008). *Occupational Self-Assessment. Model of Human Occupation Clearinghouse*. University of Illinois.

Bissessur, S. W., Geijteman, E. C. T., Al-Dulaimy, M., Teunissen, P. W., Richir, M. C., Arnold, A. E. R., & de Vries, T. P. G. M. (2009).

Therapeutic reasoning: from hiatus to hypothetical model. *Journal of Evaluation in Clinical Practice, 15,* 985–989.

Bonsall. A. (2012). An examination of the pairing between narrative and occupational science. *Scandinavian journal of occupational therapy, 19,* 92–103.

Bowyer, P., Munoz, L., Tkach, M. M., Moore, C. C., & Tiongco, C. G. (2019). Long-term impact of Model of Human occupation training on therapeutic reasoning. *Journal of Allied Health, 48*(3), 188–193.

Bundy. A. C. (1993). Assessment of play and leisure: Delineation of the problem. *American Journal of Occupational Therapy, 47,* 212–222.

Bundy. A. (2010). Test of playfulness manual. Bolder, CO: Colorado State University.

Carson. N. (2020). Psychosocial theories. In N. Carson (Ed.), *Psychosocial Occupational Therapy* (pp. 76–91). Philadelphia, PA: Elsevier.

Cherry, K. (2020). What is cognition? Retrieved from www.verywellmind.com/what-is-cognition-2794982.

Cheung, T., Clemson, L., O'Loughlin, K., & Shuttleworth, R. (2018). Ergonomic education on housework for women with upper limb repetitive strain injury (RSI): a conceptual representation of therapists' clinical reasoning. *Disability and Rehabilitation, 40*(26), 3136–3146.

Dunn, L., & Dunn, L. (1998). *Peabody Picture Vocabulary Test – revised.* American Guidance Services, Inc.

During, S., Artino, A. R., Pangaro, L., van der Vleuten, C. P. M., & Schuwirth, L. (2011). Context and clinical reasoning: understanding the perspective of the expert's voice. *Medical Education, 45,* 927–938.

Fisher. A. G. (1998). Uniting practice and theory in an occupational framework. *American Journal of Occupational Therapy, 52*(7), 509–517.

Gibson, D., Velde, B., Hoff, T., Kvashay, D., Manross, P. L., & Moreau, V. (2000). Clinical reasoning of a novice versus an experienced occupational therapist: A qualitative study. *Occupational Therapy in Health Care, 12*(4), 15–31.

Gillen. G. (2013). Eleanor Clarke Slagle lecture: A fork in the road: An occupational hazard? *American Journal of Occupational Therapy, 67*(6), 643–652.

Glaser, R., & Chi, M. (1988). Overview. In M. T. H. Chi, R. Glaser, & M. J. Far (Eds.), *The Nature of Expertise (pp. xvi-xxviii).* Mahwah, NJ: Lawrence Erlbaum.

Hagedorn. R. (1996). Clinical decision making in familiar cases: A model of the process and implications for practice. *British Journal of Occupational Therapy, 59,* 217–222.

Holmqvist, K., Kamwendo, K., & Ivarsson, A. B. (2009). Occupational therapist' descriptions of their work with persons suffering from cognitive impairment following acquired brain injury. *Scandinavian journal of occupational therapy, 15,* 13–24.

Kielhofner, G., & Forsyth, K. (2008). Therapeutic reasoning: Planning, implementing, and evaluating the outcomes of therapy. In G. Kielhofner (Ed.), *A Model of Human Occupation: Theory and Application* (4ᵗʰ ed., pp. 143–154). Baltimore, MD: Williams & Wilkins.

Kielhofner, G., Mallenson, T., Crawford, C., Novak, M., Rigby, M., Henry, A., et al. (2004). *Occupational Performance History Interview -II (OPHI-II; Version 2.1). Chicago Model of Human Occupation Clearinghouse.* University of Illinois.

Law, M., Baptiste, S., Carswell, A., McColl, A., Polatajko, H., & Pollock, N. (2015). *Canadian Occupational Performance Measure (COMP)* (5ᵗʰ ed.). Ottawa: COMP Inc.

Mahaffey. L. (2009). Using theory and the therapeutic reasoning process to guide the occupational therapy process for older adults with mental illness. *OT Practice, 14*(5), CE1–8.

Mattingly. C. (1994). The narrative nature of clinical reasoning. In C. Mattingly & M. H. Fleming (Eds.), *Clinical Reasoning: Forms of Inquiry in a Therapeutic Practice* (pp. 239–269). Philadelphia, PA: FA Davis.

Merriam-Webster. (n.d.). Conceptualize. In *Merriam-Webster.com dictionary.* Retrieved from: https://www.merriam-webster.com/dictionary/conceptualize.

Merriam-Webster. (n.d.). Creativity. In *Merriam-Webster.com dictionary.* Retrieved from https://www.merriam-webster.com/dictionary/creativity.

Missiuna. C., et al. (2001). Cognitive orientation to daily occupational performance (CO-OP): Part I: theoretical foundations. *Physical and Occupational Therapy in Pediatrics, 20*(2–3), 69–81.

Mitchell, R., & Unsworth, C. A. (2004). Role perceptions and clinical reasoning of community health occupational therapists undertaking home visits. *Australian Occupational Therapy Journal, 51,* 13–24.

Montgomery, A. A., Harding, J., & Fahey, T. (2001). Shared decisions making in hypertension: the impact of patient preferences on treatment choice. *Family Practice, 18*(3), 309–313.

O'Brien, J., Asselin, E., Fortier, K., Janzegers, R., Lagueux, B., & Silcox, C. (2010). Using therapeutic reasoning to apply the Model of Human Occupation in pediatric occupational therapy practice. *Journal of Occupational Therapy, Schools, & Early Intervention, 3*(4), 348–365.

O'Brien, J., & Patnaude, M. (2022). *Occupational therapy students' self-assessment of therapeutic reasoning following a case-based integration course. Unpublished manuscript.* University of New England.

Oakley, F., Kielhofner, G., Barris, R., & Reichler, R. K. (1986). The Role checklist: Development and empirical assessment of reliability. *Occupational Therapy Journal of Research, 6,* 157–170.

Parkinson, S., Forsyth, K., & Kielhofner, G. (2008). *The Model of Human Occupation Screening Tool (Version 2.0). Chicago Model of Human Occupation Clearinghouse,.* University of Illinois.

Persson, D., Erlandsen, L. K., Eklund, M., & Iwareson, S. (2001). Value dimensions, meaning, and complexity in human occupation – a tentative structure for analysis. *Scandinavian journal of occupational therapy, 8,* 7–18.

Rassafiani, M., Ziviani, J., Rodger, S., & Dalgleish, L. (2009). Identification of occupational therapy clinical expertise: decision-making characteristics. *Australian Occupational Therapy Journal, 56,* 156–166.

Rogers, J. C., & Holm, M. B. (1991). Occupational therapy diagnostic reasoning: a component of clinical reasoning. *American Journal of Occupational Therapy, 45*(11), 1045–1455.

Royeen, C., Mu, K., Barrett, L., & Luebben, A. (2001). Pilot investigations: Evaluation of a clinical reflection and reasoning before and after workshop intervention. In P. Crist (Ed.), *Innovations in Occupational Therapy Education* (pp. 107–114). North Bethesda, MD: American Occupational Therapy Association.

Schaaf. R. C. (2015). Creating evidence for practice using data-driven decision making. *American Journal of Occupational Therapy, 69,* 6902360010.

Schell, B. A., & Cervero, M. (1993). Clinical reasoning in occupational therapy: an integrative review. *American Journal of Occupational Therapy, 47,* 605–610.

Skarpaas, L. S., Jamissen, G., Kruger, C., Holmberg, V., & Hardy, P. (2016). Digital storytelling as poetic reflection in occupational therapy education: an empirical study. *The Open Journal of Occupational Therapy, 4*(3), 5. Article.

Sorman, D. E., Hansson, P., Pritshke, I., & Ljungberg, J. K. (2019). Complexity of primary lifetime occupation and cognitive processing. *Frontiers in Psychology, 10,* 1–12.

Stav, W. B., Hallenen, T., Lane, J., & Arbesman, M. (2012). Systematic review of occupational engagement and health outcomes among community dwelling older adults. *American Journal of Occupational Therapy, 66*(3), 301–310.

Taylor. R. (2017). *Kielhofner's Model of Human Occupation* (5th ed.). Philadelphia, PA: Wolters Kluwer.

Ward. J. D. (2003). The nature of clinical reasoning with groups: A phenomenological study of an occupational therapist in community mental health. *American Journal of Occupational Therapy, 57,* 625–634.

Weinstock-Zlotnick, G., & Mehta, S. (2018). A systematic review of the benefits of occupation-based intervention for patients with upper extremity musculoskeletal disorders. *Journal of Hand Therapy, 32,* 141–152.

Worksheets

WORKSHEET 9.1: CASE ANALYSIS

Complete an analysis of another case from Mahaffey (2009) and O'Brien et al. (2010).

Case Analysis		
Steps of Therapeutic Reasoning	**Examples of Process with Older Adults with Mental Illness (Mahaffey, 2009)**	**Examples with Children (O'Brien et al., 2010)**
Setting		
Case		
Generate clinical questions based on theory	Occupational identity: Occupational competence: Volition: Habituation: Performance capacity: Environment:	Volition: Habituation: Performance capacity: Environment:
Gather information		
Conceptualize (identify occupational challenges)	Habituation: Performance: Volition: Environment: Summary:	Volition: Habituation: Performance capacity: Environment: Summary:
Create the intervention plan (goals)		
Implement the plan		
Evaluate outcomes		
Key reasoning concepts		

WORKSHEET 9.2: TASKS, TYPES, AND THOUGHT PROCESSES

Use Worksheet 9.2 to provide examples (different from those in Table 9.2) to illustrate the types of reasoning and thought processes that may occur at each stage of therapeutic reasoning.

Tasks, Types, and Thought Processes			
Steps	**Tasks**	**Type of Reasoning**	**Thought Processes**
Generate questions			
Gather data			
Identify occupational challenges			
Create an intervention plan			
Implement intervention plan			
Assess outcomes			

WORKSHEET 9.3: IDENTIFY OCCUPATIONAL CHALLENGES

Use Worksheet 9.3 to identify hypotheses describing occupational challenges for selected case examples (see Evolve learning site).

Identify Occupational Challenges
Client's name:
Brief description of client:
Occupational strengths:
Occupational challenges:
Hypotheses regarding occupational challenges:
Describe your rationale for the hypotheses:
Model of Practice or Frame of Reference to guide intervention:
Describe why you selected the Model of Practice or Frame of Reference:

WORKSHEET 9.4: STRATEGIES AND PRINCIPLES OF FRAMES OF REFERENCE

Use Worksheet 9.4 to provide descriptions of the principles and strategies of each frame of reference. Use Table 3.1 and Table 3.2 for a list of principles of frames of reference.

Strategies and Principles of Frames of Reference		
Frame of Reference	**Principles**	**Strategies for Intervention**
Biomechanical		
Cognitive behavioral therapy		
Model of Human Occupation		
Motor control/motor learning		
How does this information inform intervention planning?		

WORKSHEET 9.5: RESEARCH NOTE: EVIDENCE

Complete Worksheet 9.5. Summarize the findings from a research article that examines a principle of a selected frame of reference.
- Based on this article, how would you apply the principle in practice?
- Describe some strategies and activities that follow this principle.

Research Note: Evidence
Reference: [Do not use theoretical papers, systematic reviews, or studies from non-peer-reviewed sources for this assignment.]
Frame of Reference: [Briefly describe the frame of reference you selected to review.]
Overview: [Synthesize information to concisely describe purpose of study and what the authors did.]
Intervention Principle: [Describe the intervention principle that the study examines.]
Findings: [Describe the key findings that relate to the specific principle you are examining. Describe the results clearly and concisely.]
Implications for OT: [Describe how the findings inform the principle and influence occupational therapy practice decisions.]
Application of Principle: [Describe how you would apply this principle in practice based on this study.]
Strategies: [Describe some strategies and activities that follow this principle.]

WORKSHEET 9.6: ACTIVITY ANALYSIS: CREATIVITY

Complete Worksheet 9.6. Design an interesting activity that could be used in occupational therapy intervention.
- Identify the materials, steps, and sequence for completing the activity.
- Describe the performance skills required.
- Identify contextual (personal and environmental factors) related to the activity.
- How would you change the activity?

Activity Analysis: Creativity
Activity description
Sequence of steps [List sequence of steps to complete.]
Materials/supplies and their properties [Identify materials and their properties (i.e., texture, consistency; size; purpose; shape; color; and sensory properties).]
Performance skills
Motor skills [Describe actions related to moving and manipulating objects.]
Process skills [Describe actions related to selecting, interacting, and using objects (e.g., problem solving).]
Social interaction skills [Describe actions related to communicating and interacting with others.]
Contexts
Environmental Factors [Describe physical, technology, social, and institution systems.]
Personal Factors [Describe culture, social, habits and routines, as related to activity.]
Describe variations of this activity.

WORKSHEET 9.7: CREATIVITY AND FLEXIBILITY IN PRACTICE

Since intervention sessions do not always go as planned, OT practitioners often have "back pocket" activities readily available, such as a balloon, deck of cards, beach ball, pen, or paperclips. Use Worksheet 9.7 to list the items you might use as back up intervention ideas. Identify 10 activities that you could use from one of the items that address different performance skills. (For example, given a beach ball you can throw it for UE strength, pick it up for dynamic standing, blow it up for pacing/energy conservation, hold with 2 hands for bimanual coordination).

- Gather the item and demonstrate the activities to peers.

Creativity and Flexibility in Practice	
List readily available items that you might use for "back up" intervention ideas:	
Activities	**Performance skills**
1.	
2.	
3.	
4.	
5.	
6.	
7.	
8.	
9.	
10.	

TEMPLATE 9.1 A: APPLY THEORY IN PRACTICE

Use Template 9.1 A to complete a case analysis on a sample case (see Evolve learning materials), showing your reasoning throughout the process. Template 9.1B does not include the descriptions.

Template 9.1 A: Occupational Therapy Intervention Plan (with descriptions)

Client's Name:

Date of report:

Date of referral:

DOB:

Primary intervention diagnosis/concern: [main reason for referral]

Secondary diagnosis/concern: [anything contributing to client's condition or performance]

Precautions/contraindications: [medicine, health or movement precautions]

Setting: [place of occupational therapy]

Reason for referral to OT: [who referred client to OT and why]

Therapist: [names of therapist(s) writing report]

Findings
Occupational Profile: [client's background medical and social "story"; may include what brought them to hospital or clinic; brief background information]
Concerns: [client's concerns, reason for coming to OT or getting services]
Description of Assessments: [Briefly describe the assessments and how they are scored; describe the client's performance and make a judgment of the validity of the findings if necessary]
Table of Results: [Include a table of the findings and interpretation of the scores]
Volition: [client's interests, values, personal causation; what motivates client]
Habituation (habits and roles): [roles, role expectations, habits, routines, patterns]
Occupational participation: [briefly describe client's occupational performance and participation]
Performance capacity:
- *Subjective experience* [how does the client view his/her performance, situation; includes "lived body" experience]
- *Performance skills:* [briefly describe client's performance skills; see OTPF]
- *Performance patterns:* [briefly describe client's performance patterns; see OTPF]
- *Client factors:* [describe client factors that are important to the client's situation and relate to the condition for which he/she is receiving OT; see OTPF] [Be sure and prioritize here – do not list all client factors]
Environment (contexts): [Briefly describe the client's environment, including social, physical, financial, and community resources]

Interpretation
[This is the place where the OT synthesizes all above information and makes a hypothesis about what is going on. Be sure and pull it all together here, do not just list things from above.]
Analysis of occupational performance: [Brief statement regarding what exactly is interfering with client's desired occupations. Use terms from model of practice.]

Strengths: [What are the client's strengths? Look at all areas. This may be a bulleted list, but needs to completely convey the strength. For example instead of writing "Friends" as a strength, state it completely, like:

- Friends support client by helping him grocery shop weekly.
- Family visits often.]

Weaknesses: [What are the client's challenges? Look at all areas. This may be a bulleted list, but be specific. For example, "ROM" is not clear enough, rather state "ROM R UE interferes with client's ability to perform bimanual tasks."]

Plan

Long term goal: [include link to theory; be sure this is focusing on an occupation; you only have to pick one goal. There are many for each client. Be sure goal is relevant, understandable, measureable, observable and achievable. It should be a meaningful goal that targets an occupation.]

Short-Term Goals (2)	Intervention Approach/Methods
[These are steps to the LTG; Be sure they are things that you will accomplish in therapy and not a therapy activity.]	[How will you specifically address the STG? What will you do in therapy session? What intervention approach will you use and how? Be specific here. How does what you are doing in the session make a difference?]

Description of Rationale for goals and how they related to client's needs (include theory): [Why did you select your goals? Use terminology from model to explain your reasoning.]

Description of Frame of Reference/Principles to address goals: [What frame of reference (such as biomechanical, rehabilitation, motor control and motor learning, cognitive behavioral) are you using to address goals. Describe it and state the principles of the FOR.]

Rationale for FOR(s): [Why did you select this FOR? How does it address the client's issues?]

Intervention session:

- **Expected frequency, duration, and intensity:** [How many days a week and for how long will you see client? This is an estimate, but think about the setting.]
- **Location of intervention:** [Where is OT being provided? Hospital, community, inpatient, outpatient?]
- **Anticipated discontinuation environment:** [Where do you think the client is being discharged to? Home, family, group home, rehabilitation unit?]
- **Role of the therapist in the intervention session (link to OTPF or theory):** [What is the OT's role in the intervention session? Refer to OTPF, FOR or Model for specifics.]
- **Intervention activities (specific along with sequence):** [Describe the intervention session to address one short-term goal in a 45-minute session. Provide an estimate of the time for each activity and put things in sequence.]

Signature and date [all teammates sign to acknowledge their work on this report]

Template 9.1B Occupational Therapy Intervention Plan (with no descriptions)

Client's Name:
Date of report:
Date of referral:
DOB:
Primary intervention diagnosis/concern:
Secondary diagnosis/concern:
Precautions/contraindications:
Reason for referral to OT:
Setting:
Therapist:

Findings

Occupational profile:
Concerns:
Description of Assessments:
Table of Results:
Volition:

Habituation (habits and roles):
Occupational participation:
Performance capacity:
- *Subjective experience:*
- *Performance skills:*
- *Performance patterns:*
- *Client factors:*

Environment (contexts):

Interpretation

Analysis of occupational performance:
Strengths:
Weaknesses:

Plan

Long term goal: [include link to MOHO theory]

Short-Term Goals (2)	Intervention Approach/Methods

Description of Rationale for goals and how they related to client's needs (include theory):
Description of Frame of Reference/Principles to address goals:
Rationale for FOR (s):
Intervention session:
- Expected frequency, duration, and intensity:
- Location of intervention:
- Anticipated discontinuation environment:
- Role of the therapist in the intervention session (link to OTPF or theory):
- Intervention activities (specific along with sequence):

Signature and date

10

Reflection and Assessment: Measuring Outcomes

Jane O'Brien

GUIDING QUESTIONS

1. How does therapeutic reasoning influence the art and science of occupational therapy?
2. What are the observable behaviors of therapeutic reasoning?
3. What strategies and behaviors support therapeutic reasoning and professional growth?
4. How does reflection, assessment, and self-awareness promote therapeutic reasoning skills and behaviors?

KEY TERMS

Art of therapy
Attitudes
Attributions
Cognitive biases
Opinions
Preparatory reflection

Reflection in action
Reflection on action
Reflective practice
Self-awareness
Self-efficacy
Values

INTRODUCTION

Therapeutic reasoning is a complex process that involves more than just the application of knowledge. It involves ongoing assessment, problem-solving, self-awareness, and reflection. The OT practitioner learns to question the client, observe behaviors, and refine hypotheses to design and adapt intervention activities. The interactive and dynamic nature of human occupation requires that the OT practitioner understand their role in the process and be aware of the changing nature of the client and situation. This process requires skills in assessment, intervention planning, and implementation, while also requiring OT practitioners be aware of their therapeutic use of self and factors influencing the client and practitioner. OT practitioners integrate knowledge of practice and human occupation with the art of therapy as they make decisions and engage clients in therapeutic activities. This complex process requires the practitioner to be aware of themselves and carefully reflect upon all aspects of the therapeutic process. The **art of therapy** refers to blending one's knowledge with therapeutic use of self and is considered essential to therapeutic effectiveness (Turner & Alsop, 2015).

In this final chapter, the author describes the art of therapy and techniques to enhance therapeutic reasoning, emphasizing methods to develop one's self-awareness and ability to critically reflect upon practice. The author reviews a variety of critical reasoning tools to assess one's decisions and support growth in practice. Descriptions of therapeutic reasoning behaviors operationalized through a variety of assessments provide further explanation of therapeutic reasoning concepts. Case examples and learning activities are interspersed throughout the chapter to reinforce concepts.

ART AND SCIENCE OF PRACTICE

The art of therapy involves building a therapeutic relationship with a client and reading and responding to the client's cues. Creating activities that are meaningful and motivating to the client is one step in the process, although the art of therapy involves much more. It involves listening and responding to the client, providing information as the client is able to hear it, and challenging the client. The art of therapy requires practitioners to anticipate and respond to the client's behaviors and understand their own biases, background, and experience and how they influence decisions and interactions.

The art of therapy includes incorporating active listening, empathizing, building a therapeutic alliance, observing cues, clarifying meaning, and giving and receiving information, into the therapeutic relationship (Falk-Kessler & Ciavarino, 2006; Schwartzberg, 2002). The Intentional Relationship Model (IRM; Taylor, 2020) provides a structured way to view and examine one's therapeutic relationships (see Chapter 4). The IRM addresses communication styles, termed modes (i.e., advocating, instructing, empathizing, problem-solving, collaborating, encouraging). Communication includes body language, use of touch, and providing physical support.

The science of the profession refers to the knowledge (such as neurological, musculoskeletal, human performance, frames of reference, research evidence) and processes (such as assessment, procedures, handling, protocols, experiences) that inform practice. While the science of the profession provides a framework (e.g., frame of reference, model of practice) based on evidence that outlines the principles, techniques, and strategies to use in practice, the OT practitioner engaging in the art of therapy applies the techniques adding in their interaction style, personality, and attitude. The following case example illustrates the art and science of therapy.

Case example: Graham is a student on his first fieldwork rotation completing an initial evaluation in an acute care setting. The client is a 70-year-old man who received a hip replacement. Graham's grandfather is also 70, so Graham feels comfortable interviewing the client. Prior to the session, Graham pictures a frail elderly man (like his grandfather). Graham organizes the assessment with these expectations in mind. The client, however, is a physically active man who injured his hip while mountain climbing. The client does not respond well when Graham speaks loudly (assuming the client is hard of hearing) and asks generic questions. Furthermore, Graham keeps comparing the client to his grandfather. He selects activities from the protocol for hip replacement but does not engage the client in conversation.

This example shows the importance of being prepared (e.g., knowing the science of hip replacement assessment and rehabilitation). However, Graham did not listen or observe the client and, consequently, Graham did not build the therapeutic relationship. He assumed the client was "like his grandfather" and did not adjust his interaction style to relate to this active 70-year-old man. The client, who was discouraged already and in pain, felt unheard and undervalued. He was not motivated to attend the next occupational therapy session.

Graham and his supervisor discussed the session and reflected upon the outcomes. Graham acknowledged that he was nervous and expected the client to act more like his grandfather. Together, they brainstormed ways for Graham to build the relationship during the next session. They discussed the importance of seeing each client as an individual and taking time to interact with the client as an essential part of the occupational therapy process. The supervisor noted that being aware of one's cognitive biases and reflecting on things that went well and those things that need improvement are important skills for OT practitioners to develop.

Reflective practice involves considering therapy decisions by examining knowledge, science, and experiences in relation to the client. Reflective practice is not always regularly facilitated through supervision, which may limit the development of professional reasoning and clinical skills in the early stages of one's career (Guy et al., 2020). Furthermore, supervisors reported that they had limited knowledge, skill, or confidence using reflective practice models (such as Gibbs, 1998), although they understood the benefits of being a reflective practitioner (Guy et al., 2020).

LEARNING ACTIVITY: THE ART AND SCIENCE OF THERAPY

Use Worksheet 10.1 to identify aspects of the art and science of therapy after reading the following case example.

Case example: A 55-year-old schoolteacher and mother of 3 teenagers is experiencing a severe exacerbation of multiple sclerosis, requiring hospitalization. She is receiving occupational services in an acute rehabilitation setting.
- Provide examples of the art and science of therapy.
- Describe the interaction between the art and science of therapy as related to this case.

COGNITIVE BIASES AND ATTRIBUTIONS

Therapeutic relationships occur between clients and OT practitioners, and each brings their own experiences, background, and beliefs to the process. Understanding one's own cognitive biases, attitudes, attributions, values, and opinions allows OT practitioners to address issues that may interfere with therapeutic reasoning.

Cognitive biases refer to one's predisposition to reach a decision based on limited information. Cognitive biases may interfere with clinical and professional reasoning, so it is important for OT practitioners to be aware of them. A summary of the common cognitive biases is provided in Table 10.1. For example, a practitioner may decide that a client's lack of progress is due to a lack of motivation for carrying out the home program and fail to explore other reasons for the lack of progress. Making decisions based on one's cognitive biases before gathering all the information or refusing to consider new information impedes the therapeutic process.

Another cognitive bias is referred to as the "rule of thumb," which refers to following a familiar intervention or rule without considering the client. For example, an OT practitioner addresses balance issues using t-stool exercises, without examining the specific child's abilities. While t-stool exercises

TABLE 10.1   Common Cognitive Biases

Cognitive bias	Description
Early decision-making	Locking into a clinical judgement or decision early on and failing to reconsider alternate ways of thinking after receiving contradictory information.
Rule of thumb	Relying on familiar clinical presentations, interventions, or "rules of thumb."
Recent exposure	Detecting a condition more often because of recent exposure.
Lack of evidence	Making rapid clinical decisions without enough evidence or information.
Ignoring alternatives	Not challenging or considering other alternatives when a situation has been labeled.

(From Lapointe, J., Craik, J., & Loiselle, C.G. (2017). Appraising potential cognitive biases impeding clinical and professional reasoning in occupational therapy practice. *Occupational Therapy Now*. Vol. 19, Iss. 6, 8–10. Used with the permission of CAOT Publications ACE.)

challenge balance, some children have more dynamic balance issues that are not addressed with generic t-stool exercises. OT practitioners may detect conditions or symptoms and use similar intervention activities because they were recently successful. For example, an OT practitioner may decide that an adult client is experiencing anxiety due to a medication change without exploring other possibilities (such as change in job, physical status). This prevents the OT practitioner from exploring other strategies that may be addressed within OT intervention. Ignoring additional information that may suggest a different intervention approach can lead to lack of progress towards goals.

> ## LEARNING ACTIVITY: COGNITIVE BIASES
>
> Use Worksheet 10.2. Create a personal example of each of the types of biases.
> * What other biases might influence decision-making?

Attitudes are one's position or emotion toward a fact (Merriam-Webster, n.d.). An OT practitioner's position (e.g., positive, negative) towards a client may influence the reasoning process. For example, an OT practitioner who approaches the session with a positive attitude believing that the client can succeed in reaching their goals makes different decisions than a practitioner who holds a negative attitude of the client. Being aware of one's attitudes makes it possible for OT practitioners to understand how the attitude may influence therapeutic decisions. Learning about one's attitude from experiences and thoughtful reflection promotes growth and professional development, which benefits future clients.

Attributions refer to the meaning given to an event or behavior (Kwaitek, 2005). For example, a child who is non-verbal and having difficulty feeding himself "spits out his food." The family reports he does not like the food. The OT practitioner does not explore other possibilities and creates an intervention plan based on the parents' interpretation of the child's behavior. During the next session, the OT practitioner realizes that the child has oral motor difficulties resulting in him spitting out the food. This example shows the importance of carefully analyzing and reflecting upon the meaning of events and behaviors in therapy.

Values are a person's acquired beliefs and commitments, derived from culture, about what is good, right, and important to do (Kielhofner, 2008). They include principles, standards, or qualities considered worthwhile (AOTA, 2020, p. 15). OT practitioners may work with clients who have opposing or different values. This requires that the practitioner respect the client–therapist relationship and not impose one's value system upon others.

Opinions include one's thoughts about events and situations, which may be based upon personal experiences, culture, or background history. One's opinions do not have to be based upon the best possible evidence. Therefore, when engaging in therapeutic reasoning, the OT practitioner backs up their opinions with evidence for practice.

> ## LEARNING ACTIVITY: ATTITUDES, ATTRIBUTIONS, VALUES, AND OPINIONS
>
> Complete Worksheet 10.3 to identify your attitudes, attributions, values, and opinions on a certain topic.
> * How might you use this knowledge in practice?

SELF-AWARENESS AND REFLECTIVE PRACTICE

Self-awareness refers to knowledge of one's own personality or character (Merriam-Webster, n.d.). Self-awareness includes becoming aware of one's internal factors (e.g., values, beliefs, strategies, interaction styles, emotional strengths, and challenges) and external factors (e.g., setting, peers, support persons, culture) that may influence behaviors. OT practitioners who enter situations with an open mind and curiosity explore and uncover important information for intervention planning. OT practitioners reflect throughout the entire therapeutic reasoning process as they consider their actions, questions, activity selection, and hypotheses regarding client behaviors. Research shows the importance of reflection to promote reasoning skills for practice (Carrier et al., 2012; Coker, 2010; Guy et al., 2020).

Reflective practice is the process of examining and exploring issues to improve and shape decisions and activities for the future (Spalding, 1998). There are several models for reflective practice, but Gibbs (1998) resembles the therapeutic reasoning process described in this textbook (see Figure 10.1). In summary, the reflective process requires the OT practitioner to describe the event and associated thoughts and feelings; evaluate the situation; analyze what happened; develop alternative possibilities for actions; and identify an action plan for the next time (Gibbs, 1998). Working through this reflective process facilitates learning and promotes professional growth. It requires honest reflection and self-awareness.

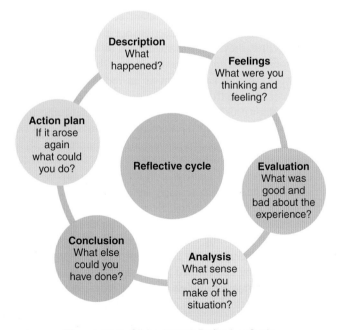

Figure 10.1 Gibbs (1988) Reflexive Cycle.

"Reflection is about learning and developing from experience, resulting in a changed perspective" (Andrews, 2000, p. 396). Three stages of reflection have been identified: preparatory reflection; reflecting in action; and reflection on action (Boud & Walker, 1990). See Figure 10.2 for a definition of each stage and an example.

Preparatory Reflection

Preparatory reflection includes understanding the client, using knowledge from one's experience, and considering factors related to the context (such as practice setting, client's discharge environment, culture) to plan assessment and intervention. This stage of reflection includes reviewing information about a new diagnosis or reviewing one's model of practice or frame of reference for new insights. The practitioner may gather assessment items, consider information from team members, and develop questions during this stage. In this stage, the practitioner may reflect on one's strengths and challenges as they relate to the client and context.

LEARNING ACTIVITY: PREPARATORY REFLECTION

Case Example: Javier is a 35-year-old man who experienced a cardiac event, requiring triple bypass surgery 24 hours ago. He is a patient in an acute care hospital where you are the OT.

Use Worksheet 10.4 to engage in preparatory reflection as you prepare to meet Javier.
- Describe your style, experience, and knowledge.
- Identify questions that you have regarding the case and context.

Reflection in Action

Reflection in action is "mindful awareness enabling the therapist to act intentionally and with immediacy within a scenario" (Yazdani et al., 2020, p. 2). While interacting with the client, the OT practitioner reflects upon the client's communication style and considers their own style or modes of communication. The practitioner notices and responds to the client's responses and behaviors and reflects on the reasons for behaviors, drawing upon theory to make sense of occupational performance challenges. Reflection in action requires the OT practitioner to respond to perceptions about behaviors or use one's intuition during the session. For example, the OT practitioner working with an adult client moves closer to a client to provide hand-over-hand assistance as she perceives the client struggling with a difficult task. However, as the practitioner approaches, the client seems to "pull away or flinch" when the OT practitioner reaches for his hand. The OT practitioner perceives this as a cue that the client wants to try to do the task on his own. The practitioner surmises that the client wants to challenge himself and moves away.

LEARNING ACTIVITY: REFLECTION IN ACTION

Complete Worksheet 10.5 as you observe an intervention session (see Evolve learning site Videos 10.1 and 10.2).
- Describe the practitioner's actions and the client's responses.
- Describe possible reasons for the actions and responses.

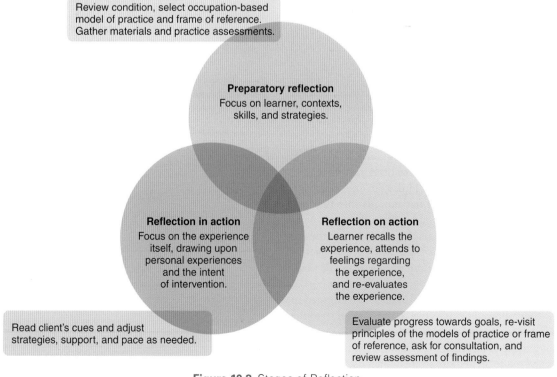

Review condition, select occupation-based model of practice and frame of reference. Gather materials and practice assessments.

Preparatory reflection
Focus on learner, contexts, skills, and strategies.

Reflection in action
Focus on the experience itself, drawing upon personal experiences and the intent of intervention.

Reflection on action
Learner recalls the experience, attends to feelings regarding the experience, and re-evaluates the experience.

Read client's cues and adjust strategies, support, and pace as needed.

Evaluate progress towards goals, re-visit principles of the models of practice or frame of reference, ask for consultation, and review assessment of findings.

Figure 10.2 Stages of Reflection.

Reflection on Action

Reflection on action involves thinking about an event that has happened and planning a future response (Yazdani et al., 2020). This stage occurs after the session as the practitioner reflects upon the experience as it occurred. The OT practitioner considers those things in the session that went as planned and those things that did not go as planned. The practitioner evaluates their decisions within the context of the session and the client's responses. When reflecting on action, the practitioner analyzes the reasons for decisions and contemplates the reasons for actions.

For example, the OT practitioner examines the strategies from a frame of reference in relation to how he used those in practice and the client's responses. He reviews the client's actions to judge the effectiveness of the methods used and decides to continue with this approach or find an alternative approach to intervention. During this stage, the OT practitioner may explore additional frames of reference, activities, strategies, or approaches.

Reflection on action may be facilitated by a supervisor, educator, or peer. For example, Seif et al. (2014) found that the therapeutic reasoning of students engaged in an interprofessional service-learning class improved after debriefing sessions. During debriefing sessions with faculty, students felt safe to discuss their reasoning, decisions, and intervention options.

LEARNING ACTIVITY: REFLECTION ON ACTION

Use Worksheet 10.6 to reflect upon the intervention session (see video clips 10.1 and 10.2 on Evolve learning site).
- Identify the model of practice or frame of reference used during the session.
- Describe the reason for the selection.
- What strategies worked? Why?
- What strategies did not work? Why?
- How did the client respond to the session? (Give specifics)
- Why do you think the client responded in that way?
- What else could the therapist have done?

Reflective Writing

Reflection involves a high level of metacognition to be aware of what is happening, analyze it, link it to other factors related to the event, interpret the response according to one's behavior, indicate what has worked and what has not, identify the next step, and check the action again (Boud, 2001). The act of writing down one's thought process helps a practitioner synthesize information, analyze findings, and learn concepts. Reflective writing helps practitioners learn and apply knowledge and skills (Yazdani et al., 2020).

Yazdani et al. (2020) found that participants who engaged in an IRM workshop followed by reflective writing appreciated the time to reflect in this way and develop action plans. The participants felt that writing about their experiences in practice clarified concepts and made them more aware of their use of the IRM concepts in practice. Almost all participants identified the need

for deeper learning via supervision or collegial discussion. More experienced participants used more reflection in action, while less experienced therapists reflected on action (Yazdani et al., 2020). They mentioned time limitations and heavy workloads as barriers to reflective writing. OT practitioners may want to set aside time each day to reflect upon practice. This may involve a 30-minute writing or discussion with a peer or colleague. Setting time aside to reflect facilitates reasoning and may result in improved client outcomes. Box 10.1 lists some strategies to incorporate reflection and reflective writing into practice.

Reflective writing is an effective tool to promote therapeutic reasoning. Box 10.2 presents tips to facilitate reflective writing. Reflective writing may begin with an open-ended question or prompt, such as "Describe an OT intervention session." The writer completes a free-writing response with no qualifiers for

BOX 10.1 Strategies to Incorporate Reflection and Reflective Writing into Daily Routines

- Add a component of reflective writing as part of the annual performance review process.
- Attend a continuing education course on reflective writing.
- Set an annual performance goal to complete reflective writing once a quarter.
- Meet with a mentor or colleague and regular intervals throughout the year to reflect on practice.
- Read professional journal articles on reflective writing and hold a journal club with colleagues.
- Create guidelines or a template for staff inservices or onsite CEU and ensure a reflective component is always completed as part of the presentation.
- Hold a staff inservice on reflective writing and share case study examples of reflection on action. Create dyads of experienced and novice therapists to facilitate mentorship.
- Encourage reflective writing in fieldwork assignments for students at the clinical site, especially as part of weekly supervision meetings.

BOX 10.2 Tips for Reflective Writing

Provide an open-ended question.	Consider the audience and the goal of the learning experience.
Write during a non-distracting time.	Do not analyze writing at the beginning, but rather get the thoughts on the paper.
Allow for short responses.	Respond to short probing questions to facilitate thinking.
Ask questions.	List questions throughout.
Return to writing samples and provide deeper prompts.	Clarify, elaborate, and answer specific questions related to the experience.
Discuss concepts and explore.	Refine responses and provide details on aspects of writing or process. Support concepts with evidence and theory.
Describe options (include self-awareness).	Summarize alternatives along with rationale for using them in practice. Address self in the process.
Summarize lessons learned.	Summarize how the process may inform occupational therapy practice.

page length, grammar, spelling, or content. The writer returns to the prompt with further short probing questions (e.g., What went well? What was difficult?). Throughout the writing process, the writer is encouraged to list questions that arise (e.g., Why did the client respond like that? Why does he have a tremor today? Did I miss something?). Next the writer clarifies, elaborates, and analyzes concepts related to the experience. They investigate the aspects of their writing more deeply (e.g., describe the principles of the frame of reference and their rationale for using it) and identify alternative options. The OT practitioner is encouraged to reflect upon their role in the process. The final step is to summarize the lessons learned and describe how this information informs future practice decisions.

LEARNING ACTIVITY: REFLECTIVE WRITING

Complete Worksheet 10.7 to practice reflective writing to promote therapeutic reasoning. Select one of the following prompts:
- Describe a recent experience with a friend.
- Describe a learning experience of which you are proud.
- Describe a therapy session (evaluation or intervention) with a client.

Theory Application Assessment Instrument

Reflective writing may also include short case examples to promote reasoning. The Theory Application Assessment Instrument (TIAA; Ikiugu & Smallfield, 2010) was created "to measure competency in combining multiple theoretical conceptual practice models in client evaluation and treatment planning" (p. 253). The Instrument consists of Part 1: Assessment and Intervention Planning, whereby respondents answer questions based on a short case example. In Part 2, respondents are interviewed to explain their choices and how they used the models to guide assessment and intervention planning. Part 3 of the instrument is the scoring guidelines.

This instrument promotes therapeutic reasoning by providing a structure and avenue for explaining and reflecting upon one's decisions. It shows promise of being an effective tool to enhance therapeutic reasoning (Ikiugu & Smallfield, 2010).

LEARNING ACTIVITY: REFLECTING ON THEORY IN PRACTICE

Review Video 10.1A/B or 10.2A/B (on the Evolve learning site) and then complete Worksheet 10.8 questions from the Theory Application Assessment Instrument (Ikiugu & Smallfield, 2010).

ASSESSMENTS OF THERAPEUTIC REASONING

Assessing therapeutic reasoning allows OT practitioners to evaluate their own learning and reasoning needs for practice (Cheung et al., 2018; Falk-Kessler & Ciaravino, 2006; Ghysels et al., 2017; Keiller & Hanekom, 2013; Popova & Taylor, 2020a; Popova & Taylor, 2020b; Popova et al., 2020; Scaffa & Wooster, 2004; Seif et al., 2014; Sladyk & Sheckley, 2001). Table 10.2 lists assessments used to measure critical thinking and therapeutic reasoning. Not all the assessments listed have been used

in occupational therapy research, but they may provide useful information for reflection.

A brief discussion of each of the assessments used in occupational therapy research is provided in the following sections.

Clinical Reasoning Case Analysis Test (CRCAT)

The Clinical Reasoning Case Analysis Test (CRCAT; Sladyk & Sheckley, 2001) was developed to measure three types of reasoning: procedural, interactive, and conditional. Three experts in occupational therapy reviewed it for face and content validity. Reliability was established using Cronbach's alpha; inter-item alpha ranged from .98 to .99 and inter-rater reliability was .98 (Sladyk & Sheckley, 2001). The authors found that clinical reasoning improved after 12-week fieldwork experiences.

The researchers (Sladyk & Sheckley, 2001) found that clinical reasoning scores on the CRCAT were lower as clinical activities for which students were engaged increased. Clinical activities included journal writing, videotaping, case studies, probing questions, supervisor modeling, supervisor stories and seeing a steady population. The authors suggest that involvement in too many activities may interfere with the development of clinical reasoning skills as students may not be able to focus on the assignments or go in depth into reasoning (Sladyk & Sheckley, 2001). Engaging in some of these activities and delving deeply into the reasoning supports therapeutic reasoning.

Evidence-Informed Professional Thinking (EIPT)

The Evidence-Informed Professional Thinking (EIPT; Benfield & Johnston, 2020) includes 32 items measuring critical clinical reasoning and evidence-informed practice behaviors. The EIPT operationalizes clinical reasoning concepts for practice. The authors completed a literature review of assessments measuring the concepts to design the scale, and the scale was reviewed by experts. Sample items indicate behaviors that promote clinical reasoning and evidence-informed practice. Box 10.3 lists sample items from both subscales. Items are rated by frequency per month (except "Prior to acting, I consider various solutions," which is rated yes/no). Rasch analysis showed that items represented a range of degree of difficulty and those respondents fell along the continuum of performance. The EIPT is a strong, interpretable, two-dimension measurement tool.

The EIPT may be useful in identifying areas for OT practitioners to explore to improve therapeutic reasoning behaviors. The initial development of the EIPT showed that the two scales within the measure identified different aspects of therapeutic reasoning (critical clinical thinking and evidence-informed practice). Since the EIPT lists behaviors associated with clinical reasoning and evidence-informed practice, OT practitioners may find value in using it as a self-evaluative tool.

The Hasselt Occupational Performance Profile (H-OPP)

The digital Hasselt Occupational Performance Profile (H-OPP) was created to enhance occupational therapy reasoning from the International Classification of Functioning (ICF) perspective. The tool considers the client's and therapist's perspective at

TABLE 10.2   Clinical Thinking and Therapeutic Reasoning Assessments

Name of Test	Description	Subscales/Categories	Scoring
California Critical Thinking Disposition Inventory (Insight Assessment, 2013)	75 Likert scale items Measures one's attributes that contribute to the disposition to engage in critical thinking.	Truth seeking Open-mindedness Systematicity Confidence Inquisitiveness Maturity	Score of 30 or below on each individual scale demonstrates weakness; 40 is minimal agreement; 50 or above indicates strength in that disposition.
California Critical Thinking Skills Test (Insight Assessment, 2016).	Examines one's critical thinking abilities in the workplace.	Analysis Inference Evaluation Deduction Induction	Low scores indicate no critical thinking; scores above 25 indicate superior skills.
Clinical Decision-Making Nursing Scale (Jenkins, 1985)	40-item self-assessment scale (5-point Likert scale) Measures one's perceived decision-making abilities in 4 processes.	1. Search for alternatives or options 2. Canvassing of objectives and values 3. Evaluation and reevaluation of consequences 4. Search for information and unbiased assimilation of new information	Total scores range from 40 to 200. The higher the score, the greater perceived decision-making ability.
Clinical Reasoning Case Analysis Test (Sladyk & Sheckley, 2001)	Measure types of reasoning used during case study analysis.	Procedural Interactive Conditional	Case study to determine types of reasoning used in practice.
The Diagnostic Thinking Inventory (Bordage et al., 1990)	Self-assessment tool that consists of 41 questions. Measures diagnostic reasoning.	Flexibility in thinking Structure of memory	
Evidence-Informed Professional Thinking (Benfield & Johnston, 2020)	32 items (rated on frequency during month) that measure behaviors that promote clinical reasoning and evidence-informed practice.	Critical clinical reasoning Evidence-informed practice	
Hasselt Occupational Performance Profile (Ghysels et al., 2017)	Digital occupational performance profile that includes template for reasoning and collaboration with client and integrates ICF with OT terminology.	• Occupational performance profile • Client and therapist views • Diagnoses translated to occupational performance • Realistic intervention plan	Results in an occupation-based client-centered occupational profile and plan that integrates ICF and OT terminology.
Health Sciences Reasoning Test (Insight Assessments, 2013).	33-item multiple choice test administered to assess clinical thinking in health professions education.	Analysis Induction Inference Evaluation Deduction	Norms exist for health professions students: scores >26 indicate superior clinical thinking skills, 21–25 strong skills, 15–20 moderate skills and <14 indicates clinical thinking is not manifested.
Lasater Clinical Judgment Rubric (Lasater, 2007)	Rubric completed by observer during nursing simulation. 11 items, rated on 4-point Likert scale of expertise: beginning, developing, accomplished and exemplary.	Noticing Interpreting Responding Reflecting	Used for clinical simulation program; has excellent reliability.
Self-Assessment of Clinical Reasoning and Reflection (Royeen et al., 2001)	26-item Likert scale questionnaire that measures one's perceptions of performance on behaviors of clinical reasoning and reflection.		Has been used with occupational therapy students to measure changes in perceptions of clinical reasoning over time (Coker, 2010; Seif et al., 2014; Scaffa & Wooster, 2004)
Yoon's Critical Thinking Disposition Tool (Yoon, 2008)	Self-assessment 27-item scale with 7 subscales that is scored on a Likert scale ranging from 0 (strong disagreement) to 5 (strong agreement).	• Objectivity • Prudence • Systematicity • Intellectual eagerness & curiosity • Intellectual fairness • Healthy skepticism • Critical thinking confidence	Scale has good reliability and demonstrates longitudinal validity in Korean nursing students.

all stages (Ghysels et al., 2017). The authors linked occupational therapy terminology with the ICF and professional reasoning to create the tool. A panel of experts determined that the most crucial features of the H-OPP include:

- The occupational performance problems and possibilities should be inventoried together with the client by analyzing the occupational performance components, abilities, and skills to create an occupational performance profile.
- Both the client's and therapist's point of view should be included in the assessment.
- Based on the assessment, a medical or psychiatric diagnosis (if present) is translated into a functional or occupational performance diagnosis.
- The H-OPP findings allow the practitioner to create a realistic intervention plan that corresponds with the client's goals and possibilities.

The H-OPP is a digital assessment tool that incorporates the reasoning process in practice. For example, Figure 10.3 outlines each of the steps and information included in the Hasselt Tool (H-OPP). The tool emphasizes a client-centered and occupation-based approach by including clients in the decision-making process. The H-OPP is used to improve or facilitate the OT reasoning process along the biopsychosocial model as it incorporates different aspects of human functioning and different steps of the reasoning process (Ghysels et al., 2017).

Self-Assessment of Clinical Reasoning and Reflection (SACRR)

Royeen and colleagues (2001) created the Self-Assessment of Clinical Reflection and Reasoning (SACRR) which measures practitioners' perceptions of their clinical reflection and reasoning. The questionnaire consists of 26 statements rated on a 5-point Likert scale (5 [strongly agree] to 1 [strongly disagree]). Box 10.4 lists sample items representing behaviors associated with clinical reasoning and reflection.

Scaffa and Wooster (2004) used the SACRR to examine occupational therapists' perceptions of their clinical reasoning before and after a PBL course. The researchers found statistically significant increases from pre- and posttest scores for 11 of 26 items on the SACRR and the total score increased from 96.88 to 102.55 (p <.01). Coker (2010) used the SACRR and the California Critical Thinking Skills Test (CCTST) to measure effects of a 1-week, experiential hands-on learning program on critical thinking and clinical reasoning skills of occupational therapy students. Coker (2010) reported significant improvements on 22 of the 26 items of the SACRR from pretest to posttest (p < .05) and for the CCTST (p < .05).

Seif et al. (2014) found that students who participated in an interprofessional service-learning course and volunteered at a student-run free clinic showed improved perceptions of clinical reasoning skills when compared to a control group (p = .0002). Specifically, students showed significantly higher SACRR ratings on items regarding making judgments, comparing, and contrasting information about a client's problems, using frames of reference for planning, identifying assumptions underlying differing views, and considering what would make a strategy work (Seif et al., 2014). The authors suggest that the changes in pre to post scores is due to the clinical reflections (students completed 5 reflections with feedback from the instructor after an experience at the student-run free clinic).

O'Brien and Patnaude (2019) found statistically significant increases for two consecutive cohorts of occupational therapy students (n = 90) in pre- to posttest total scores (p < .05) on the SACRR following a semester-long case-based integration course.

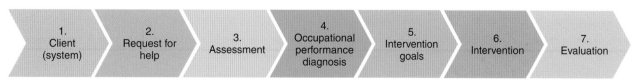

Figure 10.3 Stages of the Hasselt Occupational Performance Profile (From Ghysels et al., 2016.)

ASSESSMENTS OF THERAPEUTIC RELATIONSHIPS

The Intentional Relationship Model (IRM; Taylor, 2020) provides a variety of assessments to examine one's therapeutic use of self. Being aware of one's therapeutic communication strengths and challenges informs practitioners of how they interact with a variety of clients. The assessments are available on the IRM clearinghouse. These assessments are currently undergoing research for psychometric properties and clinical utility. See Table 10.3 for a summary of the assessments.

The Self-Assessment of Modes Questionnaire (SAMQ; Taylor et al., 2013) identifies a therapist's preferred mode use. The therapist completes the questionnaire by indicating how they would most likely respond to interpersonal issues that arise in therapy. This assessment provides therapists with the pattern of mode use that they prefer so that therapists can understand how to maximize use of preferred modes and develop less preferred modes. For example, the OT practitioner's results on the SAMQ indicate strong preferences for instructing, encouraging, and problem-solving modes. The practitioner may benefit from developing skills in advocating, collaborating, and empathizing modes. Gaining skills outside of their comfort zone may help him/her be more effective with all clients.

The Clinical Assessment of Modes (CAM) (Fan & Taylor, 2016; Taylor & Popova, 2019a) questionnaires come in four variations and assess the communication between the client and therapist. The questionnaires include CAM-Client Time 1 which is administered to the client prior to therapy to determine the client's preferred mode of communication. CAM-Client Time 2 is administered after a designated time to assess the client's perception of what modes the therapist used. The CAM-Therapists version is administered after a designated period to assess the therapist's perceptions of what modes the therapist believed they used during the observation period. The CAM-Observer is completed by an observer to get an objective opinion from someone else of therapeutic modes used.

The Clinical Assessment of Therapeutic Response (CATR) (Taylor, 2008) comes in observer and provider versions. The CATR-Observer version measures the patient–provider interaction from an observer's perspective. The CATR-Provider version measures the patient–provider interaction from the provider's perspective.

Clinical Assessment of Sub-optimal Interactions (CASI) (Taylor & Popova, 2019b) measures the frequency and type of sub-optimal interactions present within the therapist–client communication. This assessment comes in provider, observer, and client forms. It also comes in 36-item or 15-item formats. *Sub-optimal interactions* are those that interfere with, slow down, or impede the therapeutic relationship. For example, a practitioner may make a humorous comment that is misinterpreted by the client. The client may feel distant from the therapist and not as trusting. Box 10.5 provides sample items. Items are rated on a four-point rating scale (0 = never; 1 = rarely; 2 = occasionally; 3 = frequently); the versions include a 15-item and 36-item scale.

Self-efficacy of the Therapeutic Use of Self

Self-efficacy refers to a person's belief that they have the skills and abilities to do those things they want to do (Bandura, 1997; Kielhofner, 2008). Taylor (2020) suggests that practitioners can develop and nurture therapeutic relationships by increasing their awareness and competency in using a variety of modes (Bonsaksen & Carstensen, 2018). While understanding a

TABLE 10.3 Assessments Based on the Intentional Relationship Model

Assessment	Description
Self-Assessment of Modes Questionnaire (SAMQ) (Version 11) Taylor et al. (2013)	Designed to assist therapists in identifying preferred mode use during therapy sessions. It is self-administered to determine preferential mode use as a therapist during interactions with a client.
Clinical Assessment of Modes (CAM) Fan & Taylor (2016) Taylor & Popova (2019a)	Designed to estimate the communication styles used between the client and therapist, and to provide an opinion of a third-party observer. CAM assessments are self-report questionnaires with 30 items, using a 5-point Likert scale.
Clinical Assessment of Therapeutic Response (CATR) Taylor (2008)	Designed to better understand the different ways that healthcare providers communicate with their patients in therapy. CATR measures patient–provider interactions based on the IRM.
Clinical Assessment of Sub-optimal Interactions (CASI) Taylor & Popova (2019b)	Designed to measure the frequency and type of sub-optimal interactions present within provider–client communication. Three distinct assessments to capture the perspectives of the client, provider, or a third-party observer. Comes in original (30 items) or short form (15 items).

BOX 10.5 Sample Items on the CASI

The therapist was emotionally distant, too formal and/or was not fully present for the child.

The therapist focused too much on the child's problems and not enough on his or her feelings or experience of treatment.

The therapist used technical language or did not speak to the child in a way the child fully understood.

The therapists said things in a way that made the child feel anxious or pessimistic about his or her situation/condition.

The therapist talked over the child, interrupted the child, and/or did not stop to hear what the child was saying.

BOX 10.6 The Self-efficacy for Therapeutic Use of Self Scale

Self-Efficacy for Therapeutic Mode Use

When I work with clients I am confident in my ability to:

1. Advocate
2. Problem-solve
3. Instruct
4. Encourage
5. Empathize
6. Collaborate

Self-Efficacy for Recognizing Interpersonal Characteristics

I am confident in my ability to recognize my clients':

1. Preference for communication style
2. Capacity for trust
3. Need for control
4. Capacity to assert needs
5. Response to change or challenge
6. Affect
7. Predisposition to giving feedback
8. Predisposition to receiving feedback
9. Response to human diversity
10. Orientation towards relating
11. Preference for touch
12. Capacity for reciprocity

Self-Efficacy for Managing Interpersonal Events

When I work with clients I am confident in my ability to manage:

1. Expression of strong emotion
2. Intimate self-disclosure
3. Power dilemmas
4. Non-verbal cues
5. Crisis points
6. Resistance and reluctance
7. Boundary testing
8. Empathic breaks
9. Emotionally charged tasks and situations
10. Limitations of therapy
11. Contextual inconsistencies

All items are scored between 1 (lowest possible self-efficacy) and 10 (highest possible self-efficacy).

From Hussain, R.A., Carstensen, T., Yazdani, F., Ellingham, B., & Bonsaksen, T. (2018). Short-term changes in occupational therapy students' self-efficacy for therapeutic use of self. *British Journal of Occupational Therapy, 81*(5), 276–284.

---

practitioner's preferred mode use provides important information, Bonsaksen and Carstensen (2018) suggest that it is also important to understand how one feels about their ability to use the modes.

The self-efficacy scales consist of a 3-part self-report questionnaire based on Yazdani and Tune (2016 questionnaire) (see Box 10.6) (Hussain et al., 2018). All sections require respondents to rate statements on a scale of 1 (lowest possible self-efficacy) and 10 (highest possible self-efficacy). The Self-Efficacy for Therapeutic Mode Use (SETMU) was designed to measure the practitioner's confidence in using each of the 6 modes. The Self-Efficacy for Recognizing Interpersonal Characteristics (SERIC) consists of 12 statements referring to communication (e.g., preference for communication style, capacity for trust, need for control, affect, response to change or challenge), and the Self-Efficacy for Managing Interpersonal Events (SEMIE) consists of 11 statements referring to managing interpersonal events, such as power dilemmas, crisis points, boundary testing, empathetic breaks.

These scales have been translated into Norwegian and used with students (Bonsaksen et al., 2016; Bonsaksen & Carstensen, 2018; Ritter et al., 2018). Students (n = 89) improved self-efficacy for therapeutic mode use, for recognizing clients' interpersonal characteristics, and for managing interpersonal events from time 1 (after a use of self-workshop) to 3 months and maintained at 10 months (Schwank et al., 2018).

ACTIVITIES TO PROMOTE REFLECTION AND THERAPEUTIC REASONING

Figure 10.4 illustrates some activities to promote therapeutic reasoning. Reflection on shared practice through community of practice group, supervision, or mentorship supports practitioners in identifying dilemmas around therapeutic activity and clarifying concepts and reasoning (Marcolino et al., 2019). By applying a systematic and synthesizing framework to evaluation and intervention planning that requires the practitioner to describe their rationale and support for decisions, the reasoning process becomes more routine. The habitual nature of this process makes it easier for practitioners to put into words what they are doing. Some OT practitioners report they "just do it automatically" when in fact they learned the reasoning skills through the systematic process. Experienced practitioners use this intuitive knowledge to guide practice decisions whereas beginner professionals rely on facts, procedures, and protocols (Adam et al., 2013; Marcolino et al., 2019). Therefore, engaging in mentorship or supervisory discussions allows the experienced therapist to revisit theory and explicitly define his/her rationale for decisions, which strengthens their practice decisions. It allows the novice therapist the opportunity to work through the reasoning process more effectively. Both professionals benefit by reflecting on actions, exploring the reasons, beliefs, values, cultures, and theoretical conceptions of their actions, evaluating if there is coherence between what they think and do, and explaining their understanding of concepts (Marcolino et al., 2019).

Writing reflective journals about therapeutic experiences allows students and practitioners to examine their own thinking

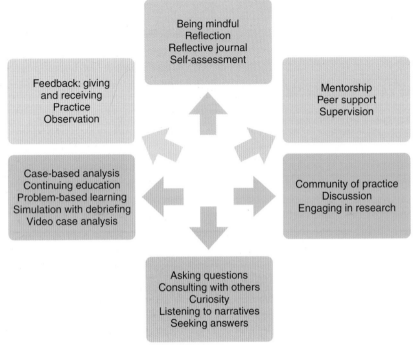

Figure 10.4 Activities to Promote Therapeutic Reasoning.

process to gain insight regarding their clinical reasoning skills (Falk-Kessler & Ciaravino, 2006). Recognizing the importance of the narrative helped students appreciate another person's experience, integrate ideas about how people cope, ask other questions, and gain a deeper understanding of the experiences of the client's situation. Students who wrote reflective journals showed greater self-awareness, recognized the importance of individuals telling their stories, learned to identify and to ask questions for clarification, and described greater insight into conditions (Falk-Kessler & Ciaravino, 2006).

Engaging in experiential activities such as simulation, problem-based learning, team-based learning, and case-based analysis requires students and OT practitioners to provide evidence for their decisions and reflect upon outcomes, which enhances reasoning for future cases (Giles et al., 2014; Macauley et al., 2017; Seif et al., 2014). As students and practitioners engage in this process repeatedly, they learn the process and can complete it more easily with more depth of thought. The key to therapeutic reasoning is to engage in it mindfully, be receptive to giving and receiving feedback, and keep searching for answers.

Video cases provide additional opportunities for students and practitioners to enhance their observation and reasoning skills. Working through the case by observing the client and OT practitioner interact provides additional information that is not found in written cases and can model different intervention strategies (see video cases on the Evolve learning site). Practitioners and students can also observe themselves in a video and reflect upon their performance. This has been found to be an effective teaching tool for simulation experiences (Giles et al., 2014). The following Learning Activity by Dr. Patee Tomsic provides an example of how to structure a video case study to promote therapeutic reasoning and reflection.

LEARNING ACTIVITY: VIDEO CASE STUDY BY DR. PATEE TOMSIC

Answer the Guiding Questions while viewing the video clip (available on the Evolve learning site).

Learning objectives

1. Identify theories or frameworks that are used to justify occupational therapy intervention in stroke rehabilitation.
2. Apply aspects of the occupational therapy domains (e.g., occupations, contexts, performance patterns, performance skills, client factors) of the *Occupational Therapy Practice Framework*, 4th edition, to stroke rehabilitation.
3. Justify the use of appropriate evaluation methods in stroke rehabilitation.
4. Produce objective and measurable documentation with accuracy in clinical detail, format, grammar, and spelling.
5. Demonstrate therapeutic use of self and professional communication skills to participate in therapeutic interactions with clients.

In preparation for the scenario seen in this case study and its accompanying critical thinking questions, review of the following skills and information is recommended:

- Stroke and indications, contraindications for OT intervention
- Diabetes mellitus and indications, contraindications for OT intervention
- Safety considerations for OT intervention in clients with hemiparesis
- Transfers with stroke
- Frames of reference for stroke intervention
  - Task-oriented training
  - Biomechanical frame of reference
  - Model of Human Occupation (MOHO)
- Documentation in the inpatient rehabilitation setting
- Goal-writing in the inpatient rehabilitation setting

Introduction

The video begins with an occupational therapist greeting her client, Mr. Conway Dean, and explaining their first treatment intervention for the day. Mr. Dean is currently admitted to an inpatient rehabilitation unit and the two talk at his bedside, where he is already dressed and ready for the day.

Continued

Patient Information

Name: Conway Dean

DOB: 3-18-1957

Age: 64 years

Reason for referral to OT: Mr. Conway Dean demonstrates right hemiparesis secondary to left ischemic stroke presenting with decreased independence in ADL and IADL. Prior to his stroke, Mr. Dean was independent with all occupations.

Client history: Conway Dean is a 64-year-old male who presents to occupational therapy following L CVA. Medical history is significant for diabetes mellitus, well controlled with medication and lifestyle (e.g., diet, physical activity).

Guiding Questions

1. What did you observe in the video case study that went well?
2. What did you observe in the video case study that could have gone better or that you would have done differently?
3. In the first activity seen in the video, Mr. Dean participates in a strengthening activity targeting his core muscles. What does the OT do to tie this activity to function?
4. Why does the OT use a bedsheet to assist with this intervention?
5. At the end of this activity, Mr. Dean transfers to sitting edge of bed moving toward his affected side. How might this transfer look different if he transferred toward his non-affected side?
6. In the context of the *Occupational Therapy Practice Framework 4*, what performance skills are being targeted while Mr. Dean sorts his tools sitting at the edge of the bed?
7. Did this activity provide the "just-right challenge" for Mr. Dean? How could the activity be graded up to increase the challenge? How could it be graded down to decrease the challenge?
8. What intervention approach or method is the therapist utilizing in this activity? Justify your answer.
9. After watching the activity where Mr. Dean puts away the meal preparation items, using the OTPF 4, identify client factors that would potentially impact his performance in this task.
10. What safety considerations should the therapist be considering for this sit-to-stand activity with Mr. Dean?
11. Why does the therapist instruct Mr. Dean to bend his elbow when weight-bearing through his right arm?
12. After watching the entire video, what evaluation tools (e.g., client interview, standardized assessments, client checklists, etc.) could have been used to evaluate Mr. Dean?
13. Write at least two potential goals that could have been written for Mr. Dean based on the treatment interventions and activities observed.

The Importance of Feedback

Receiving feedback regarding one's therapeutic reasoning and interactions with clients from clients, supervisors, and through self-reflection is part of occupational therapy practice. Students and OT practitioners who are aware of their own strengths and challenges, may be more open to feedback. Constructive feedback from a trusted professional may be easier to hear. Examining one's feelings and addressing those feelings to improve one's therapeutic use of self and reasoning in practice benefits clients and their families.

Students and OT practitioners may want to seek out feedback by asking their supervisor for specific feedback on something they want to improve. For example, an OT student received feedback from her supervisor that her initial evaluation with a client was insufficient since she did not "connect" with the client or put the client at ease. The student, known for her excellent social skills, was devastated. However, upon reflection, the student recognized she was extremely nervous and wanted to make sure she completed the initial evaluation form carefully and accurately. Based on this feedback, the student practiced asking open-ended questions and familiarized herself with the evaluation format (moving some things around to fit her style). She practiced with a peer and then asked her supervisor to observe her. The student stated, "I have been working on ways to improve my connections with clients during the initial evaluation. Could you let me know if the changes I made in the flow of the evaluation and my opening comments help?"

In this example, the student is more likely to receive constructive feedback on her performance that will help her in practice. The student is showing her supervisor she heard the feedback, reflected upon it, and would like more feedback. The supervisor will look at the student's opening comments and flow of the evaluation. Being specific about the feedback you want to hear helps both parties.

LEARNING ACTIVITY: FEEDBACK

Use Worksheet 10.11. Describe feedback you received from someone about your performance.
- Describe how you addressed the feedback.
- Describe an alternate way to address the feedback.
- How might you reframe the feedback?

LEARNING ACTIVITY: REFLECTION FROM THERAPISTS AND EDUCATORS

Review the short video clips 10.4–10.11 (on the Evolve learning site) from therapists and educators discussing reflection in occupational therapy. Complete Worksheet 10.12. Summarize the presenters' thoughts upon reflection in practice.

SUMMARY

Therapeutic reasoning involves processing information and making decisions by combining the art and science of therapy. OT practitioners consider the person, occupation, and environment when determining how to intervene to enable clients to engage in meaningful activities. This process requires blending knowledge, evidence, and processes with the OT practitioner's personality style, communication, and use of self to match the client's personality, communication style, and interactive nature. Therapeutic reasoning is a complex process that can be observed in practice as the OT practitioner engages in generating questions based on theory, gathering data, identifying occupational challenges, creating intervention plans, and assessing outcomes. At each step of the process, the OT practitioner engages in reasoning. Assessments of clinical reasoning and critical thinking describe strategies and behaviors throughout the process (i.e., I question how, what, and why I do things in practice; sought information from peers to help solve a clinical dilemma). Experiential learning activities, such as problem-based learning, case-based analysis, and simulation experiences provided with opportunities to discuss reasoning support professional growth. Reflective writing, mentorship, supervision, and receiving and responding to feedback are all strategies to enhance reasoning skills. OT practitioners who engage in reflection, assess their own abilities, value self-awareness, critically analyze evidence, and remain curious life-long learners develop advanced therapeutic reasoning skills to benefit clients and their families.

REFERENCES

Adam, K., Peters, S., & Chipcase, I. (2013). Knowledge, skills, and professional behaviors required by occupational therapist and physiotherapist beginning practitioners in work-related practice: a systematic review. *Australian Occupational Therapy Journal*, 60(2), 75–84.

American Occupational Therapy Association (AOTA). (2020). *Occupational Therapy Practice Framework: Domain and Process* (4th ed.). North Bethesda, MD: AOTA.

Andrews, J. (2000). The value of reflective practice: a student case study. *British Journal of Occupational Therapy*, 63(8), 396–398.

Bandura, A. (1997). *Self-efficacy: the exercise of control*. New York: W.H. Freeman and Company.

Benfield, A. M., & Johnston, M. V. (2020). Initial development of a measure of evidence-informed professional thinking. *Australian Occupational Therapy Journal*, 67, 308–319.

Bonsaksen, T., Kvarsnes, H., Eirum, MN., Torgrimsen S., & Hussain, R.A. (2016). Developemtn and content validity of the Norwegian Self-Assessment of Modes Questionnaire (N-SAMQ), *Scandinavian Journal of Occupational Therapy*, 23(4), 253–259.

Bonsaksen, T., & Carstensen, T. (2018). Psychometric properties of the Norwegian self-efficacy for therapeutic mode use (N-SETMU). *Scandinavian Journal of Occupational Therapy*, 25(6), 475–480.

Bordage, G., Grant, J., & Marsden, P. (1990). Qualitative assessment of diagnostic ability. *Medical Education*, 24(5), 413–425.

Boud, D. (2001). Usng journal writing to enhance reflective practice. *New Directions for Adult and Continuing Education*, 90, 9–17.

Boud, D., & Walker, D. (1990). Making the most of experience. *Studies in Continuing Education*, 12, 67.

Carrier, A., Levasseur, M., Bedard, D., & Desrosiers, J. (2012). Clinical reasoning process underlying choice of teaching strategies: a framework to improve occupational therapists' transfer skill interventions. *Australian Occupational Journal*, 59, 355–366.

Cheung, T. W. C., Clemson, L., O'Loughlin, K., & Shuttleworth, R. (2018). Ergonomic education on housework for women with upper limb repetitive strain injury (RSI): a conceptual representation of therapists' clinical reasoning. *Disability and Rehabilitation*, 40(26), 3136–3146.

Coker, P. (2010). Effects of an experiential learning program on the clinical reasoning and critical thinking skills of occupational therapy students. *Journal of Allied Health*, 39(4), 280–286.

Falk-Kessler, J., & Ciaravino, E. A. (2006). Student reflections as evidence of interactive clinical reasoning skills. *Occupational Therapy in Health Care*, 20(2), 75–88.

Fan, C.W., & Taylor, R.R. (2016). Assessing therapeutic communication during rehabilitation: The Clinical Assessment of Modes. *American Journal of Occupational Therapy*, 70, 7004280010.

Ghysels, R., Vanroye, E., Westhovens, M., & Spooren, A. (2017). A tool to enhance occupational therapy reasoning from ICF perspective: The Hasselt Occupational Performance Profile (H-OPP). *Scandinavian Journal of Occupational Therapy*, 24(2), 128–135.

Gibbs, G. (1998). *Learning by doing: a guide to teaching and learning methods*. Oxford Brookes University.

Giles, A. K., Carson, N. E., Breland, H. L., Coker-Bolt, P., & Bowman, P. J. (2014). Conference Proceedings – Use of simulated patients and reflective video analysis to assess occupational therapy students' preparedness for fieldwork. *American Journal of Occupational Therapy*, 68, 557–566.

Guy, L., Cranwell, K., Hitch, D., & McKinstry, C. (2020). Reflective practice facilitation within occupational therapy supervision processes: a mixed method study. *Australian Occupational Therapy Journal*, 67, 320–329.

Hussain, R. A., Carstensen, T., Yazdani, F., Ellingham, B., & Bonsaksen, T. (2018). Short-term changes in occupational therapy students' self-efficacy for therapeutic use of self. *British Journal of Occupational Therapy*, 81(5), 276–284.

Ikiugu, M., & Smallfield, S. (2010). Interrater, intra-rater and internal consistency reliability of the Theory Application and Assessment Instrument. *Australian Occupational Therapy Journal*, 57, 253–260.

Insight Assessment. (2013). Health sciences reasoning test. http://www.insightassessment.com/

Insight Assessment. (2016). California critical thinking skills test. http://www.insightassessment.com/

Jenkins, H. M. (1985). A research tool for measuring perceptions of clinical decision making. *Journal Professional Nursing*, 1(4), 221–229.

Keiller, L., & Hanekom, S. D. (2013). Strategies to increase clinical reasoning in physiotherapy education. *Journal of Physiology*, 70(1), 8–12.

Kielhofner, G. (Ed.), (2008). *Model of Human Occupation: Theory and application* (4th ed.). Baltimore, MD: Lippincott Williams & Wilkins.

Kwaitek, E. (2005). Self-awareness and reflection; exploring the 'therapeutic use of self'. *Learning Disability Practice*, 8(3), 27–31.

Lapointe, J., Craik, J., & Loiselle, C. G. (2017). Appraising potential cognitive biases impeding clinical and professional reasoning in occupational therapy practice. *Occupational Therapy Now*, 19(6), 8–10.

Lasater, K. (2007). Clinical judgement development: Using simulation to create an assessment rubric. *Journal of Nursing Education*, 16(11), 496–503.

Macauley, K., Brudvig, T. J., Kadakia, M., & Bonneville, M. (2017). Systematic review of assessments that evaluate clinical decision making, clinical reasoning, and critical thinking changes after simulation participation. *Journal of Physical Therapy Education*, 31(4), 64–75.

Marcolino, T. Q., Von Poellnitz, J. C., Silva, C. R., Villares, C. C., & Reali, A. M. M. R. (2019). "And a door opens": reflections on conceptual and identity issues on clinical reasoning in occupational therapy. *Cadernos Brasileiros de Terapia Occupacional*, 27(9), 403–411.

Merriam-Webster (n.d.). Attitude. In Merriam-Webster.com dictionary. Retrieved from https://www.merriam-webster.com/dictionary/attitude.

Merriam-Webster (n.d.). Self-awareness. In Merriam-Webster.com dictionary. Retrieved from https://www.merriam-webster.com/dictionary/self-awareness.

O'Brien, J., & Patnaude, M. B. (April 5, 2019). Scholarship of teaching and learning: Creative strategies to promote and measure clinical reasoning in occupational therapy students. [poster]. New Orleans: AOTA Annual Conference.

Popova, E. S., & Taylor, R. R. (2020a). Reliability and validity of the Clinical Assessment of Sub-optimal Interaction in outpatient pediatric rehabilitation. *Occupational Therapy in Mental Health, 36*(2), 176–187.

Popova, E. S., & Taylor, R. R. (2020b). Evaluating students' use of therapeutic communication in entry-level education: The observer version of the Clinical Assessment of Modes (CAM-Observer). *American Journal of Occupational Therapy, 74*(5), 7405205130.

Popova, E. S., Ostrowski, R. K., Wong, S. R., & Taylor, R. R. (2020). Reliability and validity of the Pediatric Clinical Assessment of Modes in outpatient pediatric rehabilitation. *British Journal of Occupational Therapy, 83*(8), 516–523.

Ritter, V. C., Yazdani, F., Carstensen, T., Thorrisen, M. M., & Bonsaksen, T. (2018). Psychometric properties of an instrument derived from the Intentional Relationship Model: The Self-Efficacy for Recognizing clients; Interpersonal Characteristics (N-SERIC). *The Open Journal of Occupational Therapy, 6*(2), 7. Article.

Royeen, C., Mu, K., Barrett, K., & Luebben, A. J. (2001). Pilot investigation: evaluation of clinical reflection and reasoning before and after workshop intervention. In P. Crist (Ed.), *Innovations in Occupational Therapy Education* (pp. 107–114). North Bethesda, MD: American Occupational Therapy Association.

Scaffa, M. E., & Wooster, D. M. (2004). Brief report- effects of problem-based learning on clinical reasoning in occupational therapy. *American Journal of Occupational Therapy, 58*, 333–336.

Schwank, K., Carstensen, T., Yazdani, F., & Bonsaksen, T. (2018). The course of self-efficacy for therapeutic use of self in Norwegian occupational therapy students: a 10-month follow-up study. *Occupational Therapy International, 2018*, 2962747.

Schwartzberg, S. (2002). *Interactive reasoning in the practice of occupational therapy*. Upper Saddle River, NJ: Prentice Hall.

Seif, G., Coker-Bolt, P., Kraft, S., Gonsalves, W., Simpson, K., & Johnson, E. (2014). The development of clinical reasoning and interprofessional behaviors: service-learning at a student-run free clinic. *Journal of Interprofessional Care, 28*(6), 559–564.

Sladyk, K., & Sheckley, B. (2001). Clinical reasoning and reflective practice: Implications for fieldwork activities. *Occupational Therapy in Health Care, 13*(1), 11–22.

Spalding, N. J. (1998). Reflectionin professional development: a personal experience. *British Journal of Therapy and Rehabilitation, 5*(7), 379–382.

Taylor, R. (2008). *The intentional relationship: Occupational therapy and use of self*. Philadelphia, PA: FA Davis.

Taylor, R. (2020). *The intentional relationship: Occupational therapy and use of self* (2nd ed.). Philadelphia, PA: FA Davis.

Taylor, R. R., Ivey, C., Shepherd, J., Simons, D., Brown, J., Huddle, M., … Steele, R. (2013a). *Self-assessment of modes questionnaire – version II*. Chicago, IL: University of Illinois at Chicago.

Taylor, R.R. & Popova, E. (2019a). Clinical Assessment of Modes-Therapist. Version 2.0. Chicago, IL: University of Illinois at Chicago.

Taylor, R.R. & Popova, E. (2019b). Assessment of Sub-optimal Interaction. Version 1. Chicago, IL: University of Illinois at Chicago.

Turner, A., & Alsop, A. (2015). Unique core skills: Exploring occupational therapists' hidden assets. *British Journal of Occupational Therapy, 78*(12), 739–749.

Yazdani, F., Stringer, A., Nobakht, L., Bonsaksen, T., & Tune, K. (2020). Qualitative analysis of occupational therapists' reflective notes on practicing their skills in building and maintaining therapeutic relationships. *Journal of Occupational Therapy Education, 4*(4). Available at. https://encompass.eku.edu/jotevo4/iss4/14.

Yoon, J. (2008). The degree of critical thinking disposition in nursing students and the factors influencing critical thinking disposition. *Journal of Korean Academy of Nursing Administration, 14*, 159–166.

Worksheets

WORKSHEET 10.1: THE ART AND SCIENCE OF THERAPY

Use Worksheet 10.1 to identify aspects of the art and science of therapy after reading the following case example.

Case example: A 55-year-old schoolteacher and mother of 3 teenagers is experiencing a severe exacerbation of multiple sclerosis, requiring hospitalization. She is receiving occupational services in an acute rehabilitation setting.

- Provide examples of the art and science of therapy.
- Describe the interaction between the art and science of therapy as related to this case.

The Art and Science of Therapy	
Name:	
	Examples related to case
Science of Therapy	
Art of Therapy	
Describe the interaction between the art and science of therapy as related to this case.	

WORKSHEET 10.2: COGNITIVE BIASES

Use Worksheet 10.2. Create a personal example of each of the types of biases.

- What other biases might influence decision-making?

Cognitive Biases	
Name:	
Cognitive bias	**Personal Example**
Early decision making	
Rule of thumb	
Recent exposure	
Lack of evidence	
Ignoring alternatives	
What other biases might influence decision-making?	

WORKSHEET 10.3: ATTITUDES, ATTRIBUTIONS, VALUES, AND OPINIONS

Complete Worksheet 10.3 to identify your attitudes, attributions, values, and opinions on a certain topic.
- How might you use this knowledge in practice?

Attitudes, Attributions, Values, and Opinions
Name:
Describe a specific topic:
Attitudes:
Attributions:
Values:
Opinions:
How might you use this knowledge in practice?

WORKSHEET 10.4: PREPARATORY REFLECTION

Case Example: Javier is a 35-year-old man who experienced a cardiac event, requiring triple bypass surgery 24 hours ago. He is a patient in an acute care hospital where you are the OT.

Use Worksheet 10.4 to engage in preparatory reflection as you prepare to meet Javier.
- Describe your style, experience, and knowledge.
- Identify questions that you have regarding the case and context.

Preparatory Reflection
Name:
Interaction style:
Experience:
Knowledge:
Questions regarding the client and context:
What do you want to know about the client?
How will you organize the session? Why?

WORKSHEET 10.5: REFLECTION IN ACTION

Complete Worksheet 10.5 as you observe an intervention session (see Evolve learning site).
- Describe the practitioner's actions and the client's responses.
- Describe possible reasons for the actions and responses.

Reflection in action		
Describe the setting		
List 3 Tasks	**OT practitioner's action**	**Client's response**
Describe possible reasons for the actions and responses.		
List 3 Tasks	**Client's action**	**OT practitioner's response**
Describe possible reasons for the actions and responses.		

WORKSHEET 10.6: REFLECTION ON ACTION

Use Worksheet 10.6 to reflect upon the intervention session (see video clip on Evolve learning site).

Reflection on action
Name:
Brief description of intervention session:
Identify the model of practice or frame of reference used during the session.
Describe the reason for the selection.
What strategies worked? Why?
What strategies did not work? Why?
How did the client respond to the session? (Give specifics)
Why do you think the client responded in that way?
What else could the therapist have done?

WORKSHEET 10.7: REFLECTIVE WRITING

Complete Worksheet 10.7 to practice reflective writing to promote therapeutic reasoning. Select one of the following prompts:
- Describe a recent experience with a friend.
- Describe a learning experience of which you are proud.
- Describe a therapy session (evaluation or intervention) with a client.

Reflective Writing
Name:
Prompt:
Describe what happened.
Who was there?
How did you feel?
How do you think the others felt?
What supported this?
What interfered with this event?
Would you change any of your actions?
What other things could have been done?
Describe the setting.
What resources were needed for this event?
Describe personal factors influencing the event.
Describe environmental factors (such as time, cultural, expectations, attitudes) associated with the event.

WORKSHEET 10.8: REFLECTING ON THEORY IN PRACTICE

Review videos (such as 10.1A, 10.1B, 10.2A on the Evolve learning site) and then complete complete Worksheet 10.8 questions from the Theory Application Assessment Instrument (Ikiugu & Smallfield, 2010).

Theory Application Assessment Instrument (Ikiugu & Smallfield, 2010)
a. Describe the instruments and procedures that you would use to assess the client to determine her occupational performance issues of concern.
b. Identify the occupational performance issues that need to be addressed in occupational therapy intervention based on assessment using the instruments and procedures identified above.
c. Establish short- and long-term goals to address identified issues.
d. Describe the activities, procedures, and strategies that you would use to address the identified issues so that the client's goals are achieved.
e. Please identify the occupational therapy theoretical conceptual practice model(s) that you used to guide the assessment and intervention planning to address the client's occupational performance issues. List them.
Please explain why you chose each of the theoretical conceptual practice models listed above.
Explain how you used each of the models to guide client assessment and treatment planning.

From Ikiugu, M., & Smallfield, S. (2010). Interrater, intra-rater and internal consistency reliability of the Theory Application and Assessment Instrument. *Australian Occupational Therapy Journal, 57,* 253–260.

WORKSHEET 10.9: SELF-ASSESSMENT

Select one of the therapeutic reasoning assessments from Table 10.2. Complete the assessment on yourself and describe your findings (strengths and challenges).

Self-Assessment
Name:
Date:
Brief description of assessment:
Findings (scores):
Interpretation of findings (indicate your strengths and challenges)
Were the findings what you expected?
How might you use the findings in practice?
Other comments and reflections:

WORKSHEET 10.10: THERAPEUTIC COMMUNICATION ASSESSMENTS

Complete the Observer version of one of the following: Clinical Assessment of Modes (CAM); Clinical Assessment of Therapeutic Responses (CATR); or Clinical Assessment of Sub-optimal Interactions (CLASI) by watching a video clip (from the Evolve site).

    Reflect upon the findings using Worksheet 10.10 as your guide.

- Describe your findings.
- How do the findings guide therapeutic reasoning decisions?

Therapeutic Communication Assessments
Name:
Date:
Brief description of video clip:
Brief description of assessment:
Findings (scores):
Observations:
Interpretation of findings (indicate strengths and challenges):
How do the findings guide therapeutic reasoning decisions?
Other comments and reflections:

WORKSHEET 10.11: FEEDBACK

Use Worksheet 10.11. Describe feedback you received from someone about your performance.
- Describe how you addressed the feedback.
- Describe an alternate way to address the feedback.
- How might you reframe the feedback?

Feedback
Describe the feedback you received.
Describe the situation in which you received feedback.
Describe how you addressed the feedback.
Why did you address it in that way?
Describe an alternative way to address the feedback.
How might you reframe the feedback?
How could you use the feedback to make positive changes?

WORKSHEET 10.12: REFLECTION FROM THERAPISTS AND EDUCATORS

Review the short video clips (10.4–10.11 on the Evolve learning site) from therapists and educators discussing reflection in occupational therapy. Complete Worksheet 10.12. Summarize the presenter's thoughts upon reflection in practice.

Reflection from Therapists and Educators	
Presenter	**Thoughts on Reflection/Lessons Learned**
Write one paragraph summarizing the overarching themes that emerged from hearing the speakers.	

A

Abstract thought: ability to think about things that are not actually present (Merriam-Webster, n.d).

Adjourning: signals an end to the team or case.

Advanced beginner: level of development where practitioners develop their comfort with procedures, see more clients, and reflect upon their work; they recognize additional cues and see clients as individuals.

Art of therapy: blending one's knowledge with therapeutic use of self, considered essential to therapeutic effectiveness (Turner & Alsop, 2015).

Assessment: specific tools used during the evaluation process to understand the client's occupational profile, client factors, performance skills, performance patterns, personal and environmental factors, and provide measurements (Hinojosa & Kramer, 2014).

Attitude: one's position or emotion toward a fact (Merriam-Webster, n.d.).

Attributions: meaning given to an event or behavior (Kwaitek, 2005).

B

Biomechanical frame of reference: approach that emphasizes the role of range of motion, muscle strength, and endurance on movement.

Brainstorming: technique that facilitates creativity; allows students and practitioners to think through multiple solutions and scenarios.

C

Case–control study: exploratory study that compares two groups of people: those with the disease or condition under study (cases) and a very similar group of people who do not have the disease or condition (controls).

Case series: type of study that tracks subjects who have received a similar treatment or examines their medical records for exposure and outcome.

Case report: a retrospective in-depth analysis describing an individual, single group, or event.

Cognitive biases: one's predisposition to reach a decision based on limited information.

Cognitive processes: making sense of information through one's thoughts, experiences, and senses (Cherry, 2020).

Cognitive strategy: "mental plan of action that helps a person to learn, problem-solve, and perform. The use of cognitive strategies can improve an individual's learning, problem-solving, and task performance in terms of efficiency, speed, accuracy, and consistency" (Toglia et al., 2012, p. 227).

Cohort study: exploratory longitudinal study that follows a cohort (group of subjects that share similar characteristics) that is exposed to treatment or diagnosis and compares effects to a comparison group not exposed to treatment to describe potential relationships.

Competent: level of reasoning whereby the practitioner has a broader understanding of the client's problems and is likely to individualize intervention (using narrative reasoning); they see more facts and observe more so they can prioritize goals and intervention. However, they have difficulty with flexibility and creativity.

Complementary models: two models of practice or frames of reference that are used together for one client; the models may shift throughout the OT process as the practitioner focuses on different goals and priorities (Ikiugu et al., 2009).

Conceptualization: formation of an idea of something (Merriam-Webster, n.d.), which may include creating hypotheses regarding what is influencing behaviors.

Conceptual practice models: diverse concepts organized into unique occupational therapy theory that provides a rationale and guide to practice (Kielhofner, 2004).

Context: construct that constitutes the complete makeup of a person's life as well as the common and divergent factor that characterize groups and populations. Context includes environmental factors and personal factors (AOTA, 2020).

Conditional reasoning: involves examining multiple aspects and using multiple types of reasoning (e.g., narrative, pragmatic, scientific, interactive, ethical) to evaluate the client's strengths and challenges to create and implement an intervention plan.

Context-dependent decisions: use knowledge of the context (e.g., practice setting, environment) to design individually tailored interventions that benefit the client (Kristensen & Petersen, 2016).

Creativity: the skill and imagination to create new things (Merriam-Webster, n.d.).

Critical thinking: the ability to analyze, examine, and evaluate information to make decisions, synthesize information, and prioritize (Sahamid, 2014).

D

Deductive reasoning: involves determining if logical conclusions follow a given set of premises that are based on prior beliefs, observations, and/or suppositions that are not explicit in the initial premise (Stephens et al., 2018; Wang et al., 2020).

Descriptive study: observes a group of interest at a specific time point to classify and document characteristics, explore factors that influenced an outcome, and define patterns.

Dynamic systems theory: complex, non-linear processes associated with occupation (Aldrich, 2008; Bird & Strachan, 2020; Ramshaw, 2020).

E

Eclecticism or eclectic reasoning: use of multiple models or frames of reference together, also referred to as *multimodal* (Ikiugu et al., 2009).

Emotional intelligence: awareness and understanding of one's own emotions (Howe, 2008) and includes the propensity to allow emotions to drive cognition and action (Palmer & Stough, 2001 in Chaffey et al., 2010).

Environmental factors: physical, social, and attitudinal surroundings of client (AOTA, 2020).

Ethical dilemma: situation that requires a person to choose between conflicting alternatives.

Ethical distress: feelings of discomfort when prevented from doing what is believed to be right.

Ethical reasoning: thinking through what needs to be accomplished in relation to what should be done (Boyt-Schell, 2019).

Evaluation process: opportunity for the therapist to discover the client's desires and past experiences to identify supports and barriers to health, well-being, and participation in desired occupations (AOTA, 2020, p. 25).

Evidence-based intervention: The process of critically appraising research and information available that both support and describe limitations of interventions to provide the best possible intervention.

Evidence-based practice: synthesizing knowledge from available research, clinical experience, and client priorities.

Evidence-informed practice: use of intellectual habits and beneficial professional activities to examine evidence (from multiple sources) to practice effectively (Benfield & Johnston, 2020).

Expert: practitioners who recognize and understand the rules of practice and settings to creatively address client issues, synthesize information from multiple sources; they identify relevant cues along with knowledge of the client's medical, physical, and psychosocial factors to make practice decisions and design intervention. Expert practitioners can justify their choices and articulate the evidence to support their decision.

External factors: those things that influence occupational performance, such as the environment, attitudes, political and social institutions

F

Formal communication: communication dictated by institutional policies (e.g., documentation, team meetings, or morning rounds).

Formal Operations Stage: stage in cognitive development where adolescents imagine different possibilities, make judgments, analyze problems, and determine solutions to a variety of situations (deCarvalho et al., 2017, Sahamid, 2014).

Forming: stage in group that begins by establishing the vision, values, and purpose of the teamwork which helps members work together towards the same goals. Teams begin in the *forming stage* by identifying the roles of each member and defining the purpose or practices of the team.

Frames of reference: structure-based theory that provides information based on research to guide evaluation and intervention planning. Includes descriptions of population, nature of function and dysfunction, role of the therapist, assessment tools, principles, strategies and techniques.

G

Group therapy: intervention where there is more than one client and at least one practitioner.

Guided discovery: approach whereby the supervisor or educator encourages the learner to find their own solutions (Overholser, 2018).

I

Inductive reasoning: process by which individuals make sense of the world by creating rules about the situations they encounter, remembering the instances to which the rule applies, and developing new hypotheses related to the rules (Babcock & Vallesi, 2015).

Inevitable events: situations that require the therapist change their mode of communication to support the client's engagement in activities and achieving their occupational goal.

Informal communication: communication that includes check-ins with team members or short updates.

Intentional Relationship Model (IRM):   model developed by Taylor (2020) to conceptualize the process (communication styles) and describe the approaches OT practitioners use when engaged with clients.

Interactive reasoning: the ability to therapeutically engage in interactions by giving and receiving cues about how to respond to one another (Boyt-Schell, 2019); how the client indicates their needs, makes eye contact with others, expresses emotion, and engages in group or activity expectations for behaviors.

Interdisciplinary: *or interprofessional* teams work with each other to create intervention plans for clients, while still respecting each profession's practice domains.

Interprofessional: teams collaborate to establish goals and plan, often co-treating and working together to address client issues (see interdisciplinary).

Internal factors: person's abilities and those things related to the person that influence occupational performance (such as motivation, intention, values, beliefs).

Interpersonal events: situation that occurs during therapy and evokes an emotional response.

Interpersonal reasoning: process used to understand how to communicate to the client given the client's interpersonal characteristics.

Intuition: unconscious awareness of how to proceed during OT practice.

Intuitive knowledge: immediate knowledge accessed without a conscious awareness of reasoning (Chaffey et al., 2010)

L

Level of evidence: rating that indicates the caliber of the research design and is related to the type of research being conducted.

Lived experience: client's view of their strengths and challenges to engage in daily activities. The client's subjective view of their experience (Kielhofner, 2008; Taylor, 2017).

Locus of authority: identity of person responsible for resolving the ethical issue (Grajo & Rushanan, 2021; Purtilo, 2005).

M

Meta-analysis: similar to a systematic review, but the authors gather the results of a specific construct or measure from quantitative studies and statistically analyze the data.

Metacognition: thinking about one's thinking.

Model of Human Occupation: occupation-based model of practice developed by Dr. Kielhofner that identifies person factors as volition (one's values, interests, and personal causation); habituation (routines, habits, and roles); and performance capacity (skills, abilities, and lived experience). The model emphasizes the importance of the environment (personal, physical, social, political) in supporting or hindering one's occupational performance.

Mode shift: conscious change in one's communication style (mode) based on the interpersonal events of the session and the client.

Multidisciplinary: members from many disciplines working together, each focusing on their own discipline or professional knowledge.

Multimodal approach: use of many modes (communication style).

N

Narrative reasoning: understanding the client's story from their perspective; using the client's story to influence activity choices and intervention planning.

Non-standardized assessment: non-standardized assessments do not compare measures to a group of same-age peers. The assessments may be structured but because they are not standardized, the OT practitioner can adapt and modify tasks for the individual.

Norming: stage in team process whereby members resolve issues and positive interpersonal communication increases and group members are focused on establishing group procedures (Carson, 2022).

Novice: stage of development whereby practitioners generally use scientific reasoning or concepts from coursework to guide their decisions in practice.

O

Occupation-based models of practice: based on theory; provide structure to organize one's thinking regarding the myriad of factors influencing a client's ability to engage in desired activities (i.e., occupations) and in so doing, inform therapeutic reasoning.

Occupational adaptation: person's ability to change, adjust to, and engage in a variety of activities that are meaningful to them.

Occupational analysis: details the skills, performance patterns, sequence, activity demands, contexts, and client factors required to complete a desired occupation.

Occupational competence: one's success in performing desired occupations.

Occupational engagement: participation in physical, cognitive, social, and emotional activity.

Occupational identity: sense of self; based on what is meaningful to a person and how they view their performance.

Occupational profile: understanding what is meaningful to the client, gathering information on client's background history, getting to know the client's interests, values, routines, roles, and environment.

Opinions: one's thoughts about events and situations, which may be based upon personal experiences, culture, or background history.

Organizing models: way of viewing a client based on theory that informs OT process (Ikiugu et al., 2009).

P

Peer-reviewed: journal articles that have been evaluated by objective reviewers who examine the background, methodology, findings, results, and conclusions of a research study prior to publication.

Perceptual problem-solving: thinking on one's feet, which involves observation in connection with anticipation of how a situation may possibly develop (Hutchinson et al., 2012).

Performing: stage whereby the team problem-solves and collaborates with each other.

Personal factors: client's background and life experiences that are not part of health condition (AOTA, 2020).

Playfulness: one's approach or attitude towards activities or play (Bundy, 1993).

Practice context: aspects of the physical (natural and human-made), social, and attitudinal surroundings and setting in which the intervention is being conducted. Includes products and technology, physical space, social, services, systems and policies, policies, and procedures, supports and relations. (AOTA, 2020).

Pragmatic reasoning: making decisions considering the time, setting, resources, space, and materials available; may include consideration for how long each part of the evaluation will take when selecting assessment tools and the space required and factors that support or hinder the process.

Preparatory reflection: using knowledge of client and from one's experience, and considering factors related to the context (such as practice setting, client's discharge environment, culture) to plan assessment and intervention.

Pretest posttest: a study that measures outcomes in participants before and after the implementation of an intervention. May also include treatment and control groups.

Principles: underlying assumptions regarding how factors interact to result in the outcome being examined.

Proficient: practitioners who view the client's situation as a whole and rely on professional experience to develop goals; they can modify plans.

R

Randomized control trials: studies that include a control and intervention group with objective measurements.

Relationship-building: practices, such as establishing commonalities, listening, and responding to each other, and supporting each other to gain trust and collaborate.

Reflection: the ability to examine and analyze one's decisions and actions.

Reflection in action: mindful awareness enabling the therapist to act intentionally and with immediacy within a scenario; refers to the reflections that take place while practitioner is involved with client (Yazdani et al., 2020, p. 2).

Reflection on action: involves thinking about an event that has happened and planning a future response (Yazdani et al., 2020).

Reflective practice: considering therapy decisions by examining knowledge, science, and experiences in relation to the client.

Reflective thinking: thinking while doing, being self-aware and reflecting on both the process and outcomes

Rehabilitation approach: an approach to intervention that involves adapting tasks and methods to substitute for loss of physical abilities; includes providing assistive devices or changing the context so client can participate in desired activities (Rybski, 2012).

Reliability: knowing that the information gained at one point in time or from one particular source is likely to be replicated on another occasion (test–retest) or when provided by a different source (inter-rater) (Coster, 2006).

Role overlap: two professionals engaging in similar roles with clients (Booth & Hewison, 2002).

S

Schematic processes: Rassafiani et al. (2009) suggest that experts use *schematic processing* of which they match decisions against stored patterns of information. Schematic processing is rapid and automatic, and the expert is often not conscious of using it (Hagedorn, 1996).

Scientific reasoning: understanding the client's condition and the possible effects it may have on occupational performance (Boyt-Schell, 2019). It is based on scientific inquiry which defines and tests hypotheses; used to determine how the client's condition or diagnosis manifest for the individual.

Search processing: processing information by looking for relevant information without matching patterns

Self-awareness: understanding oneself, interpersonal strengths, and challenges, and identifying one's role in relationships; knowledge of one's own personality or character (Merriam-Webster, n.d.).

Self-efficacy: person's belief that they have the skills and abilities to do those things they want to do (Bandura, 1997; Kielhofner, 2008).

Sensitivity: the ability of the measure to detect changes. Sensitivity is the ability of the assessment to detect the condition when it is present (Asher, 2014).

Simulation: type of experiential learning in which instructor-guided scenarios provide a substitution for real world experiences in a way that immerses students in the cases and clinical scenarios of clients (Reichl et al., 2019).

Single subject design: experimental study consists of one subject or a small set of subjects where the subject serves as its own control in study design by alternating between baseline and intervention phases and observing target behavior to determine cause and effect relationship.

Socratic questioning: educational technique to challenge learners through questioning to delve more deeply into topics and find their own answers; uses questions to prompt students to think deeply about concepts (Sahamid, 2016).

Specificity: ability of the measure to detect changes. Specificity refers to the ability to rule out the condition when it is not present (Asher, 2014).

Standardized assessment: structured way to measure a client's performance in comparison to the general population.

Storming: disagreements about values, roles, goals, and actions may arise during this stage of the team process.

Sub-optimal interactions: those events between therapist and client that interfere with, slow down, or impede the therapeutic relationship.

Systematic review: review of numerous publications (peer-reviewed journal articles) on a topic of interest.

T

Tacit knowledge: skills, ideas, and experiences that people have but may not necessarily be easily expressed.

Team dynamics: the interplay and relationships between team members, the power between members, and the roles that members play.

Therapeutic modes: a specific way of relating to a client (Taylor, 2020).

Therapeutic reasoning: the process of synthesizing information about the client, occupation, and environment to evaluate the client, create hypotheses or conceptualize about the client's occupational challenges, and design creative and meaningful occupational therapy intervention.

Therapeutic use of self: practitioner's planned use of his or her personality, insights, perceptions, and judgments as part of the therapeutic process (Punwar & Peloquin, 2000).

Threshold concepts: knowledge that begins as troublesome or difficult but grasping the concept leads to learner transformation of thinking and professional growth (Meyer & Land, 2005; Nicola-Richmond et al., 2016).

Transdisciplinary: teams work closely together to provide comprehensive care to clients. All team members work on the same goals and consult with each other to reinforce each member's area of expertise.

V

Validity: evidence that the assessment adequately covers the relevant domains of the construct (Coster, 2006).

Values: person's acquired beliefs and commitments, derived from culture, about what is good, right, and important to do (Kielhofner, 2008).

REFERENCES

Aldrich, R. (2008). From complexity theory to transactionalism: Moving occupational science forward in theorizing the complexity of behavior. *Journal of Occupational Science, 15*(3), 147–156.

American Occupational Therapy Association. (2020). Occupational therapy practice framework: Domain and process (4th ed.). *American Journal of Occupational Therapy, 71*(Suppl.2), S1–S96.

Asher, I. A. (2014). *Asher's Occupational Therapy Assessment Tools* (4th ed.). Bethesda, MD: AOTA Press.

Babcock, L., & Vallesi, A. (2015). The interaction of process and domain in prefrontal cortex during inductive reasoning. *Neuropsychologia, 67*, 91–99.

Bandura, A. (1997). *Self-efficacy: the exercise of control.* New York: W.H. Freeman and Company.

Benfield, A., & Johnston, M. (2020). Initial development of a measure of evidence-informed professional thinking. *Australian Journal of Occupational Therapy, 67*, 309–319.

Bird, M., & Strachan, P. H. (2020). Complexity science education for clinical nurse researchers. *Journal of Professional Nursing, 36*(2), 50–55.

Booth, J., & Hewison, A. (2002). Role overlap between occupational therapy and physiotherapy during in-patient stroke rehabilitation: an exploratory study. *Journal of Interprofessional Care, 16*(1), 31–40.

Boyt-Schell, B. A. (2019). Professional reasoning in practice. In B. A. B. Schell & G. Gillen (Eds.), *Willard and Spackman's Occupational Therapy* (13th ed., pp. 482–497). Philadelphia: Wolters Kluwer.

Bundy, A. C. (1993). Assessment of play and leisure: Delineation of the problem. *American Journal of Occupational Therapy, 47*, 212–222.

Carson, N. (2022). Interpersonal relationships and communication. In J. OBrien & J. Solomon (Eds.), *Occupational Analysis and Group Process* (2nd ed., pp. 23–32). St Louis, MO: Elsevier.

Chaffey, L., Unsworth, C. A., & Fossey, E. (2010). A grounded theory of initiation among occupational therapists in mental health practice. *British Journal of Occupational Therapy, 73*, 300–308.

Cherry, K. (2020). What is cognition? Available at: www.verywellmind.com/what-is-cognition-2794982.

Coster, W. J. (2006). Evaluating the use of assessments in practice and research. In G. Kielhofner (Ed.), *Research in Occupational Therapy: Methods of Inquiry for Enhancing Practice* (pp. 201–212). Philadelphia, PA: FA Davis.

deCarvalho, E. C., Oliveira-Kumamura, A. R. d S., & Morais, S. C. R. V. (2017). Clinical reasoning in nursing: Teaching strategies and assessment tools. *Revista Brasileira de Enfermagem REBEn, 70*(3), 662–668.

Grajo, L., & Rushanan, S. (2021). Ethical decision-making in occupational therapy practice. In J. O'Brien & J. Solomon (Eds.), *Occupational Analysis and Group Process* (2nd ed., pp. 173). St Louis, MO: Elsevier.

Hagedorn, R. (1996). Clinical decision making in familiar cases: A model of the process and implications for practice. *British Journal of Occupational Therapy, 59*, 217–222.

Hinojosa, J., & Kramer, P. (Eds.). (2014). *Evaluation in occupational therapy: Obtaining and interpreting data* (p. 322). North Bethesda, MD: American Occupational Therapy Association, Incorporated.

Howe, D. (2008). *The Emotionally Intelligent Social Worker.* New York: Palgrave Macmillan.

Hutchinson, S. L., LeBlanc, A., & Booth, R. (2012). "Perceptual problem-solving": An ethnographic study of clinical reasoning in a therapeutic recreation setting. *Therapeutic Recreation Journal, 36*, 18–34.

Ikiugu, M. N., Smallfield, S., & Condit, C. (2009). A framework for combining theoretical conceptual practice models in occupational therapy practice. *Canadian Journal of Occupational Therapy, 76*(3), 162–170.

Kielhofner, G. (2004). The organization and use of knowledge: *Conceptual Foundations of Occupational Therapy* (pp. 10–26) (3rd ed.). Philadelphia, PA: FA Davis.

Kielhofner, G. (Ed.), (2008). *Model of Human Occupation: Theory and Application* (4th ed.). Baltimore, MD: Lippincott Williams & Wilkins.

Kristensen, H. K., & Petersen, K. S. (2016). Occupational science: An important contributor to occupational therapists' clinical reasoning. *Scandinavian Journal of Occupational Therapy, 23*(3), 240–243.

Kwaitek, E. (2005). Self-awareness and reflection; exploring the 'therapeutic use of self'. *Learning Disability Practice, 8*(3), 27–31.

Merriam-Webster (n.d.). Abstract thought. In *Merriam-Webster.com dictionary.* Retrieved from https://www.merriam-webster.com/dictionary/abstractthought.

Merriam-Webster (n.d.). Attitude. In *Merriam-Webster.com dictionary.* Retrieved from https://www.merriam-webster.com/dictionary/attitude.

Merriam-Webster. (n.d.). Conceptualize. In *Merriam-Webster.com dictionary.* Retrieved from https://www.merriam-webster.com/dictionary/conceptualize.

Merriam-Webster. (n.d.). Creativity. In *Merriam-Webster.com dictionary.* Retrieved from https://www.merriam-webster.com/dictionary/creativity.

Merriam-Webster (n.d.). Self-awareness. In *Merriam-Webster.com dictionary.* Retrieved from https://www.merriam-webster.com/dictionary/self-awareness.

Meyer, J. H. F., & Land, R. (2005). Threshold concepts and troublesome knowledge (2): Epistemological considerations and a conceptual framework for teaching and learning. *Higher Education, 49*, 373–388.

Nicola-Richmond, K. M., Pepin, G., & Larkin, H. (2016). Transformation from student to occupational therapist:Using the Delphi technique to identify the threshold concepts of occupational therapy. *Australian Journal of Occupational Therapy, 63*, 95–104.

Overholser, J. C. (2018). Guided discovery: A clinical strategy derived from the Socratic method. *Journal of Cognitive Therapy, 11*, 124–139.

Palmer, B., & Stough, C. (2001). *SUEIT: Swinburne University Emotional Intelligence Test: Interim technical manual.* Melbourne, Victoria, Australia: Swinburne University Organizational Psychology Research Unit.

Punwar, J., & Peloquin, M. (2000). *Occupational Therapy: Principles and Practice.* Philadelphia: Lippincott.

Purtilo, R. (2005). *Ethical dimensions in the health professions* (4th ed.). North Bethesda, MD: American Occupational Therapy Association (AOTA).

Ramshaw, B. (2020). Ag systems and complexity science to real patient care. *Journal of Evaluation in Clinical Practice, 26*(5), 1559–1563.

Rassafiani, M., Ziviani, J., Rodger, S., & Dalgleish, L. (2009). Identification of occupational therapy clinical expertise: decision-making characteristics. *Australian Occupational Therapy Journal, 56*, 156–166.

Reichl, K., Baird, J. M., Chisholm, D., & Terhorst, L. (2019). Measuring and describing occupational therapists' perceptions of the impact of high-fidelity, high-technology simulation experiences on performance. *American Journal of Occupational Therapy, 73,* 7306205090.

Rybski, M. (2012). Rehabilitation adaptation and compensation. In *Kinesiology for Occupational Therapy: Thorofare* (pp. 355–428). NJ: SLACK Inc.

Sahamid, H. (2014). Fostering critical thinking in the classroom. *Advances in Language and Literary Studies, 5*(6), 166–172.

Sahamid. (2016). Developing critical thinking through Socratic questioning: An action research study. *International Journal of Education & Literacy Studies, 4*(3), 62–72.

Stephens, R. G., Dunn, J. C., & Hayes, B. K. (2018). Are there two processes in reasoning? The dimensionality of inductive and deductive inferences. *Psychological Review, 125*(2), 218–244.

Taylor, R. (2017). *Kielhofner's Model of Human Occupation: Theory and Application* (5th ed.). Philadelphia: Wolters Kluwer.

Taylor, R. (2020). *The intentional relationship model* (2nd ed.). Philadelphia, PA: FA Davis.

Toglia, J. P., Rodger, S. A., & Polatajko, H. J. (2012). Anatomy of cognitive strategies: A therapist's primer for enabling occupational performance. *Canadian Journal of Occupational Therapy, 79*(4), 225–236.

Turner, A., & Alsop, A. (2015). Unique core skills: Exploring occupational therapists' hidden assets. *British Journal of Occupational Therapy, 78*(12), 739–749.

Wang, L., Zhang, M., Zou, F., Wu, X., & Wang, Y. (2020). Deductive reasoning brain networks: A coordinate-based meta-analysis of the neural signatures in deductive reasoning. *Brain and Behavior, 10,* e01853.

Yazdani, F., Stringer, A., Nobakht, L., Bonsaksen, T., & Tune, K. (2020). Qualitative analysis of occupational therapists' reflective notes on practicing their skills in building and maintaining therapeutic relationships. *Journal of Occupational Therapy Education, 4*(4), 1–18.

INDEX

Note: Page numbers followed by 'f' indicate figures those followed by 't' indicate tables and 'b' indicate boxes.